DERMATOLOGY - LABORATORY AND CLINICAL RESEARCH

SUNSCREENS

PROPERTIES, ROLE IN SKIN CANCER PREVENTION AND HEALTH EFFECTS

DERMATOLOGY - LABORATORY AND CLINICAL RESEARCH

Additional books in this series can be found on Nova's website under the Series tab.

Additional e-books in this series can be found on Nova's website under the e-book tab.

DERMATOLOGY - LABORATORY AND CLINICAL RESEARCH

SUNSCREENS

PROPERTIES, ROLE IN SKIN CANCER PREVENTION AND HEALTH EFFECTS

SEAN HENRY SHARP
EDITOR

nova publishers
New York

Library of Congress Cataloging-in-Publication Data

ISBN: 978-1-63482-160-5
Library of Congress Control Number: 2015931779

Published by Nova Science Publishers, Inc. † New York

CONTENTS

PREFACE

The skin is composed of three layers of differentiated tissues. The most external layer is the epidermis, followed by the dermis and the hypodermis, which is the most internal layer of the skin. The increasing incidence of skin cancer has led international health authorities to recommend protection measures to prevent the harmful effects of skin exposure to UV-radiation. Such measures include avoidance of sun exposure, especially at times when disease-inducing wavelengths are more intense, wearing protective clothing and use of topical sunscreens. This book discusses the various properties of sunscreens, the role sunscreens play in skin cancer, and other health effects for individuals using sunscreens.

Chapter 1 – UV radiation (UVR) exposure remains the most preventable environmental risk factor for cosmetic reasons as well for skin cancers. Aside from sun avoidance, sunscreens remain our best protection. UVR directly damages DNA and cause indirect cellular damage through the creation of reactive oxygen species, the sum of which leads to cutaneous immunosuppression as well as phenotypic changes that is referred as photoaging. The current methodology for looking at sunscreens efficacy against UVR protection is limited to very few markers at molecular level, whereas erythema is the main marker validated to current date for clinical purposes. DNA damages at the molecular level are very well understood. The markers may provide information about acute exposures, but lack the ability to determine the effect with chronic exposures. Moreover, it is not necessary that the amount of photon required for DNA damage, might not be same for some of the other sensitive markers. The correct determination of the protective ability of a sunscreen product should be a prerequisite to reliably avoid the appearance of UV-induced injuries to human health, e.g., sunburn, immunosuppression, skin aging, skin cancer and radical formation. The chapter summarizes metabolomics: a relatively new branch of omics that studies the global metabolite profiles in a given biological system (cell, tissue, or organism) under a given set of conditions. Studies have shown that metabolomic analysis of skin samples from sun-exposed and sun-protected sites; demonstrated clearly that sun exposure altered the metabolic profile in the sun-exposed skin biopsies. However, the usage of sunscreen can attenuate the effect of UV exposure and prevents change in metabolomic profile of explants treated with sunscreen followed by UV exposure.

Chapter 2 – The popularization of tanning by Coco Chanel in the 1950s heralded a new era, where the once fashionable milky complexion was quickly replaced by a darker one, achieved through baby oil and iodine. Although sunburns were undoubtedly just as painful as they are today, sunscreen was certainly not seen as a necessity, often barred to the bottom of the beach bag. As public knowledge of the scientifically proven links between excessive ultraviolet exposure from the sun and the development of skin cancer and photoaging expanded, so did the marketing and use of sunscreens. Today topical sunscreen products remain one of the most widely used forms of photoprotection for the majority of the public, and within an estimated $1 billion dollar industry, past issues of variety and availability have been erased, as current and future focus puts safety and efficacy at the forefront.

Sunscreen may not have been a common household item decades ago, but the product has a surprisingly long history. The first commercial sunscreen was introduced in the United States in 1928, a greasy emulsion containing benzyl salicylate and benzyl cinnamate. In 1946, Franz Greiter introduced the concept of SPF, and by the 1970s broad introduction of SPF on sunscreen packaging revolutionized the market, as products became comparable on a quantitative basis. In the past two decades alone, sunscreen products have undergone fundamental improvements, the most significant of which is the breadth of protection against UVA I rays. Sunscreens have come a long way since the days of greasy emulsions, as today's protection products are not only super effective at protecting against UV damage, but invisible and aesthetically pleasing to the consumer. Sun protection is no longer looked at as a product brought out for a beach-day, but considered a daily-use item, used not only for sun protection but healthy prophylaxis against aging and skin damage.

Today sunscreen can be found everywhere from daily moisturizers to lip balms, but although sales have reached an all-time high, skin cancer rates continue to climb. Wild claims of safety and efficacy together with a history of limited regulation have led to an atmosphere of consumer misconception. In 2012, more than 30 years after its first stab at sunscreen regulation, the FDA has finally set down legally binding rules on the marketing on sunscreen products. New mandates touch on areas of broad-spectrum testing, SPF capping, "waterproof" labeling, and sun safety claims, in hopes that these new rules will eliminate confusion and establish consumer power.

Chapter 3 – The benefits of the use of sunscreen have been widely presented in scientific literature. UV exposure has been related to the development of skin cancers. The use of sunscreen decreases this risk. Tanning is a social desire in many cultures. Media, fashion and social behaviors motivate people to get tan. Despite warnings about skin cancer, many individuals seek for tanning salons and natural sun exposure without adequate sun protection. Frequent tanners are psychologically and physically dependent on tanning. When an individual develops a skin cancer after using inadequate sun protection measures, feelings such as guilt, depression and anxiety may arise. This chapter will discuss the social psychological aspects related to sunscreen use, tanning and skin cancer prevention.

Chapter 4 – The main objective of this chapter is to perform a detailed review on antioxidants in sunscreens, and more specifically on Melatonin. Melatonin is a neurohormone with natural antioxidant properties. In order to understand its importance, an initial review of the structure of the skin and the ultraviolet radiation effects is carried out. Throughout the chapter the nature of products, mechanisms of action and advantages and disadvantages of the conventional and novel groups of sunscreens that protect from the ultraviolet radiation are discussed, (*i*) organic sunscreens, (*ii*) inorganic sunscreens (*iii*) DNA repair agents (*iv*) cyclooxigenase-2 inhibitors, (*v*) iron chelators (*vi*) osmolytes and (*vii*) natural antioxidant substances. Several studies have reported the benefits of Melatonin used either for ultraviolet radiation protection or in combination with traditional radiotherapy for the treatment of human cancers. For this reason, in this chapter a thorough review of the characteristics and properties of this substance is performed in order to underscore the importance of this promising active for use in sunscreens.

Chapter 5 – Sunscreens or sunscreen agents are more notoriously known as ultraviolet (UV) filters, and they are the prime components of many personal care products and pharmaceuticals. Most UV filters are organic compounds that absorb UV radiation, therefore protecting us from solar radiation and its nefarious effects on human skin and health. The protective character of UV filters regarding UV radiation, would presuppose a stable nature towards alterations in general. However, the compounds are well known to undergo degradation, and in many cases quite substantially, either by influence of UV radiation itself (by photolysis or photo-isomerization) or through contact with water disinfecting agents, such as chlorine. These degradation reactions might be quite troublesome, since they generate degradation by-products that either do not present the appropriate UV-protective capabilities, as is the case with photo-isomers, or possess toxicological profiles potentially damaging for both the human health and the environment, as is the case with free-radicals or even disinfection by-products (DBP's).

Chapter 6 – One of the major concerns about the use of sunscreens is their safety. Many investigations performed with different techniques have addressed this issue providing conflicting results. To be safe and effective, sunscreens should remain on the skin surface without penetrating into the underlying living tissue. As these products are normally applied on large skin areas, even small amounts of UV-filters permeating the skin could lead to their systemic absorption, making controversial their safety after topical application. To overcome real or perceived human health concerns arising from the use of sunscreen products, their margin of safety (MoS) can be easily estimated by assessing UV-filters skin permeation using *in vitro* techniques. At present, several *in vitro* and *in vivo* test systems that provide reliable and reproducible results are used by cosmetic and pharmaceutical industries.

In this chapter, physical and chemical parameters affecting UV-filters ability to permeate the skin will be discussed, and *in vitro* and *in vivo* skin permeation studies performed on the most commonly used UV-filters will be reviewed. Estimations of UV-filter MoS from skin permeation studies will highlight the safety of currently used sunscreen formulations.

Chapter 7 – The UV protection by textiles highly depends on large number of factors such are type of fiber, fabric surface, construction, porosity, density, moisture content, type and concentration of dyestuff, fluorescent whitening agents (FWA), UV-B protective agents (UV absorbers), as well as nanoparticles, if applied. The dyes are selective absorbers. They all absorb visible light, but some absorb light in the near ultraviolet region, as well. Even though synthetic dyes are cheaper, their usage led to such consequences as carcinogenicity and some of them are toxic to the environment. Due to increased awareness of the environmental and health hazards associated with the synthesis, processing and use of synthetic dyes, most of the commercial dyers have started to re-look to the maximum possibilities of using natural dyes for dyeing and printing of different textiles for targeting niche market. Natural dyes are usually derived from the plants, animal and mineral sources. The shades produced by natural dyes are usually soft, lustrous and soothing to the human eye, can be produced a wide range of colors by mix and match system and are usually renewable and biodegradable. However, it needs longer dyeing time and excess cost for mordants and mordanting. Applied on textiles, provide some UV blocking which depends on the structure of dye molecules, type of dye or pigment, present absorptive groups, depth of dyeing and the uniformity. According to colour physic principles, darker colors (e.g., black, navy blue and dark red) absorb UV-R much more strongly than light pastel colors. For that reason, in this chapter the UV protection by woolen fabric dyed with natural dyestuff extracted from European Ash bark (*Fraxinus excelsior)* and European black elderberry berries (*Sambucus nigra)* was researched. Since these natural dyes, as most of the natural dyes, are non-substantive and must be applied on textiles in the combination with mordants i.e., metallic salts, 4 different mordants were applied. The color parameters were measured on remission spectrophotometer. The fabric UV protection was determined according to AS/NZS 4399:1996 *Sun Protective Clothing: evaluation and classification*, by UV-A and UV-B transmission measurement on transmission spectrophotometer and calculation of Ultraviolet protection factor (UPF).

Chapter 8 – The incidence of skin cancer is increasing by epidemic proportions. Its primary cause is a long exposure to solar ultraviolet (UV) radiation crossed with the amount of skin pigmentation in the population. It is believed that in childhood and adolescence 80 % of UV-R gets absorbed, whilst in the remaining 20 % gets absorbed later in the lifetime. This suggests that proper and early photoprotection may reduce the risk of subsequent occurrence of skin cancer. Textile and clothing can show UV protection, but in the most cases it does not provide full sun screening properties. UV protection highly depends on large number of factors such are type of fiber, fabric surface and construction, type and concentration of dyestuff, fluorescent whitening agent (FWA), UV-B protective agents, as well as nanoparticles, if applied. Based on electronically-excited state by energy of UV-R (usually 340-370 nm) the molecules of FWAs show the phenomenon of fluorescence giving to white textiles high whiteness of outstanding brightness by reemitting the energy at the blue region (typically 420-470 nm) of the spectrum, what leads to better UV protection. Molecules of UV absorbers are able to absorb the damaging UV-R range of 290 nm to 360 nm, and convert it into harmless heat energy. Latest research declares that FWA's and UV absorbers can be applied in textile care – washing process as well. Therefore, the UV protective properties of cotton and cotton/polyester blend fabrics achieved by light conversion in textile finishing and care was researched in this chapter. For that purpose, three stilbene derivative fluorescent compounds were selected – fluorescent whitening agent commonly used in textile finishing, the other one used in detergent formulations, and UV absorber. In textile finishing process fluorescent compounds were applied by exhaustion procedure in wide concentration range. In textile care fluorescent compounds were applied through 9 washing cycles at 60°C with standard ECE reference detergent and commercial detergent. UV protection was determined *in vitro* through Ultraviolet protection factor, UPF. Additionally the influence to fabric whiteness was researched. Since the fabric properties change in wet state, the discrepancy in whiteness and UV protection was research in distilled water as well as Adriatic Sea water.

Chapter 9 – Strong ultraviolet (UV) radiation is one of the most lethal and carcinogenic exogenous agents that can interact with and alter the normal life processes by means of its direct or indirect damaging effects. Mycosporine-like amino acids (MAAs) are important 'multipurpose' small biomolecules that provide protection from intense UV radiation without producing the reactive oxygen species (ROS). A number of MAAs have been reported from different taxonomic groups. MAAs have great potential in photoprotection and genome maintenance by minimizing the cellular damage from UV-induced ROS and thymine dimer formation. Moreover, due to strong UV-absorbing/screening function, photo-induction, strong antioxidant properties and resistance to abiotic stressors, MAAs are considered as natural photoprotectants that may be biotechnologically exploited in cosmetics and other pharmaceutical industries. In the present article, an attempt has been made to critically review and highlight the recent updates on various MAAs with respect to their function as potential UV-sunscreens.

In: Sunscreens
Editors: Sean Henry Sharp

ISBN: 978-1-63482-160-5

Chapter 1

METABOLOMIC ASSESSMENT OF SUNSCREEN EFFICACY

Manpreeet Randhawa**[*]*****, PhD, and Michael D. Southall, PhD***
Johnson and Johnson Consumer Companies, Inc., Skillman, NJ, US

ABSTRACT

UV radiation (UVR) exposure remains the most preventable environmental risk factor for cosmetic reasons as well for skin cancers. Aside from sun avoidance, sunscreens remain our best protection. UVR directly damages DNA and cause indirect cellular damage through the creation of reactive oxygen species, the sum of which leads to cutaneous immunosuppression as well as phenotypic changes that is referred as photoaging. The current methodology for looking at sunscreens efficacy against UVR protection is limited to very few markers at molecular level, whereas erythema is the main marker validated to current date for clinical purposes. DNA damages at the molecular level are very well understood (de Gruijl FR et al., 2001). The markers may provide information about acute exposures, but lack the ability to determine the effect with chronic exposures. Moreover, it is not necessary that the amount of photon required for DNA damage, might not be same for some of the other sensitive markers. The correct determination of the protective ability of a sunscreen product should be a prerequisite to reliably avoid the appearance of UV-induced injuries to human health, e.g., sunburn, immunosuppression, skin aging, skin cancer and radical formation.

The chapter summarizes metabolomics: a relatively new branch of omics that studies the global metabolite profiles in a given biological system (cell, tissue, or organism) under a given set of conditions. Studies have shown that metabolomic analysis of skin samples from sun-exposed and sun-protected sites; demonstrated clearly that sun exposure altered the metabolic profile in the sun-exposed skin biopsies. However the usage of sunscreen can attenuate the effect of UV exposure and prevents change in metabolomic profile of explants treated with sunscreen followed by UV exposure.

[*] Corresponding author: Manpreeet Randhawa, Johnson & Johnson Consumer Companies, Inc. 199 Grandview Road, Skillman, NJ 08558; Phone: 908-904-3062; Fax: 908-874-1209; Email: MRandha1@its.jnj.com.

Conflict of interest disclosure: MK Randhawa and M Southall are employees of Johnson & Johnson Consumer Companies, Inc., the manufacturer of the Ultrasheer Helioplex® broad spectrum sunscreen SPF 70.

Funding Sources: The study was funded in full by Johnson & Johnson Consumer Companies, Inc; the preparation of this manuscript was sponsored in full by Johnson & Johnson Consumer Companies, Inc.

INTRODUCTION

Skin is the largest organ that serves as an important environmental interface providing a protective envelope crucial for homeostasis. Among environmental stressors UV radiation which spans 100-400nm of solar spectrum induces a number of phenotypic responses as a result of biological alterations. Acute exposure to UV leads to clinically perceptible signs like pigmentation (tanning) and erythema (sunburn), whereas chronic exposure to UV causes premature skin aging or photoaging and even increases the risk of skin cancer (Zastrow L et al., 2009a, 2009b). Photoaging is associated with marked cutaneous alterations clinically characterized by wrinkles, roughness, sallowness, mottled pigmentation, telangiectasia, and a variety of benign and malignant neoplasms. Histologic and ultrastructural studies have shown these changes in terms of molecular endpoints in photoaged skin, which were mainly found in dermal connective tissue (Seité S. & Fourtanier A. 2008). Skin photoaging could be explained as the consequence of solar UV exposure, where DNA damage has been shown to play an important role. As a result most of the research is focused on selective DNA related markers like p53, CPD, TTdimers (de Gruijl FR., 2001; Yamaguchi Y et al., 2008) that can provide some information, but lacks the holistic view about the photodamaged skin.

Sunscreens, the UVR absorbing chemicals attenuate the amount and nature of UVR reaching viable cells in the skin. They are selected and tested for their ability to prevent erythema. The correct determination of the protective ability of a sunscreen product should be a prerequisite to reliably avoid the appearance of UV-induced injuries to human health, e.g., sunburn, immunosuppression (Bennett MF et al., 2008), skin aging, skin cancer and radical formation (Zastro L et al., 2009). But the standard method to characterize sunscreen protection properties is through determination of the sun protection factor (SPF), which is significantly influenced by MED and is based on determination of erythema as a clinical endpoint. On the other hand at molecular level, damages linked to DNA like p53, CPD and ttdimers (Mouret S et al., 2008) are explored at the biological level to verify the efficacy of sunscreen for photodamage purposes (Wassberg C. et al., 2003). This, however, could be disadvantages; as it is taking into account of other biological processes that doesn't even need that amount of energy as required for DNA damage to get initiated. On the other hand most of the DNA related damages are able to repair itself that means it could be a marker for acute damage, but does not account for low level chronic damages.

METABOLOMICS A TOOL TO MEASURE UV INDUCED ENDPOINTS

Skin exposure to physical, chemical and environmental stressors induces alterations at genetic, protein and metabolic level. Photoaging is considered of great cosmetic concern and has been studied very thoroughly at genetic and proteomic level. Often these UV induced changes studied through these tools are limited to biological markers including DNA damage (de Gruijl FR et al., 2001), inflammation, and immune suppression (Bennett MF et al., 2008). However not much attention has been paid to the change in metabolic activities with UV exposure.

Metabolomics is a relatively new branch of omics that studies the global metabolite profiles in a given biological system (cell, tissue, or organism) under a given set of conditions. Metabolites, are the end product of a complex interplay between the changes and interactions at genomic and protein levels under a given condition are the result of the interaction of the system's genome with its environment. These biochemicals are not merely the end product of gene expression but also form part of the regulatory system in an integrated manner. These metabolites could be generated or broken down by the cells, residing in the cells, secreted by the cells or taken up from ECM (Extracelluar Matrix). A metabolomics investigation provides the ability to assess changes in the abundance of large numbers of metabolites representing multiple classes of compounds and these changes capture global shifts such as catabolic or anabolic metabolism and can present an overall physiological status such as stress or hyperactivity of the biological system. Since a metabolomic profile is the downstream product of numerous genome-wide or proteome-wide interactions, so it can be a very proximal snapshot of an organism's phenotype. Studies have shown these changes in the context of biochemical networks and pathways, can serve as a means to identify biomarkers of disease (Wang-Sattler R et al., 2012).

Studies have shown that the contribution of sun exposure to biochemical changes that result in alterations in skin metabolome have essentially been limited to a few biomolecules such as glutathione (Zhu M et al., 2006). These changes have often discussed for single classes of metabolites in relevance to their biological pathway and are described as an outcome of a particular genetic pathway, yet a holistic approach to understand the effect of a biochemically related group of metabolites is missing. However these changes can account for both negative effects like oxidative stress or hyper proliferative phases as well as modulation of positive effects like acceleration of repair mechanisms in skin.

METABOLOME ANALYSIS OF SUN EXPOSED SKIN

Metabolome analysis of 50 paired skin samples obtained from sun-exposed and sun-protected sites through principal component anlaysis; demonstrated clearly that sun exposure altered the metabolic profile in the sun-exposed skin biopsies (Figure 1) (Randhawa M et al., 2014).

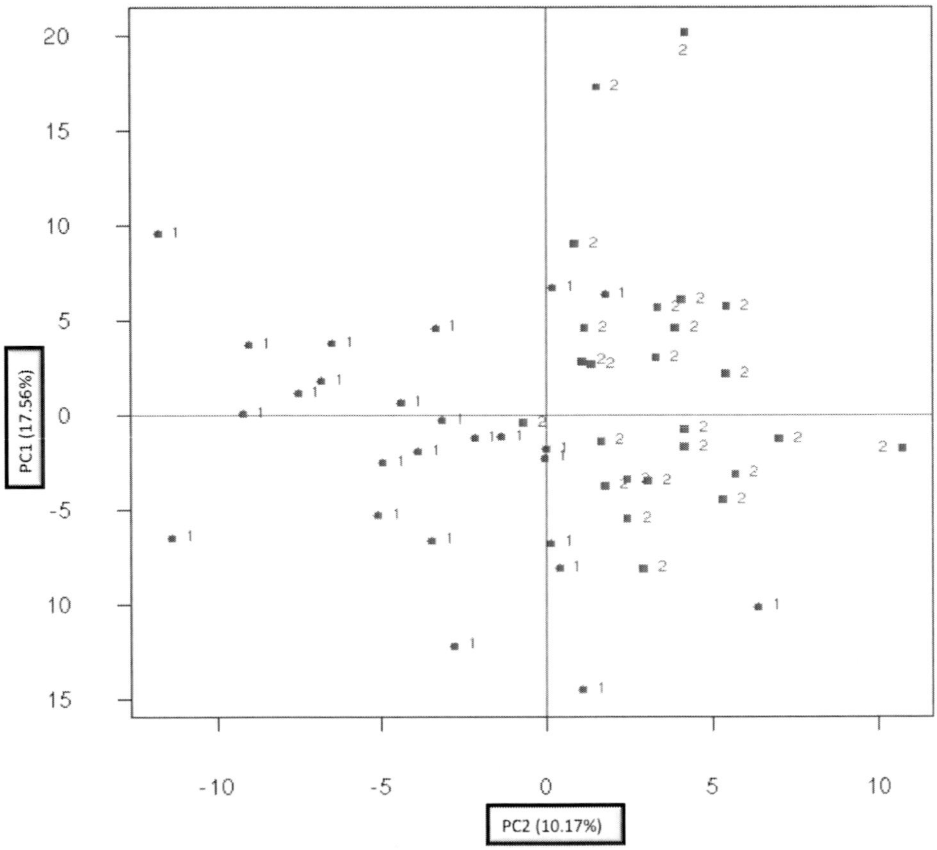

Figure 1. Principal component analysis (PCA): PCA plot showing separation of the sun exposed and sun protected skin samples. 1- unexposed inner arm. 2- exposed outer arm.

The identified metabolites belonged to a total of 52 biological pathways and a subset of 42 pathways had one or more metabolite(s) significantly different when biopsies obtained from sun-exposed regions were compared to the one obtained from sun-protected regions. These pathways spanned amino acids, nucleotides, sugars, peptides, cofactors, lipid metabolism and others (Figure 2) (Randhawa et al., 2014).

The study showed significant alterations in multiple classes of metabolites observed pointing to comprehensive alteration in the metabolic profile of sun-exposed skin. The metabolomics signature classified the sun-exposed and sun-protected skin samples with very high accuracy.

As expected, in this signature, cis-urocanate; a validated biomarker for UV damage was significantly higher in sun exposed as compared to sun protected skin. Additionally, the prioritized metabolite list presented a theme of metabolomic catabolism and oxidative stress as a result of sun exposure between the two classes, which was further corroborated when the study analyzed the three major networks. Most of these pathways suggested increased production of reactive oxygen species (ROS), which resulted in increased oxidative stress that can be held responsible for changes in the phenotypic appearance of sun-exposed skin.

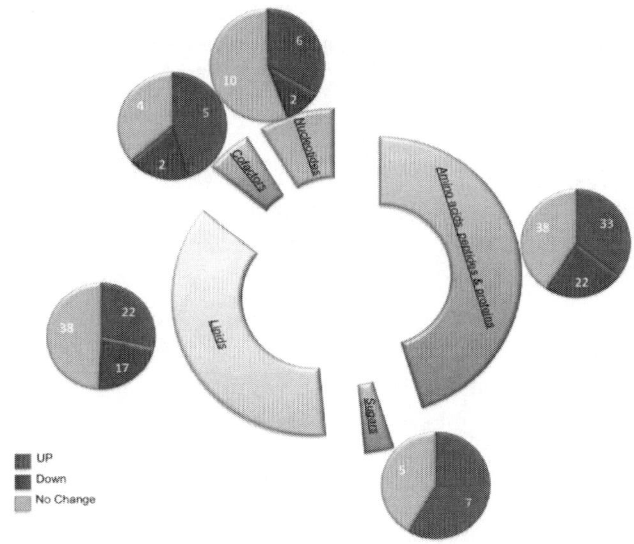

Figure 2. Distribution of the metabolomics data with colors depicting the levels of metabolites.

Urocanic Acid as a Marker of UV Exposure

The study showed decreased level of histidine and increased level of histamine that certainly pointed toward increased inflammation as well as increased catabolism for histidine. The second metabolite, urocanic acid comes from histidine metabolism represented increased isomerization from trans form to cis form (Figure 3). Trans from of urocanic acid is a major epidermal chromophore for UVR (Tabachnick, 1957), whereas cis form of urocanic acid act a mediator of the immunosuppressive effects of UVR in the skin (de Fabo EC, Noonan FP, 1983). The study validated not only one metabolite, but the whole pathway related to the natural sunscreen present in the epidermis. The various metabolites analyzed in this pathway not only played role in generating inflammation, but also in building up immunosuppression at the same time. The whole pathway suggested a very fine line between generating inflammation and building immunosuppression against generated inflammation (Randhawa et al., 2014).

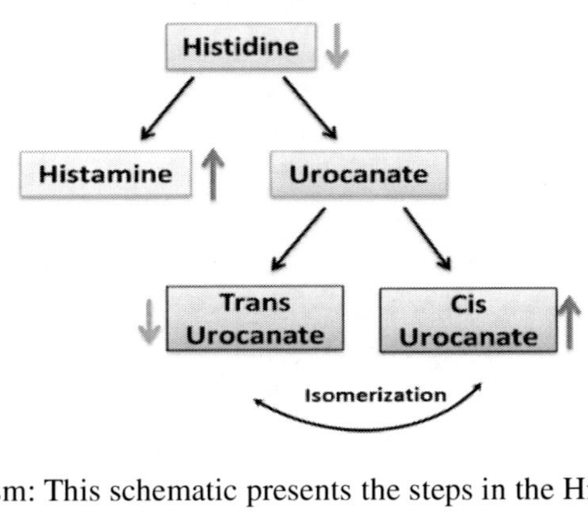

Figure 3. Histidine metabolism: This schematic presents the steps in the Histidine metabolism pathway to production histamine and urocanic acid.

Increased Oxidative Stress as a Result of Adenosine Degradation

The study represented significantly higher levels of metabolites related to adenosine pathway like inosine, inosine monophosphate, xanthine, hypo-xanthine, uric acid but without any change in adenosine. In this pathway adenosine is deaminated to form inosine that is converted into hypo-xanthine and subsequently to xanthine which gets further converted into uric acid. Another purine, guanosine's degradation can also produce xanthine however; there was no significant change in the levels of intermediate guanosine degradation metabolite: guanine when the two sets of metabolomes were compared (Figure 4). The data present in the study suggested that purine degradation is limited to adenosine and there is no contribution to purine catabolic products through guanine degradation branch of the pathway (Randhawa et al., 2014).

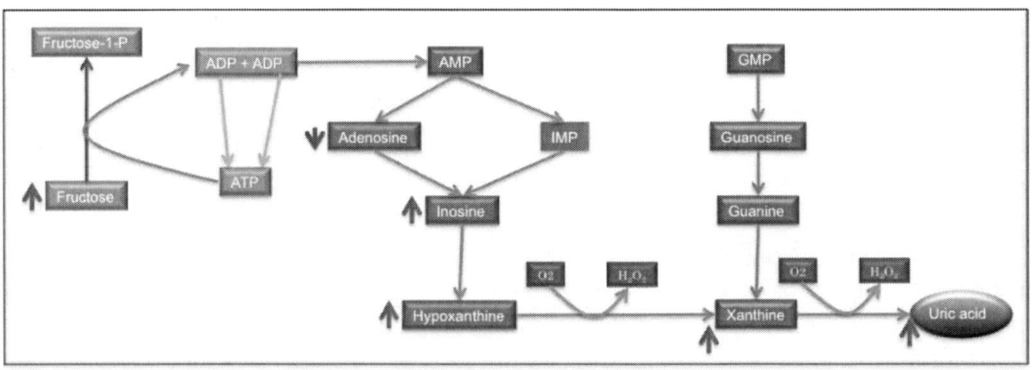

Figure 4. Adenine metabolism: This schematic presents the steps in the adenosine and guanosine pathway leading to production of uric acid. ATP – Adenosine triphosphate, GMP – guanosine monophosphate, IMP – inosine monophosphate. Red arrows – higher accumulation, green arrow – low accumulation.

Purine degradation pathway has been suggested a major biochemical source for ROS (reactive oxygen species) production (Barnes VM et al., 2009) and can be considered as one of the main pathways fueling high oxidative stress in sun exposed skin. Xanthine oxidase, the main enzyme required for degradation of xanthine to hypoxanthine and further to hydrogen peroxide has been previously shown to induce ROS (Landmesser U et al., 2007). Inhibition of this particular enzyme has also been shown to decrease ROS in the respective biological system. Increased ratio of hypoxanthine and uric acid from the data definitely suggest increased activity of xanthine oxidase, which probably contributes toward phenotypic appearance of sun exposed skin.

Interestingly, significantly higher levels of fructose were also measured in the exposed skin samples. Brosh et al. reported that higher consumption of fructose could lead to higher degradation of adenosine in the liver. Whether fructose plays role in adenosine catabolism in skin is ascertain, but cannot be ignored and needs to be evaluated further, especially the role of enzymes and fructose in the catabolic pathway. The source of a simple sugar such as fructose in this study could not be ascertained. A higher accumulation of fructose could be the result of carbohydrate degradation through UV exposure or could be contributed by diet (Randhawa et al., 2014).

Taken together, these measurements suggested that UV exposure is leading to degradation of adenosine and potentially contributing towards a more oxidized state in the cell. However finding the exact mechanism and the role of different enzymes and interestingly the role of diet needs further investigation.

ALTERED HOMOCYSTEINE PATHWAY LEADING TO ALTERED RATIO OF GLUTATIONE

Methionine and glutathione pathways are connected by the transsulfuration pathway in which methionine cycle provides sulfur for cystathione formation through homocysteine (Figure 5) (Ratnam S et al., 2012).

The study represented no significant change in the levels of methionine, S-adenosylmethionine and homocysteine in methionine pathway. Only S-adenosylhomocysteine had a significantly higher accumulation in the sun exposed skin samples as compared to sun protected skin samples. However, metabolites further than the transsulfuration pathway such as cysteine, GSH, GSSG were measured significantly different between the sun exposed and sun protected skin samples. The ratio of glutathione (GSH) to oxidized glutathione (GSSG) was lower in the sunprotected samples, suggesting increased oxidative stress. High levels of Cysteine-glutathione disulfide and the low ratio of GSH to GSSG reflect prevalence of oxidizing conditions in the samples that were photo exposed. Additionally, high levels of cysteine, glycine (not statistically significant) and glutamate, gamma-methyl ester were also detected. These metabolites are part of the glutathione biosynthesis pathway, which further indicated the pervasiveness of oxidative stress in the exposed samples (Randhawa M et al., 2014).

A biological system can also utilize an alternate pathway to generate glutathione. In this pathway, glutathione biosynthesis is achieved through γ-glutamylaminoacids, 5-oxoproline and glutamate. Levels of various γ-glutamylaminoacids (γ-glutamylalanine, γ-glutamylleucine, γ-glutamylisoleucine, γ-glutamylphenylalanine and others) were detected at low levels in the sun exposed skin samples as compared to the sun protected skin samples. These findings indicate that the alternate pathway involving γ-glutamylaminoacids is working at a lower level as compared to the pathway involving cysteine and glycine (Randhawa M et al., 2014).

Collectively, ratio of glutathione (GSH) to oxidized glutathione (GSSG) definitely points towards increased ROS as well as oxidative stress and has been documented before in context of photoaging (Randhawa M et al., 2013). According to the free radical theory of aging, ROS increases with aging due to the reduced activity of the antioxidant defense enzymes (Harman D 1956; 1968; 1981), similarly in this case it could be speculated that enzymatic machinery might be modulated resulting in high oxidative stress.

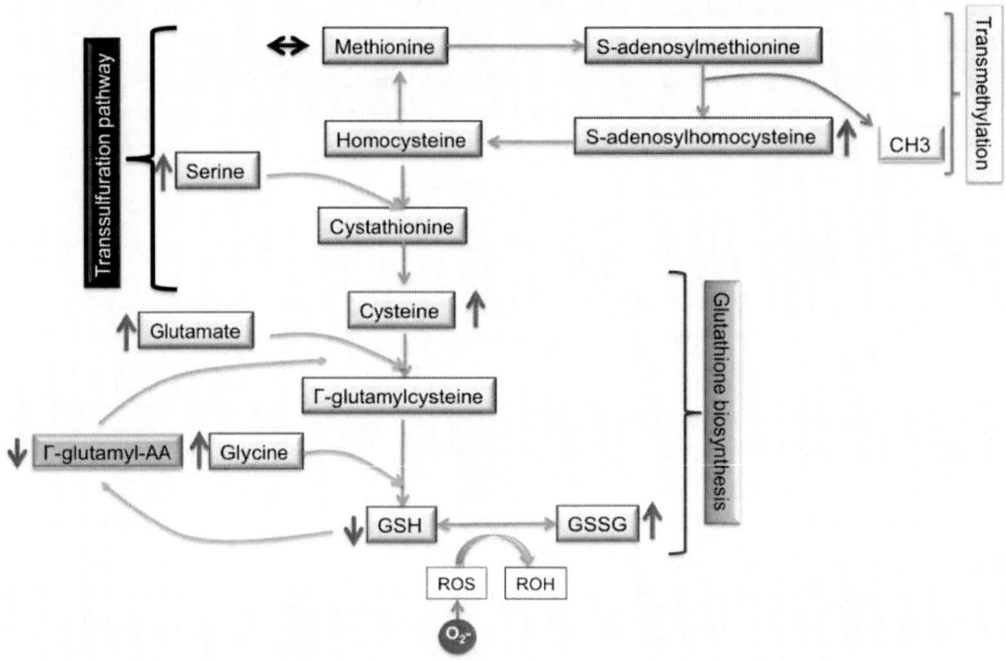

Figure 5. Methionine-Glutathione metabolism: This figures details the levels of various metabolites that were detected in the pathaway. Red arrow indicates higher levels, green arrow indicates lower levels and black arrow indicates no change in the levels of the metabolite.

Nicotinamide Pathway Suggests Pathway Suggests Skin Is Using Salvage Pathway as Compared to *de Novo* Production to Consume the Damaged Nicotinamides

In NAD+ metabolism pathway six metabolites were quantified out of which three metabolites; nicotinamide adenine dinucleotide (NAD), nicotinamide ribonucleotide (NMN) and nicotine riboside (NR) were observed at significantly higher levels. NR had highest fold change (2.69) in the exposed samples as compared to the unexposed. All of these metabolites belong to the salvage pathway and their higher accumulation indicates hyperactivity of NAD salvage pathway in the cells of the sun exposed skin samples. The biosynthesis of NAD+ occurs through salvage and/or de novo pathways.

In the de novo pathway, NAD is synthesized from tryptophan through six steps and in the salvage pathway NAD+ is synthesized by reclaiming degradation products of metabolites having nicotinamide ring NAD (Lin SJ 2003). Quinolinic acid, nicotinic acid mononucleotide which are critical intermediates in the de novo synthesis of NAD were not detected in the dataset. Their absence might indicate hypoactivity or no activity of NAD production through de novo synthesis.

Nicotinamide pathway has been studied very well and its respective metabolites has been shown the potential to influence cellular processes including DNA repair, genomic stability, the immune system, stress responses, signaling, transcription, apoptosis, metabolism, differentiation, chromatin structure and life span (Khan JA et al., 2007). In addition to its well-known redox functions in energy metabolism, NAD and NADP are also required for the synthesis of cyclic ADP-ribose and NADP, which are two major mediators of intracellular calcium signaling pathways (Khan JA et al., 2007).

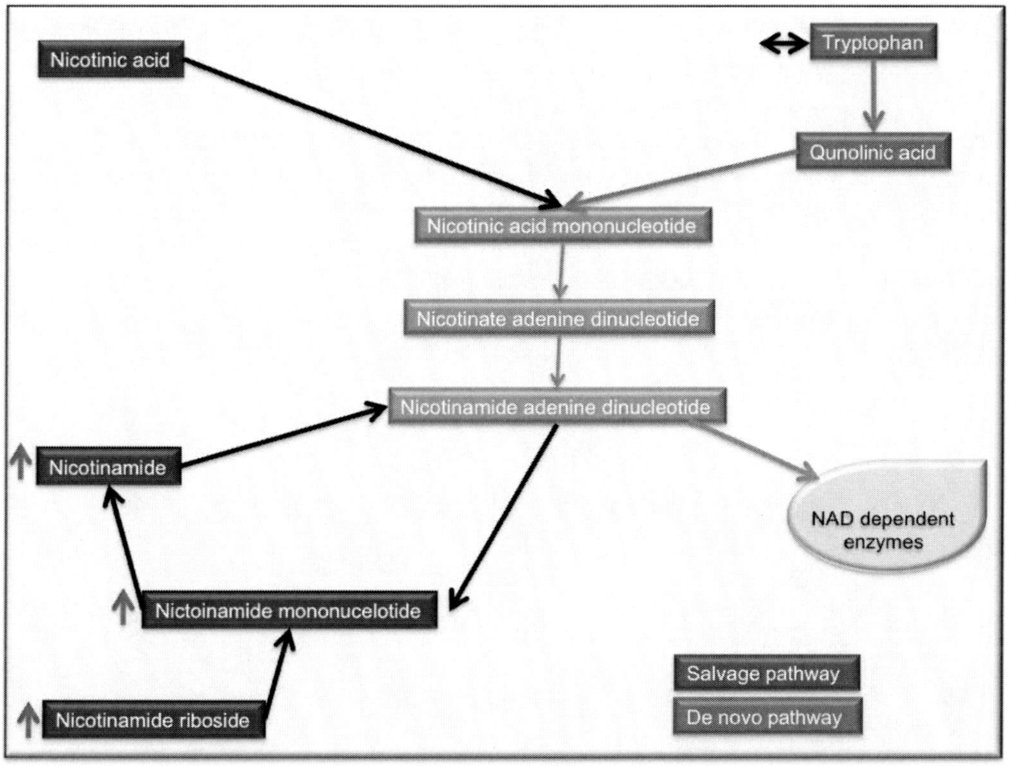

Figure 6. Nicotine metabolism pathway: This schematic presents the de novo and salvage pathways through which the NAD can be generated. Red arrow indicates higher accumulation and black arrow indicates no change.

These measurements indicate a theme of degradation in the cell because the salvage pathway recycles the degraded products of nicotinamide containing metabolites. Despite higher biosynthesis of NAD+, no significant change in the NAD+ levels between the two sets of samples. These data indicate that all the NAD+ produced through salvage pathway is siphoned to produce raw materials for DNA, proteins and other cellular processes. Besides UV induced cutaneous proliferation does justify the need for increased amount of genetic material for new multiplying cells (El-Abaseri TB et al., 2005). However the increased demand of energy by the respective biological system cannot be ignored at the same time, hence salvage pathway being more energy efficient and meets the current needs of the biological system. Moreover this information completely agrees with previously published studies that reported an increased glycolytic pathway for energy production instead of TCA cycle in sun exposed skin.

System Biology a New Approach to Investigate the Efficacy of Sunscreen

A second study performed on explants obtained from abdominal plasticity from females of Caucasian background was analyzed for global metabolomics profile. Metabolome analysis of explants treated with a photostable UVA/UVB broad spectrum Ultrasheer Helioplex® sunscreen (Neutrogena Corporation, Los Angeles, CA) followed by UV treatment revealed that the metabolomics profile of the sunscreen treated skin was most similar to the metabolomics profile of untreated skin (non-irradiated) and very different from the metabolomics profile of UV treated skin that did not receive topical sunscreen treatment. The data analyzed in the study provides the information, which is not limited to few markers, but also provides a holistic approach about how the skin acts in terms of energy consumption, oxidative stress and inflammation and role that sunscreen plays to help maintain the system near to its basal level.

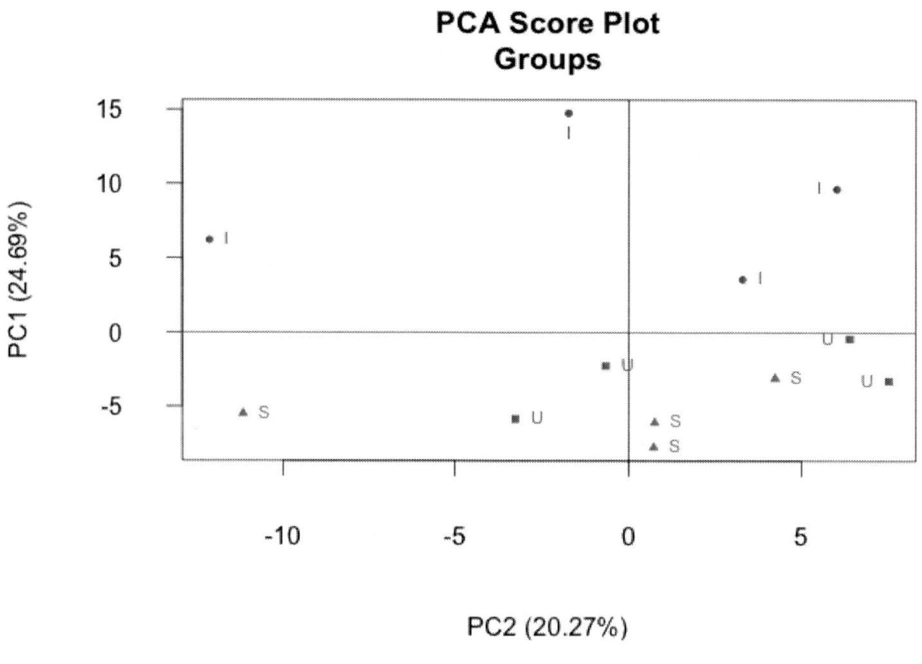

Figure 7. Principal component analysis (PCA): PCA plot showing separation of the (U) untreated, (I) UV irradiated and (S) Ultrasheer Helioplex® broad spectrum sunscreen protected explants.

In the topical sunscreen treatment study a total of 190 metabolites were measured under three conditions. When treatments were compared to the control, the radiation-exposed and Ultrasheer Helioplex® broad spectrum sunscreen-protected samples presented very different metabolomics profiles. For the radiation-exposed samples, the metabolic signature matched the metabolic signature of sun exposed skin discussed earlier. The data analysis from the respective presented convincing evidence that sunscreen protected the skin explants from the radiation. In the Principal Component Analysis (Figure 7), sunscreen-protected and unexposed clustered together and the radiation-exposed explant metabolomes were far away from this cluster. Interestingly, the photoprotective effect of Ultrasheer Helioplex® broad spectrum sunscreen was so substantial that it essentially ablated the effect of UV with the result that the Principal Component Analysis of sunscreen treated skin clustered most closely with untreated skin (non-irradiated) and was very different from UV exposed skin. These results demonstrate that even at the Principal Component Analysis level, metabolomics assessments can strongly differentiate the effects of sunscreens.

Sunscreen Application Prevents Irradiation Induced Isomerization of Urocanic Acid

The study performed on explants showed significant increase in isomerization of urocanic acid to cis form almost by 4 folds. However explants exposed to UV after sunscreen application seems to halts the isomerization of trans to cis form of urocanic acid, hence representing no change in urocanic acid. Apart from urocanic acid, histamine a marker for inflammation has also been shown to be induced by UV exposure. Increased levels of histamine were observed in explants when exposed to UV exposure, whereas no change in histamine levels was observed in explants when they were exposed to UV irradiation after sunscreen application (Figure 8). As a matter of fact UV irradiated samples in exvivo model was shown to mimic the UV irradiated skin biopsies as discussed in earlier sections.

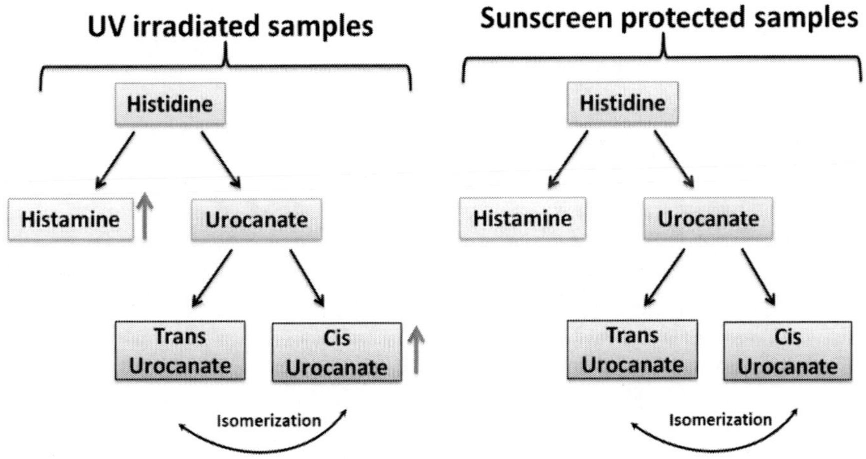

Figure 8. Histidine metabolism from UV irradiated and sunscreen protected explants: This schematic presents the steps in the Histidine metabolism pathway to production histamine and urocanic acid.

Sunscreen Application Prevents Inflammation Produced as a Result of Adenosine Catabolism Induced by UV Radiation

Metabolites belonging to Adenosine pathway followed the same metabolomics profile as discussed before for the invivo study with increased levels of Inosine, Hypoxanthine, and uric acid. Besides the adenosine pathway, guanosine catabolism was observed in exvivo model with significant increased levels of Guanosine and Guanine, which also fuels the formation of uric acid (Figure 9). The lack of imparity between the invivo and exvivo model from Guanosine pathway could be explained in terms of invivo skin is replenished with internal source of metabolites, whereas in exvivo model the skin is revived by using media with added nutrients. However the explants exposed to UV after sunscreen application did not show any increase in any of the metabolites related to adenine and guanosine pathway.

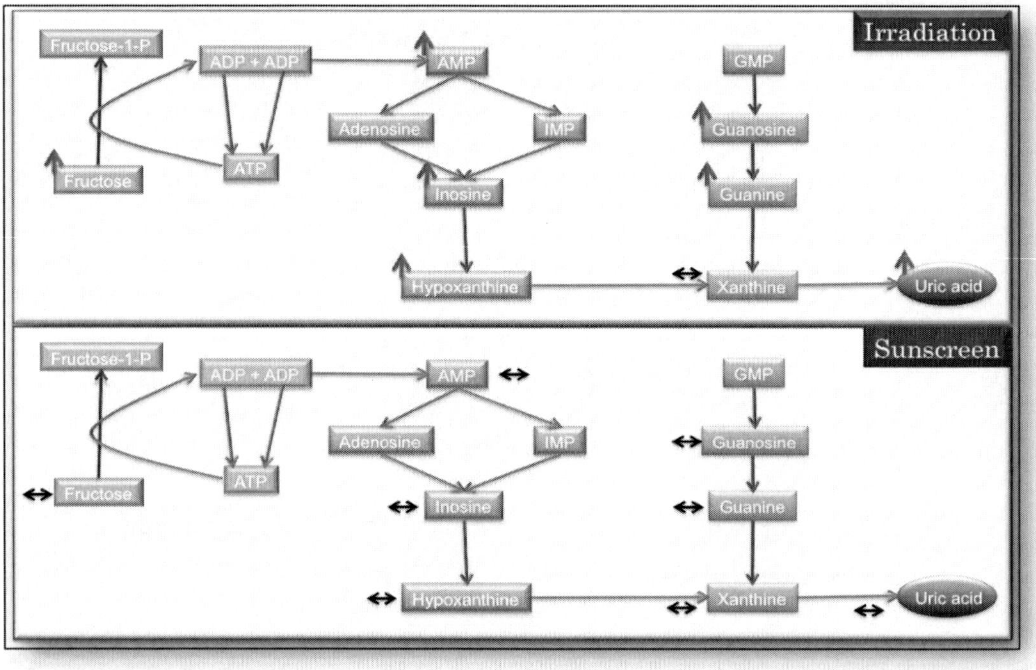

Figure 9. Adenine metabolism from UV irradiated (upper panel) and sunscreen protected (lower panel) explants: This schematic presents the steps in the adenosine and guanosine pathway leading to production of uric acid. ATP – Adenosine triphosphate, GMP – guanosine monophosphate, IMP – inosine monophosphate. Red arrows – higher accumulation, green arrow – low accumulation.

CONCLUSION

It is well established that exposure of the skin to ultraviolet (UV) light is a major risk factor for photoaging and well as developing skin carcinomas and sunfilters can provide effective photoprotection protecting skin from UV damage. Sunfilter efficacy has most commonly been demonstrated and assessed using a variety of clinical or biomarker endpoints. It has been well documented that sunscreens can provide good protection against sunburn, but other aspects of photoprotection are not simple to assess. In clinical settings the protection effectiveness of sunfilters can be assessed by the prevention of erythema or pigmentation produced as result of UVB and UVA respectively in 24hrs and expressed as sun protection factor (SPF) or pFA respectively. At the molecular level effectiveness of sunscreens has been assessed using single biomarkers such as DNA damage markers, which are also measured at 24hrs. Collectively these biomarkers provide only a small part of the information of sun damage and sunfilter efficacy and often lack a holistic view about the photoprotective effects of sunfilters on sun exposed skin. Metabolomics can assess changes in the abundance of large numbers of endogenous metabolites representing multiple biochemical pathways simultaneously. Metabolomics studies showed that markers for inflammation and oxidative stress are not limited to single biomarkers, as there are many inflammatory pathways induced in UV exposed. Moreover the effect of sun exposure and sunfilter efficacy should not be studied by only focusing on oxidative stress or inflammation since this approach may miss significant UV effects on other metabolic and biochemical process in skin. Metabolomics can assess changes in the abundance of large numbers of endogenous metabolites representing multiple biochemical pathways simultaneously. Metabolomic profiles of sun-exposed skin have demonstrated significant biochemical changes in glycolysis, oxidative phosphorylation, and lipid metabolism pathways compared to sun protected skin. Metabolomics has also identified biochemical changes in skin associated with sun exposure that were previously unknown or unclear. Thus, global metabolomics profile could serve a more useful tool to understand the physiology of skin in response to sun exposure. Sunscreens can prevent or reduce the UV-induced changes in skin metabolomics and as such may provide new approaches to investigate the efficacy of sunscreen formulations. Through providing a holistic approach to simultaneously measure biochemical pathways in skin, metabolomics may provide a more comprehensive assessment of sunscreen photoprotection than other single biomarkers. The tool can offer insight into the global metabolic profile of skin exposed to different wavelengths of UV and also offer great potential for research to assess the efficacy of sunscreens holistically through different markers.

Tool	Method	Endpoint	Advantages	Limitations
Metabolomics	Invivo: Biopsy, tape stripping, plasma, Exvivo, invitro	Urocanic acid, Adenosine metabolism, histamine, Nicotinamide metabolism, Glutathione metabolism	Number of targets can be studied at the same time and can be categorized for acute and chronic exposure. Does not only serve the purpose for target identification, but also for understanding sunscreen efficacy.	Large amount of dataset.
Molecular targets	Invitro, exvivo, invivo biopsies	p53, CPD, TTdimers	A valuable to tool understand the physiology of DNA changes.	1) Number of targets validated to date is very limited. 2) The markers usually repair itself and the information is lost about the earlier timepoints. 3) Is it a valuable tool to understand the suberythemal doses?
Clincal	Invivo	Erythema, pigmentation, sunburn	Provides information under invivo conditions, which is very relevant to the phenotype. .	1) Expensive and can be done only invivo. Usually the markers are looked at 24hrs and loses the earlier time windows to look at other markers. 2) The sunscreens test are limited to Caucasian, hence there is a gap to understand the effect and need for sunscreen in other ethnicities. 3) Not sufficient Information in generated for suberythemal doses.

Acknowledgments

The authors would like to thank Dr. Vineet Sangar, Institute for Systems Biology, Seattle, Washington, for insightful discussions on data analysis and interpretation of metabolomics. And to Dr. Curt Cole from Johnson and Johnson for extensive discussions on sunfilter efficacy studies.

References

[1] Tabachnick J (1957) Urocanic acid, the major acid soluble, ultraviolet-absorbing compound in guinea pig epidermis. *Arch Biochem Biophys* 70:295.

[2] de Fabo EC, Noonan FP (1983) Mechanism of immune suppression by ultraviolet irradiation in vivo. I. Evidence for the existence of a unique photoreceptor in skin and its role in photoimmunology. *J Exp Med* 158:84–98.

[3] Sophie Seité and Anny M.A. Fourtanier (2008) The benefit of daily photoprotection. *Journal of the American Academy of Dermatology*. Volume 58, Issue 5, Supplement 2, Pages S160–S166.

[4] Yamaguchi Y, Coelho SG, Zmudzka BZ, Takahashi K, Beer JZ, Hearing VJ, Miller SA Cyclobutane pyrimidine dimer formation and p53 production in human skin after repeated UV irradiation. (2008) *Exp Dermatol.* 17(11):916-24.

[5] Zastrow L, Groth N, Klein F, Kockott D, Lademann J, et al. (2009) [UV, visible and infrared light. Which wavelengths produce oxidative stress in human skin?]. *Hautarzt* 60: 310-317.

[6] Zastrow L, Groth N, Klein F, Kockott D, Lademann J, et al. (2009) The missing link--light-induced (280-1,600 nm) free radical formation in human skin. *Skin Pharmacol Physiol* 22: 31-44.

[7] de Gruijl FR, van Kranen HJ, Mullenders LH (2001) UV-induced DNA damage, repair, mutations and oncogenic pathways in skin cancer. *J Photochem Photobiol* B 63: 19-27.

[8] Bennett MF, Robinson MK, Baron ED, Cooper KD (2008) Skin immune systems and inflammation: protector of the skin or promoter of aging? *J Investig Dermatol Symp Proc* 13: 15-19.

[9] Mouret S, Baudouin C, Charveron M et al. (2006) Cyclobutane pyrimidine dimers are predominant DNA lesions in whole human skin exposed to UVA radiation. *Proc Natl Acad Sci USA* 103:13765–13770.

[10] Wassberg C, Ckvall H, Diffey B, Ponte F, Berne B (2003). Enhanced Epidermal Ultraviolet Responses in Chronically Sun-exposed Skin are Dependent on Previous Sun Exposure. *Acta Derm Venereol* 83: 254–261.

[11] Wang-Sattler R, Yu Z, Herder C, Messias AC, Floegel A, et al. (2012) Novel biomarkers for pre-diabetes identified by metabolomics. *Mol Syst Biol* 8: 615.

[12] Zhu M, Zhang Y, Bowden GT (2006) Involvement of mitogen-activated protein kinases and protein kinase C in regulation of antioxidant response element activity in human keratinocytes. *Cancer Lett* 244: 220-228.

[13] Barnes VM, Teles R, Trivedi HM, Devizio W, Xu T, et al. (2009) Acceleration of purine degradation by periodontal diseases. *J Dent Res* 88: 851-855.

[14] Landmesser U, Spiekermann S, Preuss C, Sorrentino S, Fischer D, et al. (2007) Angiotensin II induces endothelial xanthine oxidase activation: role for endothelial dysfunction in patients with coronary disease. *Arterioscler Thromb Vasc Biol* 27: 943-948.

[15] Brosh S, Boer P, Sperling O (1984) Effects of fructose on purine nucleotide metabolism in isolated rat hepatocytes. *Adv Exp Med Biol* 165 Pt A: 481-485.

[16] Ratnam S, Maclean KN, Jacobs RL, Brosnan ME, Kraus JP, et al. (2002) Hormonal regulation of cystathionine beta-synthase expression in liver. *J Biol Chem* 277: 42912-42918.

[17] Randhawa M, Southall M, Samaras ST (2013) Metabolomic analysis of sun exposed skin. *Mol Biosyst* 9: 2045-2050.

[18] Harman D (1956) Aging: a theory based on free radical and radiation chemistry. *J Gerontol* 11: 298-300.

[19] Harman D (1968) Free radical theory of aging: effect of free radical reaction inhibitors on the mortality rate of male LAF mice. *J Gerontol* 23: 476-482.

[20] Harman D (1981) The aging process. *Proc Natl Acad Sci U S A* 78: 7124-7128.

[21] Lin SJ, Guarente L (2003) Nicotinamide adenine dinucleotide, a metabolic regulator of transcription, longevity and disease. *Curr Opin Cell Biol* 15: 241-246.

[22] Khan JA, Forouhar F, Tao X, Tong L (2007) Nicotinamide adenine dinucleotide metabolism as an attractive target for drug discovery. *Expert Opin Ther Targets* 11: 695-705.

[23] El-Abaseri TB, Fuhrman J, Trempus C, Shendrik I, Tennant RW, et al. (2005) Chemoprevention of UV light-induced skin tumorigenesis by inhibition of the epidermal growth factor receptor. *Cancer Res* 65: 3958-3965.

[24] Randhawa M, Sangar V, Tucker-Samaras S, Southall M. (2014). *Metabolic Signature of Sun Exposed Skin Suggests Catabolic Pathway Overweighs Anabolic Pathway.* PONE DOI 10.1371.0090367.

In: Sunscreens
Editors: Sean Henry Sharp

ISBN: 978-1-63482-160-5

Chapter 2

THE HISTORY AND EVOLUTION OF SUNSCREEN

Mary Laschinger, BS, and Anna H. Chacon, MD
University of Maryland Medical Center, Dept. of Dermatology,
Baltimore, MD, US

INTRODUCTION

The popularization of tanning by Coco Chanel in the 1950s heralded a new era, where the once fashionable milky complexion was quickly replaced by a darker one, achieved through baby oil and iodine. Although sunburns were undoubtedly just as painful as they are today, sunscreen was certainly not seen as a necessity, often barred to the bottom of the beach bag. As public knowledge of the scientifically proven links between excessive ultraviolet exposure from the sun and the development of skin cancer and photoaging expanded, so did the marketing and use of sunscreens. Today topical sunscreen products remain one of the most widely used forms of photoprotection for the majority of the public, and within an estimated $1 billion dollar industry, past issues of variety and availability have been erased, as current and future focus puts safety and efficacy at the forefront. [1]

Sunscreen may not have been a common household item decades ago, but the product has a surprisingly long history. The first commercial sunscreen was introduced in the United States in 1928, a greasy emulsion containing benzyl salicylate and benzyl cinnamate. In 1946, Franz Greiter introduced the concept of SPF, and by the 1970s broad introduction of SPF on sunscreen packaging revolutionized the market, as products became comparable on a quantitative basis. [2] In the past two decades alone, sunscreen products have undergone fundamental improvements, the most significant of which is the breadth of protection against UVA I rays. Sunscreens have come a long way since the days of greasy emulsions, as today's protection products are not only super effective at protecting against UV damage, but invisible and aesthetically pleasing to the consumer. Sun protection is no longer looked at as a product brought out for a beach-day, but considered a daily-use item, used not only for sun protection but healthy prophylaxis against aging and skin damage.

Today sunscreen can be found everywhere from daily moisturizers to lip balms, but although sales have reached an all-time high, skin cancer rates continue to climb. Wild claims of safety and efficacy together with a history of limited regulation have led to an atmosphere of consumer misconception. In 2012, more than 30 years after its first stab at sunscreen regulation, the FDA has finally set down legally binding rules on the marketing on sunscreen products. New mandates touch on areas of broad-spectrum testing, SPF capping, "waterproof" labeling, and sun safety claims, in hopes that these new rules will eliminate confusion and establish consumer power. [3]

THE MILLENNIA OF PALLOR

To understand the history of sunscreen, one must first gain a good understanding of the shifting cultural beliefs and practices when it comes to tanning throughout the past twentieth century. Numerous cultural and historical factors over the past one hundred years, including social perceptions, medical knowledge, travel patterns, and fashion trends, have contributed to the popularization of tanning, dating back to as late as the early 1920s.

In the millennia preceding the twentieth century, the "porcelain beauty" was the standard, as pallor was deemed a sign of higher social status and a life of leisure spent indoors. [4] Pre-1900s through 1910, stigma was associated with tanned skin, as it was common among more working-class individuals who performed manual labor outdoors in farms and fields. This, and a general negative attitude towards dark-skinned individuals during this time, increased the appeal of a pale complexion. Fair skin was associated with both social and physical wellness, and as a result people went to great measures to protect themselves from the sun. The use of thick clothing which covered a majority of the skin's surface and parasols were considered a fashion must, while sun avoidance all together by staying indoors also played a significant role. Even swim and active wear for the outdoors was conservative, covering most of one's skin surface. [5]

Cosmetic means of achieving pale skin has a long history, dating back to the ancient Greek, Roman, and Elizabethan eras, when poisonous lead based whiteners where used to bleach the skin. [6] In addition to clothing barriers in the pre-1900s, topical sun protectants were also popular, which usually included heavy powders made up of magnesium, zinc oxide, or bismuth, designed to prevent any signs of sunburn or freckling. Up until the late 1920s, evidence of the fashionable nature of fair skin can be found in magazines and newspapers, which still widely advertised things such as bleaching creams for women. An advertisement for Elizabeth Arden's, Bleachine Cream, can be found featured in the July 1, 1920 issue of *Vogue,* marketed as *"a mild but effective preparation for removing tan. Nourishing as well as whitening. Excellent for the hands".* [7]

BEGINNING OF THE "HEALTHY TAN"

At the turn of the 20th century, new medical paradigms placed sunlight at the forefront as a both a new treatment modality for many diseases, as well as a preventative health measure, initiating a shift in social perceptions of sun exposure. The roots of this change can perhaps be traced to Downes and Blunt, who discovered that direct sunlight could inhibit the growth of microorganisms, and Palm who was the first to identify the role of sunlight in vitamin D synthesis, which later became known as the chief cause of rickets. [8] In 1903, Niels Finsen won the Nobel Prize for the use of ultraviolet radiation (UVR) in the treatment of lupus vulgaris, igniting the use of UVR phototherapy by physicians for numerous other diseases. [9] UV therapy became widespread, with physicians in both the United States and Europe advocating for its use in treating an array of cardiovascular, endocrinology, atopic, gastrointestinal, and rheumatologic diseases.

One of the most noteworthy books published in 1928 was *Ultra-Violet Rays in the Treatment and Cure of Disease* [10], on which the editorial staff at the *New England Journal of Medicine* deemed a book which they hoped did "not reach laity". [11] However, that same year *Vogue's* "Burning Question of the Summer" column featured this quote:

> "As a substitute for sun there are the ultra-violet ray lamps that have been cleverly decided to muffle heat rays and give us only the rays that tan. In addition to pleasantly modish toasting properties, actinic rays are said to stir up sluggish skin, and do all sorts of desirable things to one's internal function- reducing colds, stimulating glands, even improving the condition of such totally unexpected things such as teeth." [12]

And so was born the phase, "healthy tan".

The Industrial Revolution and the Growth of Outdoor Leisure

During the same time period that social perceptions towards sunlight and its potential health benefits were changing, so was the socioeconomics of the United States. With the introduction of the industrial revolution, lower and middle class workers were pushed indoors into factories and mines. [4] Significant changes in social class activities allowed for tanned skin to emerge as a symbol of travel, leisure, wealth, and health at this time. Leisure time shifted from the parlor room to the beaches and parks, and the allure of outdoor leisure was promoted by the new construction of thousands of athletic fields, tennis courts, baseball diamonds, and swimming pools. [13] By the 1930s, outdoor athletics to become an integral part of the American social experience, leading to a quick shift from underexposure to the sun to overexposure within the matter of decades.

Making Tan Chic

Through promotion in fashion magazines, which continued through the middle of the twentieth century, a good tan became everybody's must have accessory. In a 1929 issue of *Vogue,* CoCo Chanel endorsed tanning after coming home from a vacation in the French Rivera with a sunburn, affirming the "the 1929 girl must be tanned" and "the golden tan is the index of chic". [14] Some mark this as the beginning of the popularization of tanning from a fashion and cultural perspective. As a result, clothing became more revealing, allowing maximum sun exposure to both obtained and show off one's tanned complexion. Some of the most significant changes to American clothing around this time was the introduction of the first T-shirt allowing maximum arm exposure in 1942, and the bikini in the 1946. [15]

Throughout the late twentieth century the fad for tanning showed no signs of burning out. Celebrities and magazines maintained the allure throughout these decades continuing into present day. In 1978 tanning took on a whole new perspective when the first indoor tanning facility opened in Arkansas, allowing people to achieve a tan year round. [16] Indoor tanning today remains a major public health issue, having been linked to growing numbers of basal cell carcinoma, squamous cell carcinoma, and melanomas in young populations.

Growing Knowledge of the Dangers of UV Radiation

Despite the endorsement of UV radiation for the promotion of good health in the early twentieth century, initial warnings from within the dermatologic community did surface at this time. Chronic sun exposure as a causative agent of skin cancer was suggested as early as 1864, however, such early claims were largely ignored. [6] As a result of insufficient scientific evidence for such claims, physicians and scientists clung to clinical observation. Norman Paul was the first to make such clinical associations in his book published in 1918, *The influence of Sunlight in the Production of Cancer in the Skin.* [17] Following in his footsteps, American dermatologist James McCoy published his observations in 1920 that a disproportionately higher percentage of skin cancers occurred on sun-exposed areas including the face, neck, and hands. [18] This and other clinical observations linking UV exposure to skin cancer formation received little attention in the press, medical community at large, and public in the early 1900s. This may have occurred given the lack of knowledge when it came to the mechanisms underlying UV-induced carcinogenesis at the time, as well as widely held beliefs that skin cancer only occurred in susceptible individuals, such as those with xeroderma pigmentosum. [6]

By the 1940s, however, things changed as the pathological mechanisms of UV-induced carcinogenesis was revealed, first by George Findlay, and later Angel Roffo, who were able to produce skin tumors in animal models by subjecting them to UV radiation. [19] Segments on television, articles in lay press, and reports in non-dermatologic journals became more prevalent over the latter half of the twentieth century with focus primarily on the association between sunburns and skin cancer. [19]

The History of Sunscreen

With the increased public knowledge of the dangers of UV radiation in the 1940s came a simultaneous increased interest among consumer product industries to create novel sunscreen preparations. Although not previously a common household product by this time, topical sun protectants had been around for thousands of years. Early civilizations have been known to use plant products to protect their skin, including the use of olive oil by ancient Greeks, and rice, jasmine, and lupine extracts by ancient Egyptians. [20] Zinc oxide paste and other physical sun protectants, like titanium dioxide, had also been around for thousands of years. [21]

Early chemical sunscreens, however, were not introduced until 1928, when a blend of UVB absorbers, benzyl salicylate and benzyl cinnamate was created. [20] These newer chemical sunscreen were uniquely different in that they worked by absorbing UVB rays rather than reflecting the rays, which was the primary function of physical blockers, such a zinc oxide, with the advantage being improved aesthetics. As these new synthetic sunscreens developed, so did the market, leading to the first major, commercially sold sunscreen in 1936, created by L'Oreal founder Eugene Shueller. [20] The product was introduced under the name of Ambre Solaire and was an oil preparation made with benzyl salicylate. Other key players in the market at this same time include, chemist H.A. Milton Blake who introduced Hamilton Sunscreen in 1932, and Benjamin Green, who developed a product called Red Vet Pet for U.S. soldiers in the Pacific tropics at the height of WWII. [20, 22] The most effective modern sunscreen came out in 1946, developed by Swiss chemist Franz Greiter, called Gletscher Crème, which later became the basis of his company Piz Buin, which is still today a marketer of sunscreen products. [23]

By 1943, the FDA approved the UVB absorber p-aminobenzoic acid (PABA) for use in sunscreens. [24] PABA was believed to remain in the stratum corneum while providing UVB protection for several hours. Although PABA is still approved by the FDA for use in sunscreens, its popularity sharply declined in the mid-1980s due to its potential for causing allergies, and its yellowing staining of clothing. [23]

Evolution of Sunscreen: Aesthetics

The first commercially available sunscreens boasted the advantages of being less conspicuous and more aesthetically appealing to the consumer as compared to the otherwise incredibly effective zinc oxide pastes. The first formulations, however, where still leaps and bounds from the formulations available today, as sunscreens have come a long way from these early greasy emulsions in terms of look, feel, and effectiveness.

One of the first marketed sunscreens, Red Vet Pet, short for red veterinary petroleum, was exactly that, a red, sticky substance similar to petroleum jelly. [3] However, as demand for sunscreens grew in the latter half of the twentieth century, manufacturers worked hard to overcome these aesthetic challenges, making more appealing products by the 1950s. Green's patented Red Vet Pet was eventually sold to Coppertone who improved and commercialized the substance under the Coppertone Girl and Bain de Soleil brand in 1953. [3] This improved formula introduced cocoa butter and coconut oil into the mix, creating much more absorbable and better smelling products for consumers. The cosmetic quality of sunscreens has continued to improve over the years, with today's products being invisible and comfortable on the skin. Chemists have continued to work on sunscreens' improved look and feel, with some of the most important and recent achievements being the "micronized" versions of zinc oxide and titanium dioxide, which has eliminated the thick, streaky appearance formally associated with the highly effective sun protectants, allowing consumers to now apply them all over the body. [23]

EVOLUTION OF SUNSCREEN: EFFICACY

Many of the early sunscreen preparations introduced into the market were not only aesthetically displeasing, but vastly ineffective. The first sun protection measurement system was developed in 1934 by Friedrich Ellinger and Rudolf Schulze, which was later adopted by Greiter in 1974 and re-introduced as the "sun protection factor (SPF)". [23] The SPF quickly revolutionized the sunscreen market, as there was now a reliable means of measuring and comparing a sunscreen's effectiveness in a quantitative manner. The SPF provided the consumer with the ability to tell two things: how long they could stay out in the sun and how well the formula filtered the sun's rays.

Around this same time, the FDA reclassified sunscreens from cosmetics to over-the-counter drugs, requiring stricter and more regulated package guidelines. [3] Although their steps for regulation were limited and many were not enforced, the introduction of mandatory SPF package labeling was carried out, beginning in 1978. [3] Coppertone lead the way as one of the first manufacturers to label their products with SPF numbering, theirs being the first sunscreen with an SPF of 15, called Coppertone's Super Shade Lotion. [23] This represented quantum leaps in efficacy from earlier sunscreens, such as Franz Greiter's Gletscher Cream which only sported an SPF of two, and shifted the tone in the market towards one of safety and effectiveness. Within the last couple decades alone large increases in SPF value levels have been seen within the sunscreen market, with a twelve year cross sectional study of U.S. sunscreen products, conducted by Wang et al. noting a general increase in SPF values of products from 1997 to 2009 alone. It was also found that the percentage of low SPF products (SPF 4-14) decreased from 27% in 1997 to 6% in 2009. [1] These trends shed a positive light on the future focus of sunscreen tending towards continuing increased efficacy and safety.

In addition to the adoption of SPF as a quantitative means of standardizing sunscreen efficacy across the market, the Skin Cancer Foundation also introduced its Seal of Recommendation program in 1981. [23] This program independently assessed the safety and efficacy of sunscreen products using guidelines that were not yet monitored and regulated by the FDA. This provided consumers with an additional way to compare products on the market at the time.

Another development in sunscreen came in the late 1970s when Johnson and Johnson introduce the first "water-resistant" sunscreen. [17] The product was marketed as Sundown Sunscreen. The goal of water-resistant formulations was to allow consumers a longer-lasting, more reliable protection without the need for reapplication when enjoying outdoor sports, including swimming. Today many sunscreens claim water resistance or even water proof, however, regulations on such marketing and packaging claims have been historically lacking.

EVOLUTION OF SUNSCREEN: BREADTH OF COVERAGE

Of the tremendous fundamental improvements sunscreens have undergone in the past several decades, the most significant may be considered the increased breadth of protection to include UVA I rays. It was once thought that only UVB radiation, which is the main cause of sunburn, could cause significant damage to the skin and raise the risk of skin cancer. Research over the past twenty years, however, has unrevealed a different reality, showing that cumulative UVA exposure is the key cause of skin aging and wrinkling, while also playing a role in the development of cutaneous cancers. [23] These new findings have brought upon an urgent need for the improvement of UVA protection of sunscreens. In fact, cross sectional studies from over the past two decades show an increase in the number of products containing a UVA filter, from 5% in 1997 to 70% in 2009. [1]

UVA is considered the long-wavelength ultraviolet radiation, while UVB the short. UVA can be divided into two groups: UVA I rays with wavelengths ranging from 340-400nm and UVA II rays ranging from 320-340 nm. Different sunscreens, depending upon their formulation, either absorb or reflect parts of this ultra-violet radiation spectrum, the broad-spectrum of which cover more of the UVA wavelengths, thus providing more adequate coverage.

In the 1980s the only available UVA blockers were zinc oxide and titanium dioxide. Due to the aesthetically unappealing nature of these products however, manufacturers strived to create new formulations with different ingredients. In 1980 Coppertone sold the first UVB/UVA sunscreen, called For Faces Only. [23] This novel formulation contained oxybenzone, which offered significant although very limited UVA coverage. Following the introduction of oxybenzone, three other ingredients were created to protect against the UVA spectrum: sulisobenzone, meradimate, and dioxybenzone. [23] Sunscreens containing any of these four ingredients began to be marketed as "broad-spectrum".

Although tremendous headway in terms of increased breadth of coverage against UVR was being made with the introduction of oxybenzone, the market continued to lack a full UVA spectrum protectant. In 1988 the FDA approved the chemical avobenzone, which provided the largest UVA spectrum coverage to date. [3] Eventually concerns about avobenzone's photostability sparked interest into finding an even better UVA spectrum protectant, and within the past several years alone chemists have found ways to add stabilizing ingredients to such sunscreens, such as octocrylene. Today these photostabilized avobenzone formulations are marketed under names such as Helioplex, Active Photobarrier Complex, AvoTriplex, SunSure, and Dermaplex. [23]

CHANGING ATTITUDES OF SUN PROTECTION

Although the 1940s and 1950s heralded in an era of booming demand and sales for sunscreen products, these first lotions were definitely not viewed a necessity at the time, but rather a lotion to have handy in the beach bag to use only after the skin was burned. The first sunscreen, marketed as "suntan lotions", were promoted to be used as a means to allow longer exposure times in the sun without burning, while also allowing for the "healthy tan" so many still desired during this time. [23] Over time, due to growing evidence of harmful effects of the sun's UVR, not only in terms of increased cancer risks, but also skin aging and wrinkling, suntan lotions were eventually replaced by what we now call sunscreens, metal reflectors gave way to shade umbrellas, and visors gave way to UV-blocking sunglasses. In fact, society's perception of sun protection today is no longer thought of as something only considered on a beach-day, but rather part of one's daily routine, providing the benefits of sun protection against harmful UVR, but also the benefits of prophylaxis against skin aging and damage.

The Multi-Million Dollar Industry

Going off societal perceptions of sunscreens as part of a healthy and beautiful lifestyle, manufacturers have been able to create an estimated 700 million dollar industry. [25] The sunscreen industry has established itself as an independent industry with little direct competition, although some indirect competition does come from self-tanning lotions, sun protectant clothing, and sun protectant shelters. Topical sunscreens currently account for about 60% of the sun care market, with a predicted annual growth rate of 2.3%. [25] The average consumer is a fair-skinned woman, ages 35-44, which branding executives have capitalized on in terms of catering to this demographics health and beauty concerns. [25] The top sunscreen manufacturers today remain Coppertone and Banana Boat. Branding changes over the years have led to such manufacturers positioning themselves in the market as either a health or beauty product, while in some cases both. Issues of variety and availability are no longer present in the market as they once were. Countless different formulations can be found on the shelves of the local grocery store, drug store, or even super store. The list of products containing sunscreen has grown just as much of the number of manufacturers. Today sunscreen is advertised in moisturizers, lip balms, foundations, and make-up powders to name a few.

History of Regulation

Although sales of sunscreen have reached an all-time high, skin cancer rates continue to climb. Wild claims of safety and efficacy together with a history of limited regulation have led to an atmosphere of consumer misconception. At the root of these issues is perhaps the lack of unified FDA regulation over the past thirty years. The FDA's first stab at regulation came in 1978 when sunscreens were switched from cosmetic products to over-the-counter drugs. At this time the FDA tried to establish safety and efficacy guidelines, however, many fell to the way side, with only the mandate for SPF labeling on packaging withstanding the process. At this time the FDA did order an advanced notice of proposed rulemaking for the future stating in the document, "In the long run, suntanning is not good for the skin". [23]

Over the next 30 years FDA regulation was sparse, with the only notable legislation being the approval of avobenzone as a UVA filter in 1988, and the approval of the marketing of this ingredient by manufacturers in 1997. In 2006, the FDA missed a deadline set by Congress to approve proposed guidelines for sunscreens, and it was not until 2013 that the FDA approved legally binding rules on the marketing of sunscreen products. [3] New mandates of the regulations touch on areas of broad-spectrum testing, SPF capping, "waterproof" labeling, and sun safety claims, in hopes that these new rules will help eliminate confusion and establish consumer power.

2013 FDA Sunscreen Regulation Mandate [3]

Broad-spectrum testing: All sunscreens must now meet standardized broad-spectrum testing requirements to be labeled as such. Such testing measures the UVA protection in relation to the UVB protection, setting a minimum standard for such ratio. In addition, only sunscreens labeled "broad-spectrum" and with an SPF of 15 or greater can claim to reduce the risk of cancer and prevent premature aging of the skin.

SPF: At this point the FDA is considering the prohibition of sunscreens being labeled higher than SPF 50, given consumer misconceptions as to increased sun protection and failure to realize that protection levels are not proportional to the SPF number directly. Pushback from manufacturers has forced the FDA to negotiate this point. The FDA argues that a SPF greater than 50 has been shown to provide minimal additional protection as compared to sunscreens with SPF 50.

Waterproof terminology: The term "waterproof" will be a thing of the past as the only acceptable new terms that can be used will be "water-resistant" and "very water-resistant". The FDA claims there is no such things a waterproof sunscreen and require products to be labeled as either resistant for 40 minutes or 80 minutes. Other terms including "sweatproof" and "sunblock" will also be discarded.

Sun safety claims: Sunscreens can no longer claim immediate efficacy, nor can they claim to provide more than 2 hours of protection unless otherwise approved by the FDA. This is in hopes of reminding the consumer of proper application techniques including applying sunscreens thirty minutes before sun exposure, and the need for frequent reapplication throughout the day.

FUTURE OF SUNSCREEN

Recent industry trends involve the addition of antioxidants to sunscreens. Numerous manufacturers have begun to embrace this trend, with new marketing strategies aimed at the inclusion of vitamin C, vitamin E, and other antioxidants in products. [26] The rationale behind the additions is that such antioxidants serve as another line of protection against radical oxygen species produced by the UV, helping to diminish the harmful effects of UVR that gets past the incomplete protection of current filters.

Although the addition of antioxidants seems appealing, a recent study from Wang et al., demonstrates that the protection against ROS in sunscreens containing antioxidants still mainly is derived from the UVA filters, concluding that the action of antioxidants in sunscreens containing such filters is essential non-existent. [27] This is proposed to be due to either inadequate concentrations of antioxidants, unstable formulations, and use of the wrong active forms. [26] Studies such as these shed light on the fact that substantial progress must be made before any significant benefits will likely be seen from adding antioxidants to sunscreens.

TIMELINE

The following is a timeline outlining the key social, scientific, and regulatory events in the history and evolution of sunscreen:

1918: *Influence of Sunlight in the Production of Cancer of the Skin* is published.
1920: Elizabeth Arden's Bleachine Cream is advertised in July issue of *Vogue* magazine.

1928: First commercial sunscreen containing benzyl salicylate and cinnamate is manufactured.

1928: *Ultra-Violet Radiation in the Treatment and Cure of Disease* is published.

1929: Coco Chanel shows off tanned skin after trip to French Rivera.

1934: Ellinger and Schulze create ultraviolet protection quotient system.

1936: L'Oreal releases Ambre Solaire, the first major commercialized sunscreen on the market.

1940: Findlay and Roffo undercover pathologic mechanisms underlying UVR carcinogenesis.

1943: PABA is approved by the FDA.

1944: Green introduces Red Vet Pet for use by U.S. soliders in the Pacific.

1946: Helm and Reard introduce the bikini, ushering in an era of more revealing clothing.

1946: Greiter created Gletscher Crème, the most effective commercial sunscreen to date.

1953: Coppertone debuts Little Miss Coppertone and revolutionizes sunscreen by creating aesthetically pleasing formulations with cocoa butter and coconut oil.

1972: FDA reclassifies sunscreen from cosmetic products to over-the-counter drugs, making them subject to regulation.

1974: Greiter adapts Schulze system and coins term SPF.

1977: Johnson and Johnson release the first "waterproof" sunscreen.

1978: First indoor tanning bed facility opens in Arkansas.

1978: FDA mandates SPF labeling on sunscreen products.

1978: Coppertone releases the first sunscreen with SPF 15 labeling.

1980: Coppertone releases the first "broad-spectrum" sunscreen containing oxybenzone.

1988: FDA approves avobenzone for use as a UVA filter in sunscreen products.

2006: FDA misses deadline for approval of regulator guidelines.

2013: FDA sets legally binding regulations pertaining the marketing of sunscreen products.

REFERENCES

[1] Wang S, Tanner P, Lin H. The evolution of sunscreen products in the United States-A 12-year cross sectional study. *Photochem Photobiol Sci*. Jan 2013; 12 (1): 197-202.

[2] Jacob U. "Skin Care-Then and Now: Sunscreen". *Skin Inc*. Apr 2013.

[3] Stanfield. New trends in sunscreen testing and labeling. *Am Acad of Dermatol*. Jan 2014.

[4] Chang C MD, Muraku E, Penn L Md, et al. More Skin, More Sun, More Tan, More Melanoma. *Am Journ of Public Health*. Nov 2014; 104 (11):92-99.

[5] Martin J, Ghaferi J MD, Cummins D MD, et al. Changes in skinning tanning attitude: Fashion Articles and Advertisements in the Early 20th Century. *Am Journ of Public Health*. Dec 2009; 99 (12): 2140-2146.

[6] Albert MR, Ostheimer KG. The evolution of current medical and popular attitudes towards ultraviolet light exposure: part 1. *J Am Acad Dermatol*. 2002; 47(6):930-937.

[7] Elizabeth Arden advertisement. *Vogue*. July 1, 1920:112.

[8] Hockberger, PE. A history of ultraviolet photobiology for humans, animals, and microrganisms. *Photochem Photobiol.* 2002; 76(6):561-579.

[9] Howell J. Niels Ryberg Finsen. In: Fox DM, Rezak I, eds. *Nobel Laureates in Medicine of Physiology: A Biographic Dictionary.* New York, NY: Garland Publishing; 1990:181-183.

[10] Hall P. *Ultra-violet rays in the treatment and cure of disease.* 3rd ed. St, Louis, MO: C.V. Mosby Co; 1928.

[11] Ultra-violet rays in the treatment and cure of disease [book review]. *Bos Med Surg J.* 1928; 199:591.

[12] The burning question of the summer: *Vogue*. July 1, 1928: 100.

[13] Durant J, Bettman O. *Pictorial History of American Sports: From Colonial Times to the Present.* New York, NY: AS Barnes &Co Inc; 1952.

[14] Segrave K. *Suntanning in 20th Century America*: Jefferson, NC: McFarland &Co Inc; 2005.

[15] Whiteman, Honor. "Are changes in fashion, tanning perceptions to blame for rising melanoma rate?." *Medical News Today.* MediLexicon, Intl., 6 Oct. 2014. Web. Available at: http://www.medicalnewstoday.com/articles/283472.php. Accessed 12 Oct. 2014.

[16] Kaminester LH. Suntanning centers. *JAMA*. 1980;244(11):1258-1259.

[17] Thomas L. Lim HW. Sunscreens. *Journal of Drugs in Dermatol.*2003; 2,174.

[18] McCoy J. The solar keratosis and cutaneous cancer. *Arch Derm Syphilol.*1920;1(2):175-181.

[19] Albert M, Ostheimer KG. The evolution of current medical and popular attitudes toward ultraviolet light exposure: part 3. *J Am Acad Dermatol.*2003;49(6):1096-1106.

[20] Shaath, Nadim A., editor (2005). *Sunscreens: Regulations and Commercial Development,* Third Edition. Taylor & Francis Group.

[21] Craddock, P.T. (1998). *2000 Years of Zinc and Brass.* British Museum. p. 27.

[22] MacEachern, W.N.; Jillson, O.F. (January 1964). "A Practical Sunscreen — 'Red Vet Pet'". *Arch Dermatol* 89 (1): 147–150.

[23] Lim, Henry W. "Quantum Leaps: New, Improved Sunscreens Have Arrived". The Skin Cancer Foundation. Accessed Oct, 10, 2014.

[24] Shaath, N. *Evolution of modern sunscreen chemicals,* 3.

[25] Mosambuka B. "Sunscreen Market Presentation". Available at: https://prezi.com/ebnpw3tew10k/copy-of-sunscreen-market-presentation/. Accessed 13 Oct 2014.

[26] Wang SQ, Hu JY. "Challenges in Making an Effective Sunscreen." The Skin Cancer Foundation. Accessed 28 Sept 2014.

[27] Wang SQ, Osterwalder U, Jung K. Ex vivo evaluation of radical sun protection factor in popular sunscreens with antioxidants. Epub 2011 May 31. *J Am Acad Dermatol.* 2011; 65(3):525-30.

In: Sunscreens
Editors: Sean Henry Sharp

ISBN: 978-1-63482-160-5

Chapter 3

PSYCHOLOGY BEHIND THE USE OF SUNSCREENS, TANNING AND SKIN CANCER PREVENTION

Shailee Patel, Tulsie Patel and Katlein França*
Department of Dermatology & Cutaneous Surgery,
University of Miami Miller School of Medicine, Miami, FL, US

ABSTRACT

The benefits of the use of sunscreen have been widely presented in scientific literature. UV exposure has been related to the development of skin cancers. The use of sunscreen decreases this risk. Tanning is a social desire in many cultures. Media, fashion and social behaviors motivate people to get tan. Despite warnings about skin cancer, many individuals seek for tanning salons and natural sun exposure without adequate sun protection. Frequent tanners are psychologically and physically dependent on tanning. When an individual develops a skin cancer after using inadequate sun protection measures, feelings such as guilt, depression and anxiety may arise. This chapter will discuss the social psychological aspects related to sunscreen use, tanning and skin cancer prevention.

SUNSCREEN AND SKIN CANCER PREVENTION

Ultraviolet light is a major factor in the development of skin cancer and sunscreens can reduce the extent of photocarcinogenesis when sun avoidance is not possible [1]. The damaging effects from ultraviolet B (UVB) radiation (290-320 nm) are directed to DNA, which acts as an epidermal chromophore by undergoing conformational changes when exposed to UVB. This exposure results in the formation of pyrimidine dimers in the double helix and subsequent mutations [2, 3]. In contrast, ultraviolet A (UVA) radiation (320-400 nm) is less directly absorbed by DNA and causes most of its genotoxic effects by induction of oxidative stress that indirectly damages DNA and other critical intracellular structures [4, 5]. Without accurate and rapid repair of this damage, mutations in the genome and machinery of

* Corresponding Author: Katlein França, MD, MSc; Volunteer Faculty- Assistant Professor; Department of Dermatology & Cutaneous Surgery; University of Miami Miller School of Medicine; Miami, FL, USA.

the epidermal cells amass and lead to the development of both nonmelanoma and melanoma cancers.

Consistent and appropriate use of sunscreens has demonstrated to reduce the risk of actinic keratosis, nonmelanoma, and melanoma skin cancers [6-11]. Most of the data are based on randomized trials conducted with a pool of 1,621 patients that were followed for various amounts of time in Australia [8-11]. The researchers found a statistically significant reduction in incidence of squamous cell carcinoma at the sites of the sunscreen application compared to the no daily sunscreen group (rate ratio [RR] = 0.61; 95% confidence interval [CI], 0.46 to 0.81) [9]. Further analysis eight years after the completion of the initial trial showed a prolonged protective effect with a 35% lower incidence of squamous cell carcinoma in the daily sunscreen groups (RR = 0.65; 95% CI, 0.43 to 0.98) [10]. In terms of the incidence of basal cell carcinoma, the daily sunscreen group compared to the no daily sunscreen group was not statistically significant in either the four or eight year follow up study [9, 12]. Interestingly, a 50% reduction in the risk of melanoma was seen in the daily sunscreen group compared to the control (hazard ratio [HR], 0.50; 95% CI, 0.24 to 1.02; P = .051) [11].

These studies findings are the first to provide evidence for a reduction in the incidence of squamous cell carcinoma and melanoma after regular application of broad- spectrum sunscreen in adults. Of note, Australia has very high UV exposure thus making it difficult to generalize the data to other regions. In addition, the sunscreen used in the study was SPF 16 with inadequate UVA protection. Another factor to consider is that the control group was allowed to use sunscreen, so the defensive benefit from sunscreen may be much greater than the results suggested [9-12]. Nevertheless, there are not enough studies overall to know if sunscreen recommendations are clearly helpful but considering it has few harms, it would be reasonable to provide sunscreen counseling to patients at risk of developing skin cancer who will be exposed to excessive sunlight [13].

Initially sunscreens provided insufficient UVB protection and virtually no UVA protection, but modern formulations include novel UV filters, UV boosters, and photostabilizers that deliver substantial coverage against both UVB and UVA radiation [1]. In regards to UV protection, the main area of progress has been the expansion of coverage of the long UVA-I (340-400 nm) range with filters such as avobenzone and zinc oxide. Apart from new filters, the vehicle compounds have increased UV protective properties by using additives and film formers to ensure even coverage with every application. In addition to the advancements in superior UV protection, sunscreen technology has also enhanced the sensory profile with addition of silicones, silicas, and other slipping agents to minimize the unpleasant sticking feeling. To prevent the opaque white appearance due to the macro-sized titanium oxide and zinc oxide molecules, sunscreens now use nano-sized molecules for a better aesthetic finish [1].

The goal of photoprotection through sunscreen use is contingent on the combination of technological improvements in sunscreen preparation, the regulation of sunscreens, and proper behavior patterns by the public in regards to the use of sunscreens.

BEHAVIORAL AND SOCIAL PSYCHOLOGY OF SUNSCREEN USE

Despite improvements in sunscreen technology and regulatory changes, knowledge and behavior of the individual consumer play the most crucial role in obtaining sufficient photoprotection. Most of the research on the topic of skin cancer involves studies that focus on epidemiology, diagnosis and treatment while there is paucity in regards to behavioral research of the psychological aspects of sun exposure and protection. A better understanding of the behavioral psychology of sunscreen use would entail investigating the decision-making processes and communication strategies within and between individuals in a social system. For example, this could include assessing if fear-based versus appearance-based marketing improve sunscreen compliance. In addition, determining whether parental versus peer motivation would encourage better sun safety practices in adolescents. While social psychology of sunscreen use would evaluate the processes of a social system through impact of social organization on structural adjustment of the individual and of groups. This may include public health organizations such as the World Health Organization warning of the dangers of sun exposure and endorsing photoprotection on a global platform. Another potential social psychological intervention could address the impact of motivation by consistent health care provider recommendations of sunscreen use.

One of first studies in 1987 investigating the psychosocial factors in sunscreen use amongst beachgoers in California found that being a woman, having better skin cancer knowledge, and knowing someone who had cancer were associated with more sunscreen use. The higher usage among women may be due to anti-aging goals, association of sunscreen use with cosmetics, or that sunscreen advertisements are targeted to women. Interestingly, individuals with anxious mood were also associated with more sunscreen use. This might be explained by cancer fearing individuals may choose to use sunscreen or the use of sunscreen reminds individuals of skin cancer which results in anxiety [14]. Similarly, a study of teenagers in Virginia from 1992 found that female participants used more sunscreen than their male counterparts. In addition, having a friend who routinely used sunscreen, having parents who insisted on sunscreen use, and knowing that the maximum time for safe sun exposure is short were associated with more frequent sunscreen use. However, family history of skin cancer in this study was unrelated to sunscreen use and overall compliance was poor [15].

Unfortunately over a decade later even after improved efforts from the medical community and government agencies, less than 40% of teenagers used sunscreen and 83% reported having experience at least one sunburn in their lifetime [16]. Studies have also shown that approximately half of children do not protect themselves properly from solar UV exposure [17-20]. Continuing to empower the public with proper knowledge regarding the safety and benefits of sunscreen require a lot of effort similar to educating the public about cigarette smoke causing cancer. Thus targeting elementary school aged children and implementing basic knowledge during physical education or science class could provide better long term behavioral outcomes and save millions of lives. In term of adolescents, who are often motivated by beauty standards set by society such as having a tan can be encouraged use sunless tanning booths which are a safer alternative to artificial UV induced tanning and are increasing in popularity [21, 22].

In addition to educating specific populations, debunking myths to help reinforce healthy attitudes and motivate photoprotective behaviors are necessary. Often times sensationalized media coverage have been generated from studies that do not represent actual human usage leading to controversy about the hormonal effects of oxybenzone or phototoxicity of zinc oxide. For example, it would take 277 years of daily topical application of a sunscreen containing oxybenzone to reproduce the findings amongst the rats used in the study [23]. Another source of confusion comes from the tanning industry and its supporters trying to manipulate the public on the benefits of tanning including improved Vitamin D levels [24]. In reality, the amount of UV exposure needed to produce sufficient Vitamin D levels is small for example within 5 minutes at noon in June in Boston, Massachusetts and does not justify the use of artificial UV exposure or overlook the risk of cutaneous malignancy associated with its use [25]. Moreover, vitamin D supplements can easily avoid any risk of insufficiency even in those who practice proper photoprotection [26].

Public health interventions including the Surgeon General stance that the rise in skin cancers is associated with excessive exposure to indoor and outdoor UV is a step in the right direction but more is needed to ensure sustained momentum for prevention of skin cancer. Consumer behavior will guide the amount of photoprotection from sunscreens and other sun protective methods. Effective behavioral changes may take time to permeate through society by empowerment with knowledge and motivation.

TANNING AND SKIN CANCER

The ability for one to tan is directly related to the amount of melanin (pigment) that is present in the epidermis. The pigment itself is dependent on the number and size of the melanosomes that are released by the melanocytes in the basal layer of the skin as opposed to the actual number of melanocytes themselves [27]. This varied ability to tan is outlined most clearly by Fitzpatrick. Fitzpatrick created the gold standard classification system for detecting the degree of tanning or burning of one's skin following UV exposure [28].

Tanning is due to exposure to UVA and UVB light [29]. This exposure leads to a change in the skin such that there is a combination of immediate pigment darkening which is associated with activation of pre-existing melanin followed by tanning, which involves melanogenesis. Tanning becomes concerning for the development of cancer when the formation of DNA damage is considered [27]. For example, exposure to UVB is incredibly dangerous due to the formation of cyclobutane pyrimidine dimers that affect transcription and replication [29]. Exposure to UVA, on the other hand, may lead to the formation of oxygen free radicals that lead to breaks in DNA [30]. One innate mechanism for fighting this DNA damage is dependent on the effects of tumor suppressor, p53. P53 is essential in ensuring that replication of damaged DNA is halted until repair is complete [27]. Studies have shown that sunlight can often lead to p53 mutations that lead to unregulated cell growth due to the down-regulation of the inhibitory function of p53 [31]. It was also recently discovered that these DNA sequences that are halted by p53 play a direct role in the tanning process as they lead to tanning regardless of exposure to UV light. Further, a new study indicated that p53 is further involved in tanning as it leads to the ultimate activation of melanocortin-1 receptor, which activates melanocytes to produce melanin. In addition, mice models have shown that mice without p53 are increasingly susceptible to the effects of the damage of UV light on DNA [27].

There have been numerous studies indicating the relationship between UV light exposure and skin cancer. Solar radiation has already been deemed as "carcinogenic to humans" by the International Agency for Research on Cancer [31]. Over 50% of malignancies that are diagnosed each year in the United States are from cutaneous malignancies. Although sun safety measures are easily available, there is also an underlying misunderstanding among individuals that stems from the belief that tanning is protective against skin cancer. In actuality, not only is the original tanning behavior dangerous, but ongoing tanning is even more precarious as relatively unhealthy skin is further exposed to dangerous rays. Further, patients may be less likely to alter their behaviors given that the effects of UV exposure often take many years to develop. Childhood exposure often takes 30+ years to appear as a cutaneous malignancy, therefore making direct relationships between cutaneous injury (as a child) and the presence of skin cancer (as an adult) difficult [27]. No matter the source of exposure, whether natural sunlight or artificial sources such as tanning beds, exposure to UV light is dangerous [31].

Psychological Aspects of Tanning

Tanning, like any other behavior, can be attributed to numerous influences [32]. In popular culture, the term tanorexia has been coined to describe a person's constant desire to be excessively tan [33].

Although the term tanorexia seems to indicate a correlation between tanning and the psychology behind an eating disorder, numerous studies have shown a greater association between substance abuse disorders and addiction with a disproportionate use of tanning [32, 34]. A recent study actually found that individuals who had abused substances were more likely to participate in indoor tanning [35]. Further, those with substance abuse disorders and those who participate in excessive tanning also share other characteristics such as they both tend to be younger individuals who are negligent of the long-term consequences of their actions and who are more focused on enhancing their appearance [35-40]. Other common characteristics include the desire for pleasure in both addiction and tanning [41-43]. For example, many describe tanning as relaxing and mood boosting [41-43]. These latter effects have been associated with the concept that tanning dependence stems from the release of endogenous opioids upon UVR exposure [41, 42, 44, 45]. This idea has been further proven through the presence of withdrawal symptoms in frequent indoor tanners who were exposed to opioid blockers [42]. Overall, it has been found that indoor tanners often behave similar to those facing substance abuse and addiction as they are also more likely to be responding to social pressure, concerned about their appearance (ex. weight), and are also more likely to be smokers, drinkers, and drug users [46-48].

Skin Cancer Psychology

Many studies are being done to determine the effects of a diagnosis with melanoma or other non-melanoma conditions on the behavior of an individual and those around them. Although diagnoses with conditions as serious as melanoma are incredibly life altering, it has been found that it is actually quite difficult to change a person's behavior [49]. For example, a recent study showed that patients with dysplastic nevus syndrome, although aware of their increased risk for skin cancer, were not always willing to change their behavior [50]. Further, less than 33% of first-degree relatives of melanoma patients were willing to practice better sun safety precautions [51]. Alarmingly, even some patients with melanoma themselves, were not always willing to increase their sun safety measures despite an increased chance for recurrence [49].

However, behavior can be changed. For example, it has been shown that patients who have been diagnosed with melanoma are often more likely to change their behavior than others as they are more likely to appreciate the severity of their condition and the possible complications and results [52-54]. Patients with melanoma are more likely to experience anxiety and even fear following their diagnosis, thus leading to changes in their behavior [55]. Thus, preventative measures must be undertaken by matching the response that patients have following diagnosis to the currently limited changes that occur following simple sun safety education [49, 52-54].

CONCLUSION

There are numerous factors that influence a person's exposure to UVR. From a quest for a certain appearance to the availability of indoor and outdoor tanning, exposure to dangerous UVR is widespread in our culture. Social and psychological influences play a role in these behaviors. For example, many in our society are now classified as tanorexic due to their excessive need to tan. Although there are benefits to limited and protected sun exposure, it is greatly important that proper education be provided to all who are exposed to UVR. It is imperative that early intervention be implemented in the hopes of establishing safe behaviors that will help to prevent serious complications including melanoma.

REFERENCES

[1] Burnett ME, Hu JY, Wang SQ. Sunscreens: obtaining adequate photoprotection. *Dermatologic therapy.* 2012 May-Jun;25(3):244-51.

[2] Matsunaga T, Hieda K, Nikaido O. Wavelength dependent formation of thymine dimers and (6-4) photoproducts in DNA by monochromatic ultraviolet light ranging from 150 to 365 nm. *Photochemistry and photobiology.* 1991 Sep;54(3):403-10.

[3] Young AR, Chadwick CA, Harrison GI, Nikaido O, Ramsden J, Potten CS. The similarity of action spectra for thymine dimers in human epidermis and erythema suggests that DNA is the chromophore for erythema. *The Journal of investigative dermatology.* 1998 Dec;111(6):982-8.

[4] Mouret S, Baudouin C, Charveron M, Favier A, Cadet J, Douki T. Cyclobutane pyrimidine dimers are predominant DNA lesions in whole human skin exposed to UVA radiation. *Proceedings of the National Academy of Sciences of the United States of America.* 2006 Sep 12;103(37):13765-70.

[5] Tewari A, Sarkany RP, Young AR. UVA1 induces cyclobutane pyrimidine dimers but not 6-4 photoproducts in human skin in vivo. *The Journal of investigative dermatology.* 2012 Feb;132(2):394-400.

[6] Thompson SC, Jolley D, Marks R. Reduction of solar keratoses by regular sunscreen use. *The New England journal of medicine*. 1993 Oct 14;329(16):1147-51.

[7] Naylor MF, Boyd A, Smith DW, Cameron GS, Hubbard D, Neldner KH. High sun protection factor sunscreens in the suppression of actinic neoplasia. *Archives of dermatology*. 1995 Feb;131(2):170-5.

[8] Darlington S, Williams G, Neale R, Frost C, Green A. A randomized controlled trial to assess sunscreen application and beta carotene supplementation in the prevention of solar keratoses. *Archives of dermatology.* 2003 Apr;139(4):451-5.

[9] Green A, Williams G, Neale R, Hart V, Leslie D, Parsons P, et al. Daily sunscreen application and betacarotene supplementation in prevention of basal-cell and squamous-cell carcinomas of the skin: a randomised controlled trial. *Lancet.* 1999 Aug 28;354(9180):723-9.

[10] van der Pols JC, Williams GM, Pandeya N, Logan V, Green AC. Prolonged prevention of squamous cell carcinoma of the skin by regular sunscreen use. Cancer epidemiology, biomarkers & prevention: a publication of the American Association for Cancer Research, cosponsored by the American Society of Preventive Oncology. 2006 Dec;15(12):2546-8.

[11] Green AC, Williams GM, Logan V, Strutton GM. Reduced melanoma after regular sunscreen use: randomized trial follow-up. *Journal of clinical oncology: official journal of the American Society of Clinical Oncology.* 2011 Jan 20;29(3):257-63.

[12] Pandeya N, Purdie DM, Green A, Williams G. Repeated occurrence of basal cell carcinoma of the skin and multifailure survival analysis: follow-up data from the Nambour Skin Cancer Prevention Trial. *American journal of epidemiology.* 2005 Apr 15;161(8):748-54.

[13] Federman DG, Kirsner RS, Concato J. Sunscreen counseling by US physicians. *JAMA.* 2014 Jul 2;312(1):87-8.

[14] Keesling B, Friedman HS. Psychosocial factors in sunbathing and sunscreen use. Health psychology: official journal of the Division of Health Psychology, American Psychological Association. 1987;6(5):477-93.

[15] Banks BA, Silverman RA, Schwartz RH, Tunnessen WW, Jr. Attitudes of teenagers toward sun exposure and sunscreen use. *Pediatrics*. 1992 Jan;89(1):40-2.

[16] Geller AC, Oliveria SA, Bishop M, Buckminster M, Brooks KR, Halpern AC. Study of health outcomes in school children: key challenges and lessons learned from the Framingham Schools' Natural History of Nevi Study. *The Journal of school health.* 2007 Aug;77(6):312-8.

[17] Hall HI, May DS, Lew RA, Koh HK, Nadel M. Sun protection behaviors of the U.S. white population. *Preventive medicine.* 1997 Jul-Aug;26(4):401-7.

[18] Napier JA, Cavill I, Dunn CD, May A, Ricketts C. Oxymetholone treatment in aplastic anaemia: changes in erythropoiesis and serum erythropoietin. *British medical journa*l. 1976 Dec 11;2(6049):1426.

[19] Robinson JK, Rademaker AW, Sylvester JA, Cook B. Summer sun exposure: knowledge, attitudes, and behaviors of Midwest adolescents. *Preventive medicine*. 1997 May-Jun;26(3):364-72.

[20] Weinstock MA, Rossi JS, Redding CA, Maddock JE, Cottrill SD. Sun protection behaviors and stages of change for the primary prevention of skin cancers among beachgoers in southeastern New England. *Annals of behavioral medicine: a publication of the Society of Behavioral Medicine.* 2000 Fall;22(4):286-93.

[21] Brooks K, Brooks D, Dajani Z, Swetter SM, Powers E, Pagoto S, et al. Use of artificial tanning products among young adults. *Journal of the American Academy of Dermatology.* 2006 Jun;54(6):1060-6.

[22] Fu JM, Dusza SW, Halpern AC. Sunless tanning. Journal of the American Academy of Dermatology. 2004 May;50(5):706-13.

[23] Wang SQ, Burnett ME, Lim HW. Safety of oxybenzone: putting numbers into perspective. *Archives of dermatology.* 2011 Jul;147(7):865-6.

[24] Tangpricha V, Turner A, Spina C, Decastro S, Chen TC, Holick MF. Tanning is associated with optimal vitamin D status (serum 25-hydroxyvitamin D concentration) and higher bone mineral density. The American journal of clinical nutrition. 2004 Dec;80(6):1645-9.

[25] Wolpowitz D, Gilchrest BA. The vitamin D questions: how much do you need and how should you get it? *Journal of the American Academy of Dermatology.* 2006 Feb;54(2):301-17.

[26] Dermatology. AAo. Position Statement on VitaminD. 2009 [December 29, 2009].

[27] Ibrahim SF, Brown MD. Tanning and cutaneous malignancy. Dermatologic surgery: official publication for American Society for Dermatologic Surgery [et al]. 2008 Apr;34(4):460-74.

[28] Roberts WE. Skin type classification systems old and new. *Dermatologic clinics.* 2009 Oct;27(4):529-33, viii.

[29] Matsumura Y, Ananthaswamy HN. Toxic effects of ultraviolet radiation on the skin. *Toxicology and applied pharmacology.* 2004 Mar 15;195(3):298-308.

[30] Eller MS, Gilchrest BA. Tanning as part of the eukaryotic SOS response. Pigment cell research / sponsored by the European Society for Pigment Cell Research and the International Pigment Cell Society. 2000;13 Suppl 8:94-7.

[31] Woo DK, Eide MJ. Tanning beds, skin cancer, and vitamin D: An examination of the scientific evidence and public health implications. *Dermatologic therapy.* 2010 Jan-Feb;23(1):61-71.

[32] Heckman CJ, Egleston BL, Wilson DB, Ingersoll KS. A preliminary investigation of the predictors of tanning dependence. *American journal of health behavior.* 2008 Sep-Oct;32(5):451-64.

[33] News B. Young 'tanorexics' risking cancer. 2004.

[34] Warthan MM, Uchida T, Wagner RF, Jr. UV light tanning as a type of substance-related disorder. *Archives of dermatology.* 2005 Aug;141(8):963-6.

[35] O'Riordan DL, Field AE, Geller AC, Brooks DR, Aweh G, Colditz GA, et al. Frequent tanning bed use, weight concerns, and other health risk behaviors in adolescent females (United States). *Cancer causes & control: CCC.* 2006 Jun;17(5):679-86.

[36] Boldeman C, Jansson B, Dal H, Ullen H. Sunbed use among Swedish adolescents in the 1990s: a decline with an unchanged relationship to health risk behaviors. *Scandinavian journal of public health.* 2003;31(3):233-7.

[37] Hillhouse J, Stapleton J, Turrisi R. Association of frequent indoor UV tanning with seasonal affective disorder. *Archives of dermatology.* 2005 Nov;141(11):1465.

[38] Demko CA, Borawski EA, Debanne SM, Cooper KD, Stange KC. Use of indoor tanning facilities by white adolescents in the United States. *Archives of pediatrics & adolescent medicine.* 2003 Sep;157(9):854-60.

[39] Boldeman C, Jansson B, Nilsson B, Ullen H. Sunbed use in Swedish urban adolescents related to behavioral characteristics. *Preventive medicine.* 1997 Jan-Feb;26(1):114-9.

[40] Zeller S, Lazovich D, Forster J, Widome R. Do adolescent indoor tanners exhibit dependency? *Journal of the American Academy of Dermatology.* 2006 Apr;54(4):589-96.

[41] Feldman SR, Liguori A, Kucenic M, Rapp SR, Fleischer AB, Jr., Lang W, et al. Ultraviolet exposure is a reinforcing stimulus in frequent indoor tanners. *Journal of the American Academy of Dermatology.* 2004 Jul;51(1):45-51.

[42] Kaur M, Liguori A, Lang W, Rapp SR, Fleischer AB, Jr., Feldman SR. Induction of withdrawal-like symptoms in a small randomized, controlled trial of opioid blockade in frequent tanners. *Journal of the American Academy of Dermatology.* 2006 Apr;54(4):709-11.

[43] Poorsattar SP, Hornung RL. UV light abuse and high-risk tanning behavior among undergraduate college students. *Journal of the American Academy of Dermatology.* 2007 Mar;56(3):375-9.

[44] Levins PC, Carr DB, Fisher JE, Momtaz K, Parrish JA. Plasma beta-endorphin and beta-lipoprotein response to ultraviolet radiation. *Lancet.* 1983 Jul 16;2(8342):166.

[45] Belon PE. UVA exposure and pituitary secretion. Variations of human lipotropin concentrations (beta LPH) after UVA exposure. *Photochemistry and photobiology.* 1985 Sep;42(3):327-9.

[46] Diffey BL, Farr PM. Tanning with UVB or UVA: an appraisal of risks. *Journal of photochemistry and photobiology B, Biology.* 1991 Jan;8(2):219-23.

[47] Lazovich D, Forster J. Indoor tanning by adolescents: prevalence, practices and policies. *European journal of cancer.* 2005 Jan;41(1):20-7.

[48] Guay AT, Perez JB, Heatley GJ. Cessation of smoking rapidly decreases erectile dysfunction. *Endocrine practice: official journal of the American College of Endocrinology and the American Association of Clinical Endocrinologists.* 1998 Jan-Feb;4(1):23-6.

[49] Hornquist JO, Wikby A, Andersson PO, Dufva AM. Insulin-pen treatment, quality of life and metabolic control: retrospective intra-group evaluations. *Diabetes research and clinical practice.* 1990 Nov-Dec;10(3):221-30.

[50] Brandberg Y, Sjoden PO, Rosdahl I. Assessment of sun-related behaviour in individuals with dysplastic naevus syndrome: a comparison between diary recordings and questionnaire responses. *Melanoma research.* 1997 Aug;7(4):347-51.

[51] Azzarello LM, Dessureault S, Jacobsen PB. Sun-protective behavior among individuals with a family history of melanoma. Cancer epidemiology, biomarkers & prevention: a publication of the American Association for Cancer Research, cosponsored by the American Society of Preventive Oncology. 2006 Jan;15(1):142-5.

[52] Boggild AK, From L. Barriers to sun safety in a Canadian outpatient population. *Journal of cutaneous medicine and surgery.* 2003 Jul-Aug;7(4):292-9.

[53] Meyer N, Pruvost-Balland C, Bourdon-Lanoy E, Maubec E, Avri MF. Awareness, knowledge and attitudes towards sun protection among skin cancer-treated patients in

France. *Journal of the European Academy of Dermatology and Venereology: JEADV.* 2007 Apr;21(4):520-5.

[54] Smith BJ, Ferguson C, McKenzie J, Bauman A, Vita P. Impacts from repeated mass media campaigns to promote sun protection in Australia. *Health promotion international.* 2002 Mar;17(1):51-60.

[55] McBride CM, Emmons KM, Lipkus IM. Understanding the potential of teachable moments: the case of smoking cessation. *Health education research.* 2003 Apr;18(2):156-70.

In: Sunscreens
Editors: Sean Henry Sharp

ISBN: 978-1-63482-160-5

Chapter 4

THE ROLE OF ANTIOXIDANTS IN SUNSCREENS: THE CASE OF MELATONIN

***Ana Flo Sierra*[1], *Víctor Flo Sierra*[1], *Ana Cristina Calpena Campmany*[1] *and Beatriz Clares Naveros*[2,*]**

[1]Pharmacy and Pharmaceutical Technology Department,
Faculty of Pharmacy, University of Barcelona, Spain
[2]Pharmacy and Pharmaceutical Technology Department,
Faculty of Pharmacy, University of Granada, Spain

ABSTRACT

The main objective of this chapter is to perform a detailed review on antioxidants in sunscreens, and more specifically on Melatonin. Melatonin is a neurohormone with natural antioxidant properties. In order to understand its importance, an initial review of the structure of the skin and the ultraviolet radiation effects is carried out. Throughout the chapter the nature of products, mechanisms of action and advantages and disadvantages of the conventional and novel groups of sunscreens that protect from the ultraviolet radiation are discussed, (*i*) organic sunscreens, (*ii*) inorganic sunscreens (*iii*) DNA repair agents (*iv*) cyclooxigenase-2 inhibitors, (*v*) iron chelators (*vi*) osmolytes and (*vii*) natural antioxidant substances. Several studies have reported the benefits of Melatonin used either for ultraviolet radiation protection or in combination with traditional radiotherapy for the treatment of human cancers. For this reason, in this chapter a thorough review of the characteristics and properties of this substance is performed in order to underscore the importance of this promising active for use in sunscreens.

1. HUMAN SKIN

The skin is composed of 3 layers of differentiated tissues. The most external layer is the epidermis, followed by the dermis and the hypodermis, which is the most internal layer of the

* Corresponding author: Campus of Cartuja St, Granada 18071, Spain. Email: beatrizclares@ugr.es.

skin. Overall, it is a thick, resistant and flexible membrane that in an adult has an approximate area of 1.5 – 2 m^2 [1].

1.1. Epidermis

It is the most external layer of the skin. Its thickness varies from 0.04 mm to 1.6 mm depending on the zone of the body. The primary cell in the epidermis is the keratinocyte, but there are additional cells such as melanocytes, Langerhans cells and Merkel cells. In the epidermis there are three different appendages: the sweat glands, the pilosebaceous follicles and the nails [1].

Epidermis is composed by 4 distinct layers; *Stratum basal* is a single layer of columnar basal cells, which are attached to the basal membrane via hemidesmosomes. It is composed of epidermal stem cells that by mithosis produce new keratinocytes. These cells evolve as they move toward the surface layer. When keratinocytes mature, they become in the *Stratum spinosum*, the *Stratum granulosum* and finally the *Stratum corneum* [2]. The normal turnover rate of a healthy epidermis is about 28 days [1].

The latter layer, *Stratum corneum*, formed mainly by corneocytes (terminally differentiated keratinocytes), is the responsible for the skin barrier that acts protecting the skin, preventing water loss, maintaining the hydration of the skin and so many other protective functions [2].

1.2. Dermis

It is located between the subcutaneous and dermal-epidermal junction. It measures from 0.3 mm to 3.0 mm depending on the zone of the body. The dermis is composed in a 90% of collagen, elastic fibers, blood vessels, lymph vessels, some muscle fibers and pilosebaceous and sweat glands and a 10% of cellular components, including fibrocyte, monocyte, histiocyte, Langerhans cells, lymphocytes, and eosinophils, along with the vascular and lymphaticassociated cells [2].

1.3. Hypodermis

It is the innermost layer of the skin. It invaginates into the dermis, with which is attached by collagen and elastin fibers. It is composed by fibroblasts, adipose cells and macrophages. Its principal function is fat storage [2].

The ability of the skin to bear and react to solar radiation depends primarily on the skin phototype. In Table 1 are classified the 6 different phototypes depending on the ease of sunburning and skin pigmentation.

The skin, due to its location in the body, is the most important protective barrier against external aggressions. One of the main aggressions comes from solar radiation, causing damages such as sunburn, photoaging, skin cancer among others that we be reviewed in the next section.

Table 1. Classification of skin phototypes (adaptation from the classification created by Fitzpatrick and Bolognia [3]

Skin type classification/phototype		Sunburn	Tans after sun exposure
Melano-compromised	I	Always	Seldom
	II	Usually	Sometimes
Melano-competent	III	Sometimes	Usually
	IV	Seldom	Always
Melano-protected	V	Never	Naturally brown skin
	VI		Naturally black skin

2. Solar Radiation

The electromagnetic radiation spectrum is classified based on its wavelength in radio waves, microwaves, infrared (IR), visible light (Vis), ultraviolet light (UV), X-rays and γ radiation. However, the solar spectrum that reaches the surface of the earth only comprises wavelengths of electromagnetic energy between 300 and 3000 nm, which include UVB, UVA, Vis and NIR. The photobiological effects are higher at shorter wavelengths because they have higher energy.

The main human photobiology studies have been focused on UV but Vis light and NIR also reach the earth and have photobiological effects [4]. In Figure 1, are summarized the photobiological effects distributed depending on the wavelength. The main characteristics of each one of the solar radiations that arrive to the ground are described below.

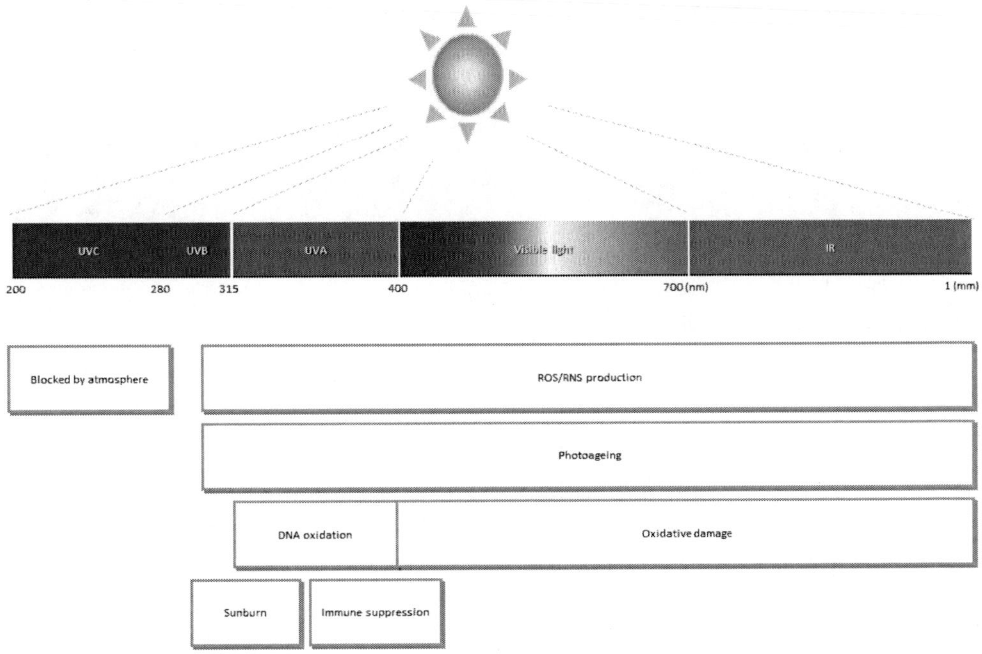

Figure 1. Solar spectrum that arrives to the Earth and photobiological effects that produces.

2.1. UVB

Wavelength: 280 – 315 nm. Wavelengths between 280 and 295 nm are filtered by the atmosphere.

Penetration: It penetrates up to the basal layer of the epidermis (Figure 2)

Effects: It generates reactive oxygen species (ROS) and reactive nitrogen species (RNS). These species create inflammation, sunburn and stimulate skin ageing. The high energy photons of UVB can be absorbed by DNA bases of the cell, causing mutagenic lesions. These lesions are normally repaired by nucleotide excision repair. However, a high accumulation of mutations in skin cells due to UVB exposition could potentially develop a UV-associated skin cancer [5]. It is responsible of the delayed tanning [6].

Endogen chromophores: Melanin [6].

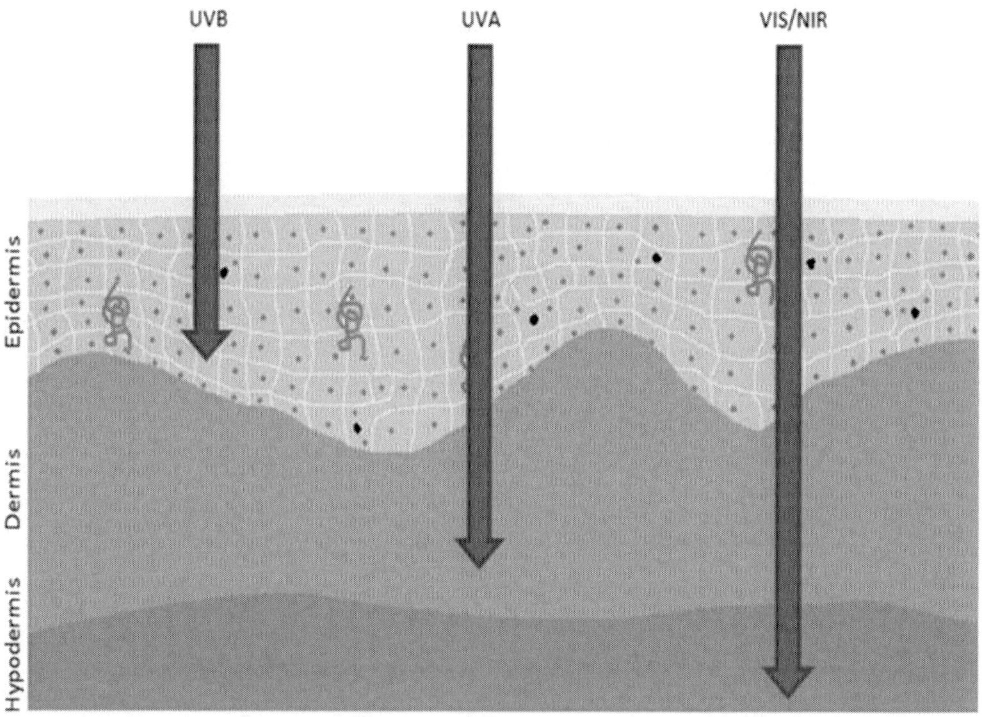

Figure 2. Penetration of solar radiation in the skin.

2.2. UVA

Wavelength: 315 – 400 nm. The biological effects of the shorter wavelengths of UVA are very similar to those of UVB, for that reason, some authors differentiates between UVA2 (315-340 nm) and UVA1 (340-400 nm) [4].

Penetration: It penetrates up to the dermis (Figure 2).

Effects: It generates ROS and RNS that alters DNA, proteins and lipids. It also generates immunosuppression. The oxidative damage that causes in the skin can increase indirectly the risk of skin cancer due to the formation of oxidized DNA bases. It also contributes to skin photoaging [5, 7, 8]. It is responsible of the immediate pigmentation [6].

Endogen chromophores: Melanin, Riboflavin-containing FAD and FMN trans-urocanic acid [9].

2.3. Vis Light

Wavelength: 400 – 700 nm.

Penetration: It is approximately the 50% of the solar spectrum [10]. It penetrates deeper than UV radiation, and a 20% reaches the hypodermis (Figure 2).

Effects: It generated ROS and it also induces inflammatory cytokines such as IL-1, IL-6, IL-8 and GM-CSF, increases the expression of matrix degrading enzymes (MMP-1 and MMP-9) and may form oxidized DNA bases [11]. It is also responsible of the pigment darkening in subjects with phototypes IV and V [12].

Endogen chromophores: Hemoglobin, Melanin, Bilirubin Riboflavin, Porphyrins [13].

2.4. NIR

Wavelength: 700 – 3000 nm.

Penetration: It is approximately the 30% of the solar spectrum, 65% penetrates up to the dermis and a 10% up to the hypodermis [10] (Figure 2).

Effects: It generates ROS and induces unbalanced gene expression of MMP. It also decreases collagen gene expression, favors angiogenesis, affects mitochondrial integrity, is involved in photoaging and it can potentially promote carcinogenesis [14-16].

Endogen chromophores: Cytochrome C oxydase of the mitochondria [15, 17].

3. Sun Exposure Effects

It is globally accepted that solar radiation has beneficial health effects. For example, it stimulates the production of cholecalciferol (vitamin D_3) [18], necessary for the proper functioning of bone metabolism and immune system. It is also recommended the controlled exposure to the sun to treat or reduce the severity of skin diseases such as psoriasis and vitiligo [19]. But it is also accepted that uncontrolled exposure to sun has harmful photobiological effects. These effects can be divided into acute or short-term effects and long-term or chronic effects.

3.1. Short Time Effects

Erythema

This is the best recognized effect of UV radiation in the skin. Commonly known as sunburn, is primarily caused by exposure to UVB and in lesser extent to UVA2. The signs of erythema are the classic of an inflammation, such as redness, tenderness, edema and warmth [20].

Free Radical Formation

Under sun exposure, the endogenous chromophores absorb the photons produced by radiation. After photon absorption these excited molecules react with oxygen, resulting in the generation of ROS. When ROS are generated in an amount that overcome the endogenous antioxidant defense, it is produced an oxidative stress. ROS include hydroxyl ($OH^{\cdot}$), singlet oxygen ($^1O_2$) and superoxide anion ($O_2^{\cdot-}$). The 2 last species are also produced by neutrophils that are increased in photodamage skin. The enzyme superoxide dismutase converts $O_2^{\cdot-}$ into hydrogen peroxide (H_2O_2). H_2O_2 can cross cell membranes and in conjunction with transitional Fe^{2+} produces the hydroxyl radical ($OH^{\cdot}$) Fe^{3+}. Both $^1O_2$ and $OH^{\cdot}$ can interact with cell membrane lipids producing lipid peroxidation that leads to inflammation [21]. ROS inactivate TIMPs, which are tissue inhibitors of matrix-metalloproteases and induce the synthesis and activation of the enzyme MMP responsible of its degradation. Both $OH^{\cdot}$ and $^1O_2$ are able to directly damage DNA. ROS also damage proteins [22].

3.2. Long Time Effects

Photoaging

ROS promote cytokine cascade producing inflammatory reactions that are the responsible of photoaging. They cause the activation of matrix metalloproteinase (MMP) and the release of proinflammatory cytokines and growth factors that modify both collagen and elastin in the extracellular matrix, ending in the degradation of skin structural integrity and causing dysfunction of the melanocytes, which leads to skin hyperpigmentation [23].

Immunosuppression

It is known that UV radiation has both effects anti- and proinflammatory on the immune system of the skin. The irradiation of the skin suppress the immunity mediated by cells because it alters the Langerhans cell migration, producing suppressor T lymphocytes and altering the skin cytokine profile [24].

Photocarcinogenesis

Solar radiation induces mutations in DNA and its immunosuppressive properties also affect host immune system which causes problems recognizing damaged malignant cells. The association between exposure to UV radiation and the development of skin cancer, including malignant melanoma, basal cell carcinoma and squamous cell carcinoma is well documented [25]. Superficial spreading and nodular melanoma are associated with intermittent and intense solar radiation exposure, while lentigo maligna melanoma and squamous cell carcinoma are linked to cumulative sun exposure [26, 27].

Ciclooxigenase-2 (COX-2) is an enzyme that is induced in the epidermis by various cytokines such as IF-γ, TNF-α, IL-1 and growth factors, in various cells and tissues. Some of these inflammatory mediators are produced in response to UV irradiation. COX-2 is the first enzyme in the enzymatic cascade that converts arachidonic acid into prostaglandins (PG) and thromboxane. A study performed by Tripp et al. [28] demonstrated that keratinocyte proliferation and apoptosis are regulated by COX-2 after acute UV exposure *in vivo*, probably by the production of PG. It suggested that COX-2 induced PG had a significant role in the pathogenesis of UV-induced epidermal neoplasia.

Photodermatoses

The exposure to UV radiation and Vis light UVR can reduce the quality of life for people with immunologically mediated photodermatoses, such as solar urticaria, photoallergic drug reactions and chronic actinic dermatitis among others [29].

4. SUN PROTECTION

Protection against this harmful radiation can be carried out by physical barriers, such as hats, sunglasses and long sleeved clothing or using photoprotective substances. In the next section is reviewed the current situation of sunscreens, what types there are, what are their advantages and disadvantages and how the use of antioxidants improve the current situation of the photoprotection. The use of sunscreens is the most popular measure of protection to prevent the undesirable effects of solar radiation. Many studies have shown that regular use of sunscreens applied correctly reduces the number of cases of actinic keratosis, squamous cell carcinoma and attenuates the development of new nevi in children. In addition, regular use of sunscreen prevents premature skin aging [30].

The development of the first sunscreens dates back to the early twentieth century, when Norman Paul first linked sun exposure with skin cancer. Shortly thereafter, it was proposed that the responsible for sunburn and skin cancer was only UVB radiation. Following this discovery, pharmacists began to develop formulations containing substances that are able to block the UVB radiation. The first sunscreen was commercialized in 1928. Later in the 60s, the Austrian scientist Franz Greiter introduced the concept of Sun Protection Factor (SPF) to determine the effectiveness of a sunscreen to suppress UV-induced sunburn. Furthermore, people began to understand that sun exposure not only caused sunburn and cancer, it also caused structural damage to the skin which favored the skin ageing. In the 70s, it was demonstrated that UVA rays also cause premature skin ageing. Therefore, cosmetic ~~so~~ companies started offering sunscreens that protected against UVA and UVB.

Since then, the use of sunscreens has spread worldwide and people are becoming more aware of the importance of protecting the skin to prevent undesirable effects of solar radiation.

Nowadays, there are many different sunscreens, with single active substances or combined with complex combinations.

It is important to take into account that in order to have a complete action preventing all undesirable effects associated with sun exposure in short and long term, it is necessary to have a sunscreen that complies with the requirements of:

(i) Providing uniform protection against all the radiation that arrives to the ground. The major part of the sunscreens that are actually in the market were studied for its utility absorbing or scattering UVA and/or UVB radiations but they have not been studied for their usefulness avoiding photobiological effects of IR and Vis light [10, 16, 31, 32].

(ii) Free radicals scavenging. The photoprotective agents included in the sunscreens should exert as scavengers of the free radicals formed after exposure to solar radiation.

(iii) Containing active ingredients that stimulate DNA repair systems. The ideal sunscreen should include a component capable of directly or indirectly repair DNA damage as a result of solar exposure.

(iv) Photostability. The substances that act absorbing UV photons, reduce the solar radiation acting as a chromophore, which absorbs the energy in form of photons when arriving to the skin during sun exposure. This absorption results in the excitation of the molecule that has absorbed the energy. The excited filter dissipates the absorbed energy generally very fast, in the form of heat or light, returning to its native state. This process, could theoretically continue repetitively, and this will lead in a photoestable filter [33].

(v) Safety. Sunscreens may be formulated to be retained in the skin, therefore and will not arrive to plasma. Moreover, they cannot produce photoallergenity.

(vi) In addition, to facilitate the user's compliance, it is important that it has pleasing sensory and tactile profiles [31].

The active substances that compose sunscreens are classified depending on how they exert its effect in: chemical or organic filters, physical or inorganic filters, antioxidants, DNA repair agents, cyclooxygenase-2 inhibitors, iron chelators and osmolytes.

4.1. Chemical Filters

Usually, this type of filters acts absorbing UV radiation through chemical reactions. Nevertheless, new developed filters such as Tinosorb M and Tinosorb S can also act reflecting UV radiation. As an advantage, organic filters are more popular than inorganic filters because they do not leave white appearance onto the skin. But they have several disadvantages:

(i) Photoinstability: Some organic filters, when absorbing UV photons can dissipate the energy by other pathways that lead to the destruction of them or to a partial or complete reduction of their capacity to absorb energy, through processes such as fragmentation, isomerization, reactivity with other molecules or free radicals production [34]. Examples of photounstable organic filters are Octyl methoxycinnamate, 2-phenylbenzimidazole-5-sulfonic acid, Benzophenone-3, and avobenzone [35].

(ii) Photodegradation: The photoinstability of some organic filters can lead to decomposition of the molecule under UV light, potentially leading to the generation of ROS and toxic derivative compounds [36]. Photodegradation, which is one of the consequences of photoinstability, can cause among other phototoxicity, photoirritation and photoallergic reactions that may occur by contact with the degradation of products formed. The use of sunscreens with photodegradable substances may increase the risk of sunburn, but it can also increase the risk of cancer. For that reason, the photostability of the filters included in a sunscreen should be always determined *in vitro*, alone and in combination, by using absorbance measures [37, 38].

(iii) Absorption through the skin: there are studies that have demonstrated that some of the most used organic filters are able to penetrate the skin and have been found in plasma, urine and even in breast women milk [39, 40].

(iv) Estrogenic effects: it has been demonstrated that some of the filters, such as, Benzophenone-3, homomethyl salicylate, Octyl methoxycinnamate, 3-(4-methylbenzylidene) camphor have estrogenic effects [35, 41].

(v) Spectrum of action: most of the organic filters absorb only UVB photons and only a few are able to absorb both UVB and UVA. For that reason, complex combinations are formulated. Nevertheless, studies have demonstrated that *per se*, organic filters do not have protective effect in the NIR range [33].

Usually, a combination of different organic UV filters is used in order to reach sufficient SPF. After several studies that demonstrated the incompatibility of some filters when are combined in a sunscreen due to reactions between the molecules that made them photounstable [33], FDA regulate the combinations of organic filters that could be used for the preparation of sunscreen and the maximum concentration that can be used for each of them [42].

4.2. Physical Filters

Inorganic filters are inert materials formed by particles that act as a barrier to UV radiation because they reflect and scatter the light and also can absorb photons. The photon absorption results in electron mobility and transitions between electronic states forming excited species. The two best known inorganic particles used in sunscreens are micronized zinc oxide (ZnO) and titanium dioxide (TiO_2). The problems arisen with ZnO and TiO_2 due to photocalatytic activity and the poor acceptance of these filters, due to the high refractive index, have led to the development of new inorganic molecules with better stability and low refractive index, one of them is $CePO_4$. This substance has shown chemical and physical stability and low interaction with organic filters [43]. Inorganic filters have some advantages:

(i) They do not degrade when exposed to UV radiation

(ii) If they are not used in a nanoparticulate size they are not able to penetrate the skin

(iii) Broad spectrum. They exert their action in UV, Vis and IR ranges

But these filters can also have some disadvantages:

(i) High refractive index: The inorganic materials with high refractive index tend to leave the skin with a peculiar white appearance that leads to a low cosmetic acceptability. It has been tried to reduce the size of the inorganic filter into nanoscale in order to avoid the undesirable white marks that they leave in the skin. But these TiO_2 and ZnO have been deeply studied because these nanoscale particles can generate highly oxidizing ROS when exposed to ultraviolet radiation [44]. Nanoparticles with a surface coating by silica and alumina and/or doping with vanadium or manganese reduce the generation of ROS.

(ii) Photocatalityc activity: Dunford et al. [45] demonstrated that both ZnO and TiO_2 can catalyze oxidative damage to DNA in vitro and in cultured human fibroblasts.

(iii) ROS generation: in a study performed by Lewicka et al. [44] eight commercial formulation containing nanoparticles of ZnO and TiO_2 were analyzed to determine the ability to generate ROS, and it was concluded that formulations containing nanoparticles of ZnO when exposed to UV radiation generate as much ROS as sunlight.

(iv) Interaction with organic unstable organic filters: The high photocatalytic activity that facilitates the generation of ROS, can oxidize and degrade other organic filters included in the sunscreen that would result in instability and unsafe reactions.

4.3. Antioxidants

In the lasts sections, it has been explained how, most organic filters do not adequately protect not only against free radicals but also generating free radicals *per se* due to lack of photostability. Also, it has been explained that conventional inorganic filters are not popular because they leave white appearance on the skin and that these filters, when incorporated as nanoparticles have some toxicological problems, one of them is the production of free radicals after sun exposure.

Consequently, in the previous years it has increased the necessity of finding new substances whose main mechanism of action was free radicals scavenging and the oxidative stress elimination. Molecules that can perform these actions are the antioxidants.

Despite the large amount of antioxidants known, are not yet widely used in commercial sunscreens. However, there are many articles that demonstrate the goodness of these substances and describe how they act at the molecular level to scavenge free radicals and prevent oxidative stress.

Table 2 shows an extensively list of antioxidants which have shown good antioxidant action against oxidative stress, as well as free radical scavenger in the presence of UV radiation. Studies also have shown that most of them also work against Vis light and IR radiation as the main damages of these radiations are oxidative stress and free radical formation, as shown in Figure 1.

One of the antioxidants that have been more studied is melatonin. Several studies give as powerful properties as free radical scavenger, oxidative stress reducer and DNA damage reduction, among others. For this reason, many authors have focused on the study of melatonin as possible photoprotective, and due to the large number of studies showing his goodness for this use, in Section 5 will be reviewed this substance in detail.

Table 2. Antioxidants which good antioxidant action against oxidative stress, and free radical scavenger in the presence of UV radiation

Aloe poly/ oligosaccharides	Aloe poly and oligosaccharide prevent immune suppression induced by exposure to UV by reducing the production of IL-10 in mice. Aloe protects against delayed-type hypersensitivity (DTH) in a stable manner over time, however it is a process that is not yet well studied.	[46,47]
Apigenin and luteolin	The use combined of apigenin and luteolin inhibits ROS production in HaCaT cells irradiated with UVA. Keratinocytes pretreated with these flavonoids also inhibit MMP-1 production induced by UVA and suppresses the expression of c-jun and c-fos, as well as the MAPK phosphorylation. Flavonoids also reduce the influx of calcium and the Ca^{2+}/CaMKs phosphorylation.	[48]
Astaxanthin	Astaxanthin is a lipid-soluble carotenoid mainly obtained from *Haematococcus pluvialis*. In humans it is administered orally and topically. It provides a significant inhibition of melanogenesis in age spots by suppressing melanocyte oxidative polymerization and inflammation of the epidermis. A treatment with astaxanthin also acts protecting keratinocyte differentiation and cornification induced by oxidative stress.	[49]
β-carotene	β-carotene inhibits UVA-induced genetic modulation in the lineages of human keratinocyte HaCaT. In unirradiated cells, gene regulation suggests that β-carotene significantly reduce stress signs and degradation of the extracellular matrix, also promotes the differentiation of keratinocytes. These effects occur through sequestration $^1O_2$.	[50,51]
Butylated hydroxitoluene	It is a synthetic antioxidant used as a preservative in products which contain lipids. It has been shown to inhibit erythema, ornithine decarboxylase activity, carcinogenesis and photoaging.	[52]
Cadmium chloride-induced MT	It is an antioxidant. In mice deficient in MT-1 and MT-2 genes occurs more sunburn and apoptosis UVB-induced.	[53]
Caffeic acid	This substance applied topically protects from UV-induced erythema in vivo and in vitro. Its protective effect comes from its ability to decrease ROS.	[54]
Caffeine	Topical application of caffeine reduces the formation of malignant and non-malignant tumors, as well as partial reduction of damage by irradiation. Some studies suggest that caffeine facilitates apoptosis in tumor tissue by inhibiting gene expression of ATR (ataxia telangiectasia and Rad3 related).	[55]
Calcitriol	Active form of vitamin D. Topical application of calcitrol in mice inhibits the sunburn cells formation due to the induction of melatotionein expression.	[56]
Calluna vulgaris L. extract	Topical application of C. vulgaris extract (4 mg of polyphenols /cm^2) in mice during the 30 minutes before exposure to UVB radiation for 10 days provides protection to the skin by reducing the levels of TNF-α and IL-6 and the formation of sunburn cells induced by UVB. Therefore, C. vulgaris extract protects skin from DNA damage caused by the sun.	[57]

Table 2. (Continued)

Cistus extracts	This genus of Mediterranean shrubs contains flavonoids that are considered oxidative chain disruptors because they react as intermediators and form stable products. The leaf extracts of Cistus have shown in rat liver microsomes the ability of free radical scavenging and inhibition of lipid peroxidation.	[58]
Cocoa powder	Volunteers who took this flavonoid for 12 weeks showed a reduction in UV-induced erythema, improved skin appearance and hydration, increased the thickness of the skin and a reduction in transepidermal water loss.	[59]
Coptis chinensis glycans	It contains arabinose, manose and galactose. It scavenges superoxide and hydroxyl radical in a dose-dependent way, and DPPH radicals. It increases significantly IL-10 and TNF-α. The glycans that compose C. chinensis absorb in IR range.	[60]
Cynaropicrin	Cynaropicrin prevents photoaging by suppression of light induction of NF-kB transactivation.	[61]
Dacryodes sp.	Leaf extract or fruit has a high antioxidant activity against DPPH radicals and hydrogen peroxide radical. This activity is produced mainly by its composition in flavonoids, phenols and anthocyanins. Ellagic acid present in these species can inhibit the growth of chemically induced tumors. It has not yet been tested for use in effects induced by UVR.	[62]
Divalent zinc ion	It is the topical form of zinc and provides antioxidant photoprotection. It can replace the redox active, such as iron and copper; on the other hand can also induce the synthesis of MT's, sulfhydryl-rich proteins that protect against free radical molecules. It has also been shown to efficiently protect mouse skin against the appearance of sunburn cells induced by UVB and UVA.	[63]
Equol (4',7-isoflavandiol)	It is a derivative of daizein isoflavonoid, metabolized by the intestinal flora in mammals. Topical application in mice protects against inflammation, immunosuppression, and the formation of cyclobutane pyrimidine dimers. However, its photoprotective effect is lower than genistein or its precursor, daidzein.	[64]
Ferulic acid	It is used as photoprotective agent in many solar creams and lotions. It is a powerful antioxidant that inhibits lipid peroxidation and oxidative deterioration of cosmetic products and food.	[54]
Fish oil	Rich in omega-3 has been shown to have photoprotective properties. Decreases the formation of sunburn cells and UVB-induced inflammation after 3 months of ingestion. Reduces response to UVA in patients with polymorphous light eruptions. However, the effects are achieved only with large doses of fish oil; therefore, their use is not widely extended.	[65]
Fucoxanthin	The antioxidant activity of flucoxanthin inhibits blood vessel formation induced by UVB exposure in hairless mice model. The expression of vascular endothelial growth factor decreases with wrinkle reduction, reducing the hypertrophy of the epidermis caused by exposure to UV.	[66]
General carotenoids	Raman spectroscopy has shown that as a defense mechanism against harmful radiation and environmental factors, topical application of carotenoids increases the potential defense of human epidermis. However, carotenoids are renowned nutricosmetics, improving the resistance and hydration of the skin.	[67]

Genistein	It is a powerful antioxidant found in soybeans. After sun exposure, it inhibits tyrosine kinase, reduces inflammation and the subsequent immunosuppression. Applied topically, it protects against radiation damage between 1 and 4 hours after application.	[68]
Green tea extract	Green tea extract contains variety of active molecules including catechins, polysaccharides, caffeine, apigenin and luteolin. Dietary intake of green tea extracts or topical application provides anti-inflammatory effects, antioxidant, and UVB-induced DNA damage reparation mechanisms. Protection against photoaging related to matrix metalloproteinase (MMP-2, MMP-9) and photoinmunology. Inhibit foto-increased lipid peroxidation. At 2.5mg/cm2 concentration on human skin before UV irradiation reduced UV-induced oxidative damage.	[69, 70]
Jacquez grapes wine extract	The extract of grape Jacquez wine efficiently prevents oxidative injury suffered by the skin induced by exposure to UVB radiation. This photoprotective effect is attributed to its high content of polyphenols. Its application, tested in *in vitro* reconstituted skin helps to maintain the redox state of the epidermis even after radiation exposure.	[71]
Kaempferia parviflora extract	It prevents the appearance of wrinkles and loss of collagen and increases the expression of catalase. The treatment with this extract significantly reduces inflammatory mediators NF-KB, IL-1β and COX-2.	[72]
L-carnosine and Rhodiola rosea extract association	The combination of these extracts modulates the levels of β-endorphin, enkephalin, CGRP, substance P, IL-1α, TNF-α and IL-10 in normal human keratinocytes in normal conditions and after punctual or chronic exposure to UV radiation.	[73]
L-epicatechin-3-gallate (ECG)	It has free radical scavenging effects. ECG inhibits keratinocytes apoptosis induced by UVA and UVB in a dose-dependent manner. For UVA, this mechanism works by inhibiting the production of hydrogen peroxide. For UVB, ECG inhibits peroxidation of membrane lipids, and also blocking the activation of ERK1 / 2, p38 and JNK in keratinocytes. Therefore, ECG has demonstrated an important antioxidant potential to prevent photodamage.	[74]
L-epigallocatechin-3-gallate (EGCG)	It is the most active polyphenol of Green tea. It induces the reduction of H2O2, iNOS, NO, LPO and MPO. It also inhibits the decrease of cell antioxidant enzymes (catalase, glutathione peroxidase, superoxide dismutase and glutathione). It has DNA repair properties through NER mechanism. EGCG promotes survival of keratinocytes and inhibits UV-induced apoptosis with the help of a dual mechanism: (1) bad phosphorylation increased via the ERK-AKT dependent pathways (2) ratio Bcl-2 / Bax increased. EGCG treatment of human HaCaT keratinocyte cultures reduces UVB-induced cytotoxicity and also inhibits the expression of p53 mRNA and p21 regulators of apoptosis, and the genes c-fos gene and blocks the secretion of IL and TNF-α. These data suggest that EGCG can be used for its anti-aging effects and as a tumor suppressor in human skin. In addition, EGCG may inhibit /regulate the action of NF-kB, iNOS gene expression and NO generation in keratinocytes after UVB exposure. This suggests that EGCG can have an inhibitory effect of the UVB photodamage caused in the epidermis.	[69,70,75]

Table 2. (Continued)

	In an in-vivo evaluation in humans, the addition of EGCG into a broad spectrum sunscreen decreased UV-induced damage compared to the cream alone.	
Lycopene	Employed in various formulations for topical use, lycopene has a high therapeutic potential for recover of epidermal antioxidants lost during UV exposure. It also acts as a skin protectant against UV damage. It has been found that lycopene also acts as a preventive agent by inhibiting the activity of ornithine decarboxylase in the epidermis, reducing inflammation and maintaining normal levels of cell proliferation, presumably by preventing DNA damage by apoptotic lock, after exposure to UVB.	[76]
Mangifera indica L. extract	Mice orally treated with mango extract showed a significant ability to modulate the effects of UV radiation by inhibiting epidermal hypertrophy.	[77]
Mangiferin	The mangiferine is a scavenger of ROS (superoxide radicals and hydroxyl radicals). In cultures of human HaCaT keratinocytes, mangiferin inhibits induction of MMP-1 produced by the hydrogen peroxide, blocking the binding of AP-1 to DNA. Furthermore, mangiferin inhibits keratinocyte death by reducing the MEK-ERK and JNK-SEK pathways.	[78]
Myricetin	Myricetin inhibits keratinocyte death UVB-induced in a dose-dependent manner, due to the inhibition of the increase of hydrogen peroxide and the inhibition of of c-jun activation induced by UVB.	[79]
N-acetil cysteine and genistein	Human skin pretreatment with N-acetylcysteine in combination with genistein, blocks UV induction of collagen, indicating the photoprotective potential of these substances.	[80]
Naringenin	The treatment of human HaCaT keratinocytes with naringenin extends the long-term survival of the cells after irradiation with UVB. Excision of PARP-1, caspase activation and the ratio Bax/Bcl2 induced by UVB are modulated after treatment with naringenin, indicating an antiapoptotic effect of this molecule. Also, when HaCaT cells are irradiated with UVB, naringenin increases CPD removal, indicating that the active ingredient has a protective effect against DNA damage.	[81]
Phellodendron amullenses glycans	It contains arabinose, xylose, glucose, galactose. It scavenges superoxide and hydroxyl radical in a dose-dependent way, and DPPH radicals. It increases significantly IL-10 and TNF-α. The glycans that compose C. chinensis absorb in IR range.	[60]
Phenylpropanoid glycosides	The phenylpropanoid glycosides (Verbascoside, forsitoside B, echinacoside and campneoside I) induce Nrf2 and cytoprotective enzymatic activity and exhibits an antioxidant activity in cultured human keratinocytes.	[82]
Phlebodium aureum L. extract (synonym - *Polypodium leucatomos* Poir./ in articles - *P. leucotomos)*	Also known as Polypodium leucotomos. Oral administration of P. aureum extract in mice for 5 days before exposure to UV and for 2 days post-irradiation reduces by 13% the number of proliferating epidermal cells, and promotes an increase in p53 positive cells and an increase of 30% in the plasmatic antioxidant capacity. The beneficial effect of the extract of P. aureum is probably due to its anti-ROS properties.	[83, 84]

Pomegranate fruit extract	The pretreatments of human HaCaT keratinocytes with this extract modulate the effects of UVB radiation, in relation to the reduction of cell viability, intracellular glutathione content and lipid peroxidation. It has also been demonstrated the ability of this extract to inhibit the increase of MMP-1, MMP-2, MMP-9 and MMP-7, the reduction of TIMP-1, and phosphorylation of MAPK and c-jun induced by UV radiation.	[85]
Proanthocyanidins	Coming mainly from grape seeds (GSP's). Human keratinocytes irradiated with UVB and treated with GSP's inhibit the formation of hydrogen peroxide, lipid peroxidation, protein oxidation and DNA damage. It also inhibits the reduction in endogenous antioxidant compounds such as glutathione peroxidase, catalase, superoxide dismutase and glutathione. GSP's also inhibit the phosphorylation of ERK1/2, JNK, p38 and MAPK family proteins, and the activation of NF-kB/p65 induced by UVB. These results suggest that GSP can attenuate oxidative stress caused by UV in human skin.	[86]
Psidium catleianum fruit extract	P. catleianum extract has a high antioxidant capacity against ROS and RNS. Its effect may be mainly due to its phenolic content and especially epicatechins and ellagic acid.	[87]
Quercetin	It is a flavonoid with powerful antioxidant properties; however it has not been extensively studied. Some formulations for topical application with quercetin inhibit UVB radiation-induced damage in animals.	[88]
Red clover	The red clover extract is a rich source of isoflavones, such as genistein, equol, isoequol and dehidroequol, which are able to reduce edema and immunosuppression caused by UV radiation.	[89]
Red orange extract	Red orange extract is able to neutralize the UVB-induced response in human HaCaT keratinocytes. In particular, the events related to apoptosis and inflammation, such as translocation of NF-kB and AP-1 and cleavage of procaspase - 3. This activity is probably due to blocking events related to oxidative stress, showing that red orange extract can be useful for the photoprotection of the skin.	[90]
Resveratrol	Resveratrol is a phytoalexin polyphenolic, which is a substance able to delay or even stop the normal course of skin aging, by blocking apoptotic mitochondrial events and malfunctions in keratinocytes. Human skin has specific unions for resveratrol. Studies with human HaCaT keratinocyte lines have shown that trans-resveratrol is capable of inhibiting the production of hydrogen peroxide. In humans, while providing a protective effect against UVA radiation, trans-resveratrol is even able to improve clinical signs of aging when used associated with β-cyclodextrin excipient.	[88, 91]
Rheum rhaponticum L. rizome extract	The rhubarb extract has anti-radical characteristics and antioxidants properties against lipid peroxidation in *in vitro* studies. The extract also reduces the activity of tyrosinase and inhibits the production of IL-1α, TNF-α, and α-MSH, and tyrosine kinase activity in human melanocytes exposed to UV radiation.	[92]
Rutin	It is a polyphenol with anti-tumor, anti-inflammatory, antioxidant, and anti-mutagenic properties. Topically applied it decreases epidermal hyperplasia and levels of 4-hydroxynonenal modified protein, which is characteristic of lipid peroxidation. It also reduces the expression of iNOS and COX-2 and inhibits the activation of AP-1.	[88, 93]

Table 2. (Continued)

Sea buckthorn fruit extract	UV irradiated mice were treated orally with a mixture of extract of fruits of sea buckthorn (SBF), blueberry extract and collagen. Oral ingestion of SBF reduces wrinkles formation and helps to maintain skin thickness. SBF treated mice exhibited inhibition of TEWL and an increase of the skin moisture content. The application of SBF also reduces expression of MMP-1 and MMP-9, and reduces the levels of SOD activity.	[94]
Silk lutein	Silk lutein protects cells exposed to UVB radiation, reducing the levels of cytotoxicity and apoptosis.	[95]
Silymarins	It is a flavonoid coming from *Silybum marianum* seed and is composed of three molecules: silibinin, silidianin and silicristin. In animal models it protects against erythema, DNA damage and radiation-induced immune suppression. It is an excellent antioxidant, anti-inflammatory and immunomodulatory.	[96]
Soybean extract	Soy extract is rich in isoflavones. It inhibits human HaCaT keratinocyte cell death UVB-induced, as well as phosphorylation of p38, JNK and ERK1/2. In mice, topical application prior to UV irradiation was found to reduce the thickness of the epidermis, the expression of COX-2 and PCNA, and increases the concentration of catalase.	[97]
T4 endonuclease V liposomes	T4 endonuclease V is a bacterial DNA repairing enzyme, which repairs cyclobutane pyrimidine dimers in DNA. When it is encapsulated in liposomes and applied topically, it can eliminate the DNA dimers formed both in animals and humans. It also prevents the upregulation of IL-10. The topical application of T4N5 for a year reduces the proportion of actinic keratosis and basal cell carcinoma. Also partially protects against formation of sunburn cells, contact hypersensitivity and DTH. However, it has no effect against edema.	[98]
Tannase-converted green tea extract	Tannase is an enzyme produced by fungi, yeasts and bacteria that hydrolyze gallates catechins (EGCG and ECG) of green tea and thus increase its potential application for the removal of free radicals such as superoxide and hydrogen peroxide. A formulation containing extract of green tea tannase-converted was used to inhibit oxidative damage in mouse epidermis induced by UV. The formulation acts to prevent the reduction of glutathione levels and controlling hydrogen peroxide. Treated mice showed significantly reduced levels of reactive substances of thiobarbituric acid by lipid peroxidation, compared to UVB-irradiated controls, suggesting that this formulation is effective in protecting the skin against photoaging.	[99]
Tectroside	This substance inhibits the production of proinflammatory cytokines (IL-6 and IL-8) induced by UVB in cultured human HaCaT keratinocytes in a dose dependent way. Also inhibits the expression of COX-2 and JNK phosphorylation. These results suggest that this component has the potential to protect the skin against UVB induced inflammation.	[100]
Coenzyme Q10 (CoQ10)	CoQ10 is an endogenous electron carrier in cellular respiration. CoQ10 is used in many creams due to its antioxidant and skin protective photoaging properties and. It is able to scavenge ROS and to protect cells from oxidative stress, both in absence and in presence of UV radiation.	[100-103]

Vitamin C	Vitamin C (ascorbic acid) reduces the effects of aging, such as superficial and deep wrinkles and increases skin elasticity, firmness and hydration. The evaluation of ascorbic acid and its derivatives, AA 2-phosphate and AA 2-glucoside, in human HaCaT keratinocytes subjected to UVB-induced cytotoxicity, showed that ascorbic acid is not able to inhibit the cytotoxicity, however, their derivatives do.	[104]
Vitamin E	The antioxidant potential of α-tocopherol, one of the forms of vitamin E, is widely known. It has been tested the inhibitory role of α-tocopherol in the regulation of the production of IL-8 and AP-1in human keratinocytes exposed to UVA, and the results show significant inhibition of NADPH oxidase activity, which is responsible for activating IL-8 and AP-1. α-tocopherol also inhibits the formation of thiobarbituric acid-malondialdehyde in cells exposed to UVA radiation.	[105]
Vitis vinifera L. shoot extract	V. vinifera sprouts extract has an *in vitro* antioxidant capacity higher than vitamin C or E. An aqueous extract of V. vinifera tendril, applied in human keratinocytes (NCTC 2544) was capable of increasing the glutathione concentration and the activity of trans-plasma membrane oxido-reductase, in a time-dose dependent manner, demonstrating that is has a significant antioxidant activity.	[106]
Xyloglucans	They prevent immune suppression induced by UV exposure by reducing IL-10 production in mice.	[107]
Zeaxanthin and lutein	An increased lutein intake improves the health of the skin when administered orally or topically (zeaxanthin and lutein), as evaluated in the following five physiological parameters: surface lipids of the skin, skin moisturizing, photoprotective activity, elasticity of the skin and lipid peroxidation. The oral or topical administration significantly improves these measures, oral administration results in better protection against changes in lipid peroxidation and photoprotective activity after UV irradiation. However, a combined oral and topical administration provides a greater degree of protection. Other studies have shown the protective effect of this combination against hyperproliferation and inflammation of the epidermis after UVB exposure in mice.	[108]
2-furildioxime	It is an iron chelator that applied topically prevents erythema, sunburn cell, thickness reduction of the skin, inflammation and induction of ornithine decarboxylase.	[109]

4.4. DNA Repair Agents

Some of the antioxidants described in Table 2, such as L-epigallocatechin-3-gallate (EGCG), T4 endonuclease V liposomes and Green tea extract, besides their antioxidant properties; they are also able to promote the reparation of damaged DNA.

There are other substances whose main mechanism of action the repair of DNA damage. Are examples of these substances Photolyase, which is a DNA repair enzyme that applied immediately after UVB exposure decreases the number of dimers of DNA between 40 and 45% in human skin [110] and Thymidine dinucleotides. Thymidine dinucleotides produce a mimic effect on the cells as which occurs after exposure to UVR. However, thymidine dinucleotides pretreatments cause that cells develop a protective response against UV by activating p53 protein, which is involved in DNA regeneration [111].

4.5. Cyclooxygenase-2 Inhibitors

The results of the study performed Tripp et al. [28] previously commented, suggest that inhibitors of COX-2 may play a role in the prevention of epidermal skin cancers development, such as squamous cell carcinoma, and for that reason, it would be interesting to include these substances in sunscreens.

Kaempferia parviflora extract, Rutin, Soybean extract and Tectroside, included in Table 2, besides their antioxidant properties, they also act inhibiting COX-2, so the use of these substances in sunscreens would be useful for their different mechanisms of action against the harmful effects of radiation.

A study performed by Orengo et al. [112] demonstrated that Colecoxib, an inhibitor of COX-2, orally administrated, inhibits the induced photocarcinogenesis in hairless mouse model of squamous cell carcinoma and basal cell carcinoma, where COX-2 is overexpressed.

4.6. Iron Chelators

Endogenous iron (Fe^{2+}), under normal conditions, is sequestered by iron-binding proteins, such as transferrin and ferritin and does not participate in ROS generation. Nevertheless, when skin is exposed to sun exposure and consequently to oxidative stress, Fe^{2+} is released from these proteins. This free Fe^{2+} catalyses hydroxyl radical generation through Fenton reaction [113]:

$$H_2O_2 + Fe^{2+} \rightarrow OH + OH^- + Fe^{3+}$$

For that reason, it has been proposed by some authors the use of iron chelators in sunscreens, which will reduce the free Fe^{2+} and thus will prevent the Fenton reaction and consequently hydroxyl radical formation through this reaction. Examples of iron chelators are 2,2′-dipyridyl, 1,10-phenanthroline and 2,2′-dipyridylamine [114].

4.7. Osmolytes

Osmolytes are compounds that protect cells from desiccation by maintaining a high intracellular osmolality. Compatible organic osmolytes, such as taurine, betaine and myoinositol are involved in maintaining the cell homeostasis and protecting the cell against oxidative stress, which could be produced by UV radiation.

An augmented osmolyte uptake has been shown in UV-irradiated keratinocytes and for that reason it has been suggested that these substances play a role in protecting keratinocytes against some of the harmful effects induced by UV irradiation [115]. Nowadays, there are not so many studies of the use of osmolytes in sunscreens.

5. Melatonin

Melatonin (N-acetyl-5-methoxytryptamine) actually known as a neurohormone is secreted primarily at night-time by the pineal gland. It is in fact, a very well conserved molecule. Its presence has been discovered in very ancient living beings such as a photosynthetic prokaryote, *Rhodospirillum rubrum* [116], unicellular organisms, marine algae, dinoflagellate *Gonuaulaz poliedra* [117] and yeast (*Saccharomyces cerevisae*) [118]. In all these organisms, the main function of melatonin was to protect against the oxidative stress. With the years, this molecule took new roles such as a chemical signal of light and dark, immunoestimulation, mediator of the seasonal physiological functions and other functions that exerts in numerous and extremely diverse biological systems.

5.1. Endogenous Synthesis

Endogenously, melatonin is synthesized from the amino acid tryptophan, not only in the pineal gland, but also in tissues such as retina [119] and skin [120], among others. Melatonin synthesis in the skin begins with hydroxylation of tryptophan by the action of the tryptophan-5-hydroxylase enzyme (TPH) in the skin cells; this process is catalyzed mainly by TPH1, which is a compound of about 50kD that is degraded to lower molecular weight species. The TPH is located in the epidermis, the hair follicle and eccrine gland, although the place of expression is melanocytes. 5-hydroxytryptophan (5-HTP) is rapidly decarboxylated by the aromatic amino acid decarboxylase (AAD). Serotonin is the product, which is acetylated by N-acetyl transferase (NAT), and it is expressed in cells of the epidermis, dermis and other associated compartments. The last step of the synthesis is carried out by the action of the HIOMT, converting the N-Acetylserotonin in melatonin, this reaction can be reversed by the action of the CYP450 (Figure 3).

5.2. Skin Metabolism

In the skin, the metabolism of melatonin involves indolic and kynuric pathways and can be catalyzed by enzymatic or non-enzymatic reactions. The multiple pathways of the metabolism of melatonin are summarized in Figure 4.

The most important metabolites are 6-hydroxymelatonin, 2-hydroxymelatonin, Cyclic-3 hydroxymelatonin, AFMK and AMK.

6-hydroxymelatonin

In the skin, melatonin can be catabolized to 6-hydroxymelatonin by enzymatic process involving CYP1B1 or by the interaction with peroxynitrite ($ONOO^-$) [121] and $^{\bullet}OH$ [122].

2-hydroxymelatonin

In the skin, this molecule is produced by the interaction of melatonin with HClO [123] and $^{\bullet}OH$ [122]. The reaction of cytochrome C with H_2O_2, uses melatonin and the metabolite obtained is also 2-hydroxymelatonin [124].

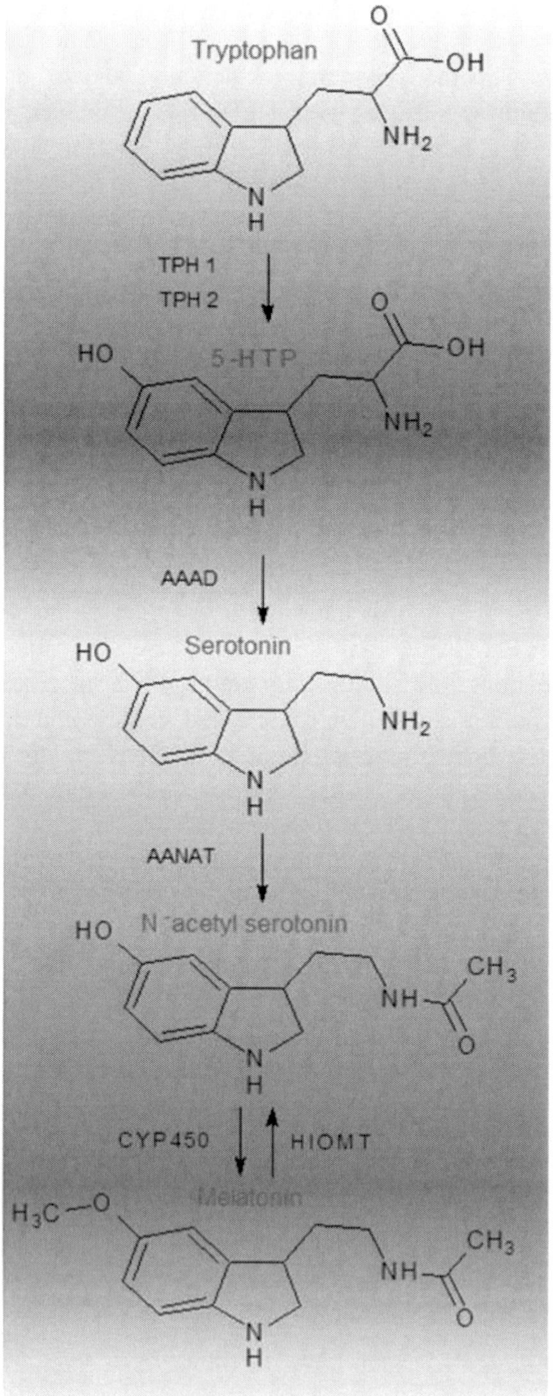

Figure 3. Biochemical synthesis of melatonin in the skin.

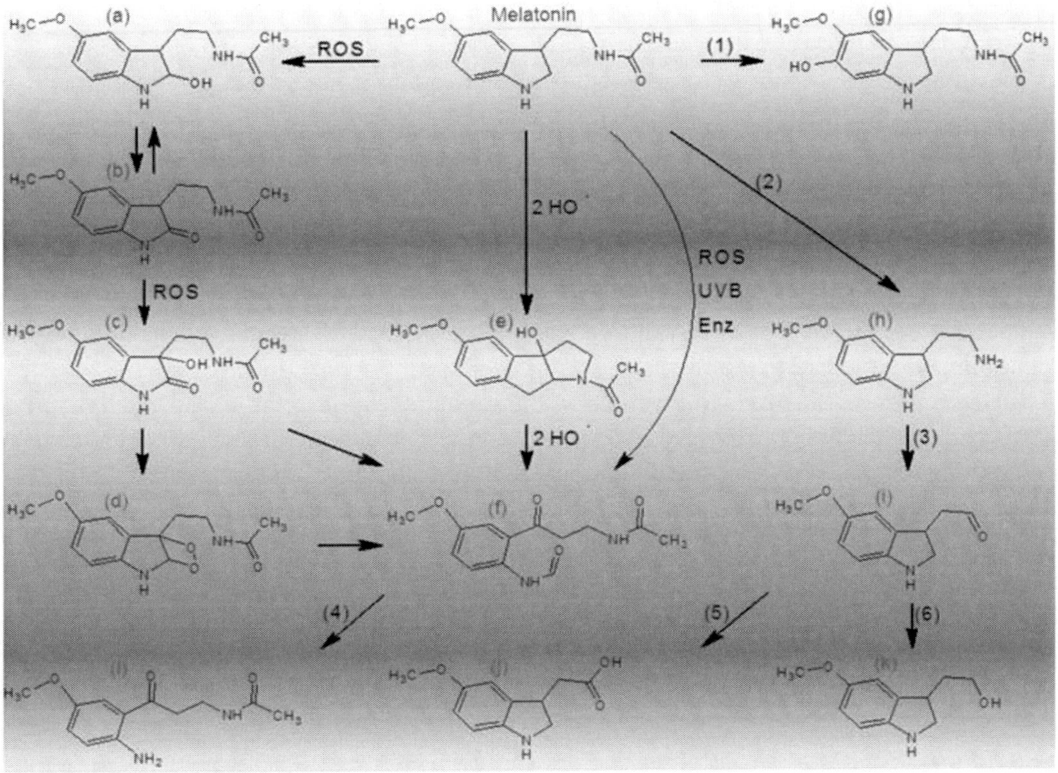

Figure 4. Melatonin metabolism. (a) 2-hydroxymelatonin (b) melatonin 2-indolinone (c) 3-hydroxymelatonin 2-indolinone (d) melatonin dioxetane (e) cyclic 3-hydroxymelatonin (f) AFMK (g) 6-hydroxymelatonin (h) 5-methoxytryptamine (i) 5-methoxyindoleacetaldehyde (j) 5-methoxyindole acetic acid (k) 5-methoxytryptophol (l) AMK. (1) CYP1A1, CYP1A2 or CYP1B1 (2) melatonin deacetylase (3) monoamine oxidase (4) arylamine formamidase, hemoperoxidase and ROS/RNS (5) aldehyde dehydrogenase (6) alcohol dehydrogenase.

Cyclic 3-hydroxymelatonin

Melatonin scavenges 2 $^{\bullet}$OH to form this metabolite [125], but can also be produced by the interaction of melatonin with $ONOO^-$ [126,127]. This molecule is readily converted to AFMK by interaction of ROS and RNS.

AFMK

The metabolite AFMK can be generated by the interaction of melatonin with multiple agents, such as H_2O_2 [128], horseradish peroxidase, myeloperoxidase [129, 130], cytochrome C [122], $^1O_2$ [131, 132], carbonate radical and $ONOO^-$ [130]. Humans cells also generates AFMK when are exposed to oxidative stress, such as UVB radiation [133].

AMK

This metabolite is generated by the interaction of AFMK with arylamine formamidase, hemoperoxidases or interaction with ROS/RNS.

5.3. Melatonin Effects

Melatonin plays a main role in the control of circadian rhythms and also participates in the regulation of reproduction, however, in this section is described only the pleiotropic effects that converts melatonin in a major skin protectant and how it counteracts the solar radiation effects. The main effects of melatonin in the skin are:

Immunomodulation

The immunoregulatory effects of melatonin represent a line of defense [134, 135]. This compound has shown to be an efficacious photoprotective agent via modulation of proinflammatory mediators [136].

Melatonin exerts a stimulating action on the immune response through the activation of various cell types as B and T lymphocytes, NK, monocytes and reticulum endothelial cells ~~86~~ [135] and the increase of IL-4 production on T helper cells (T_{CD4}) of bone marrow and stem cells of granulocytic-macrophage line [137].

Other authors have reported that melatonin stimulates the secretion of IL-1, IL-6 and INFα [138].

AFMK and AMK also have antiinflamatory and immunoregulatory properties. AFMK inhibits TNF-α and IL-8, AMK inhibit the synthesis of prostaglandins [139] and both molecules inhibit the gene expression of COX-2 [140].

Antioxidant

The antioxidant effects of melatonin occur by at least two mechanisms. The first mechanism is its direct antioxidant effects via free radical scavenging by inhibiting their generation [141]. The second is by enhancing the activity of antioxidants enzymes, which improve the endogenous antioxidant defense capacity of the organisms and induce up-regulation of gene expression, thereby increasing the first line of defense against oxidative damage of the cells [142, 143].

Free Radical Scavenger

The reaction of melatonin with free radicals occurs in all the compartments of the body due to its lipophilicity and consequently it has wide distribution capabilities. The first observation that showed that melatonin has antioxidant effects was made in 1991 by Lanas et al. [144] and was confirmed by Tan et al. in 1993 [145] that showed that melatonin neutralizes $^{\bullet}OH$. Since then, numerous papers have been published demonstrating the ability of melatonin to interact with reactive species, and thus act as an antioxidant molecule. Melatonin directly reacts with $^{\bullet}OH$, H_2O_2, $ONOO^-$, HClO, $^1O_2$ and O_2^-, obtaining the metabolites described before. Free radicals are the main responsible of lipid peroxidation, protein oxidation, caspase activation and release, apoptosis, mitochondrial instability and DNA damage. Therefore, melatonin, when scavenge free radicals, acts indirectly reducing the above processes.

Endogenous Antioxidant Defense Capacity Improvement

In addition to the intrinsic ability of melatonin to scavenge free radicals, it is also capable of stimulating the activity and expression of other antioxidant systems, thus establishing a form to reduce oxidative stress using an indirect action [146].

First, it stimulates glutathione cycle, melatonin up-regulate the activity of Gluthation peroxidase (GPx), which reduces H_20_2 to water both in rat brain [142] and in chicken tissues [147] equilibrating the balance of GSSG/GSH [148] and Glutathion reductase (GRd).

It also increases the production of glutathione by stimulating γ-glutamylcysteine synthase, which is a limiting enzyme in glutathione synthesis pathway [149], and stimulates glucose-6-phosphate dehydrogenase, which is responsible for generating the NADPH required by GRd [150]. Melatonin also stimulates other antioxidant enzymes such as SOD and catalase [151].

The nuclear factor NFkB, induced by ROS is a central and early event in the induction of inflammatory reactions [152]. NFkB is an oxidative stress sensitive factor that activates multiple target genes involved in the expression of several proinflammatory mediators. Melatonin has been reported to inhibit the NFkB activation as action of the cell protection signaling of melatonin by transcriptional response control [153].

Not only melatonin has antioxidant effects, some of its metabolites also have them. For example, 6-hydroxymelatonin reduces lipid peroxidation and protects against DNA damage [154,155] due to its direct free radical scavenging and antioxidant properties [156–158]. It has been found that cyclic 3-hydroxymelatonin is able to prevent the oxidative DNA damage produced by Fenton regents [154].

AFMK is a powerful antioxidant that can donate 4 or more electrons to interact with free radicals; it is as potent as melatonin scavenging some free radicals such as $O_2^{\cdot-}$ AFMK also reduces lipid peroxidation and oxidative DNA [156,159]. AMK is more efficient as an antioxidant than AFMK.

Melatonin As an Adjuvant in the Treatment of Cancer

It has been shown in cell studies that both in animals and humans melatonin directly suppresses and inhibits the tumor cell growth in carcinoma cell lines and inhibits the growth of colon carcinoma and breast, so it leads to a reduction in the cancer development [138, 160, 161]. Melatonin is also capable of suppressing the proliferation in melanoma cells of different dignity and growth characteristics; MT1 and RORα receptor-dependent enhance the suppressive effects [162-164]. In humans, it has been demonstrated that it has a potential efficacy against malignant melanoma in patients in stage IV [165].

5.4. Melatonin As a Photoprotective Agent

Several studies have shown the beneficial effects of melatonin counteracting the harmful effects of sun radiation. In this section are reviewed the different actions of melatonin that demonstrate its potential to be used as a photoprotective agent.

Erythema

It has been shown that the application of melatonin reduces the erythema induced by UV radiation [166] in a dose-dependent manner [167]. But this reduction is only produced when melatonin is applied before UV exposure [168]. The minimum concentration of Melatonin necessary for a statistically significant reduction in erythema is 0.5%.

Apoptosis

UV radiation increases the apoptosis by damaging cellular structures that undergo apoptosis. Cellular studies have shown that melatonin applied before UV exposure prevents apoptosis [169-177].

Generation of ROS

As it has been previously explained, sun radiation generates ROS and it has been widely demonstrated that melatonin act as a potent free radical scavenger, not only by itself but also by its metabolites [170, 172, 174, 175].

Cell Viability

It has been demonstrated in cellular cultures that UV radiation reduces the cell viability and melatonin prevents this reduction [169, 170, 172, 176, 177].

Gene Expression

When the cells are exposed to UV radiation it is up-regulated the apoptosis of controller gens, cancer related genes, and oxidative stress response genes. In the presence of melatonin these up-regulations were prevented [173, 174, 176, 178]. For example, it down-regulates the expression of genes, that play an important role in the photodamage induced by UV, such as intersticial collagen (MMP-1), stromelysin (MMP-3), stromelysin (MMP-10) and aldehyde dehydrogenase 3 type A1 [179].

Mitochondrial Membrane Potential

The exposure to UV radiation leads to a reduction of the mitochondrial membrane potential that leads to its damage and thus to the activation of the intrinsic pathway of apoptosis. Melatonin acts preventing the dissipation of the mitochondrial membrane potential [171, 172, 177, 180].

DNA Synthesis

In cellular studies, it has been shown that the exposure to UV decreases the rate of DNA synthesis and it has been demonstrated that melatonin prevents this reduction [133, 177].

DNA Damage

UV radiation causes oxidative stress, which subsequently leads to oxidative DNA damage (represented by 8-OHdG formation). Cellular studies have shown that the oxidative DNA damage induced by UV decreases when the cells are pretreated with melatonin. For example, melatonin activates the poly(DP-ribose) polymerase, which is a key DNA-repair-mediating enzyme [178, 181].

5.5. Melatonin in Sunscreens

As previously mentioned, melatonin is a lipophilic molecule with strong ability to cross cell membranes, because of this property and the multiple actions as an antioxidant, there are groups trying to formulate sunscreens containing melatonin as an antioxidant. Although there isn't currently marketed formulation, there are a few references to sunscreens containing melatonin.

Dreher et al. demonstrated in 1998 [182] that melatonin incorporated in a topical formulation combined with vitamins E and C exerts a synergistic antioxidant action.

In another study, Flo et al. [183] reported an approach on the use of melatonin in a sunscreen emulsion combined with the common used UV filters octyl salicylate (5%), octyl methoxycinnamate (5%) and benzophenone-3 (5%). The antioxidant activity assay demonstrated that the formulation possesses higher antioxidant properties that the formulation that does not contain melatonin. The *in vivo* assay demonstrated that irradiated skin areas of animals treated with this formulation were statistically equivalent to the unirradiated control areas, thus the photoprotective effect of the formulation was clearly shown.

Another study has demonstrated that melatonin formulated in creams creates a depot structure in the stratum corneum, in which a small part goes releasing to blood during 24 h [184]. Therefore, the topical administration is a good candidate for treatment with melatonin for local action but also as transdermal delivery to reach constant plasma levels.

Due to these direct and indirect antioxidant effects of melatonin and its metabolites, it is a promising photoprotective agent, acting directly as a free radical scavenger and indirectly by stimulating antioxidant enzymes [180], inducing down regulation of the gene expression of enzymes that are involved in the generation of oxidative stress and enhancing the activation of antioxidant enzyme gene expression [178].

Summarizing, melatonin is a promising photoprotective substance that complies with all the requirements described for an ideal sunscreen: it provides uniform protection against UV, Vis and IR, it is a potent free radical scavenging, it stimulates the DNA repair systems, although not being photostable its metabolites are safe and have *per se* a potent antioxidant activity, and it is safe.

REFERENCES

[1] Fore, J. (2006). A review of skin and the effects of aging on skin structure and function. *Ostomy Wound Management*, 59(2), 29–35.

[2] Menon, G.K. (2002). New insights into skin structure: scratching the surface. *Advanced Drug Delivery Reviews*. 54, Suppl 1, S3–S17.

[3] Fitzpatrick, T.B., & Bolognia, J.L. (1995). Human melanin pigmentation: Role in pathogenesis of cutaneous melanoma. In: L. Zeise, M.R. Chedekel, & T.B. Fitzpatrick (Eds.), *Melanin: Its role in human photoprotection* (239–244). Overland Park, KS: Valdenmar Publishing Co.

[4] Grether-Beck, S., Marini, A., Jaenicke, T., & Krutmann, J. (2014). Photoprotection of human skin beyond ultraviolet radiation. *Photodermatology, Photoimmunology & Photomedicine*, 30(2-3), 167–74.

[5] Svobodová, A. R., Galandáková, A., Sianská, J., Doležal, D., Lichnovská, R., Ulrichová, J., et al. (2012). DNA damage after acute exposure of mice skin to physiological doses of UVB and UVA light. *Archives of Dermatological Research*, 304(5), 407–12.

[6] Choi, W., Brenner, M., Passeron, T., & Zhang, G. (2012). The deceptive nature of UVA-tanning versus the modest protective of UVB-tanning on human skin. *National Institute of Health*, 24(1), 136–147.

[7] Moriwaki, S., & Takahashi, Y. (2008). Photoaging and DNA repair. *Journal of Dermatological Science*, 50(3), 169–76.

[8] Pfeifer, G. P., & Besaratinia, A. (2013). UV wavelength-dependent DNA damage and human nonmelanoma and melanoma skin cancer. *National Institute of Health*, 11(1), 90–97.

[9] Hanson KM, S. J. (1998). Epidermal trans-urocanic acid and the UV-A-induced photoaging of the skin. *Proceedings of the National Academy of Sciences of the United States of America*, 95(18), 10576–10578.

[10] Svobodová, A., & Vostálová, J. (2010). Solar radiation induced skin damage: review of protective and preventive options. *International Journal of Radiation Biology*, 86(12), 999–1030.

[11] Polefka, T. G., Meyer, T. A., Agin, P. P., & Bianchini, R. J. (2012). Effects of solar radiation on the skin. *Journal of Cosmetic Dermatology*, 11(2), 134–43.

[12] Mahmoud, B. H., Ruvolo, E., Hexsel, C. L., Liu, Y., Owen, M. R., Kollias, N., et al. (2010). Impact of long-wavelength uva and visible light on melanocompetent skin. *Journal of Investigative Dermatology*, 130(8), 2092–2097.

[13] Mahmoud, B. H., Hexsel, C. L., Hamzavi, I. H., & Lim, H. W. (2008). Effects of visible light on the skin. *Photochemistry and Photobiology*, 84(2), 450–62.

[14] Cho, S., Lee, M. J., Kim, M. S., Lee, S., Kim, Y. K., Lee, D. H., et al. (2008). Infrared plus visible light and heat from natural sunlight participate in the expression of MMPs and type I procollagen as well as infiltration of inflammatory cell in human skin in vivo. *Journal of Dermatological Science*, 50(2), 123–33.

[15] Krutmann, J., & Schroeder, P. (2009). Role of mitochondria in photoaging of human skin: the defective powerhouse model. *The Journal of Investigative Dermatology*. 14(1), 44–49.

[16] Zastrow, L., Groth, N., Klein, F., Kockott, D., Lademann, J., Renneberg, R., & Ferrero, L. (2009). The missing link-light-induced (280-1,600 nm) free radical formation in human skin. *Skin Pharmacology and Physiology*, 22(1), 31–44.

[17] Krutmann, J., Morita, A., & Chung, J. H. (2012). Sun exposure: what molecular photodermatology tells us about its good and bad sides. *The Journal of Investigative Dermatology*, 132(3 Pt 2), 976–984.

[18] Vanchinathan, V., & Lim, H. W. (2012). A dermatologist's perspective on vitamin D. *Mayo Clinic Proceedings*, 87(4), 372–380.

[19] Gilaberte, Y., & González, S. (2010). Update on Photoprotection. *Actas Dermo-Sifiliográficas* (English Edition), 101(8), 659–672.

[20] Jansen, R., Wang, S. Q., Burnett, M., Osterwalder, U., & Lim, H. W. (2013). Photoprotection: part I. Photoprotection by naturally occurring, physical, and systemic agents. *Journal of the American Academy of Dermatology*, 69(6), 853.e1–12; quiz 865–866.

[21] Brenneisen, P. (1998). Central role of ferrous/ferric iron in the ultraviolet B irradiation-mediated signaling pathway leading to increased interstitial collagenase (matrix-degrading metalloprotease (MMP)-1) and stromelysin-1 (MMP-3) mRNA levels in cultured human dermal fibroblasts. *Journal of Biological Chemistry*, 273(9), 5279–5287.

[22] Epe, B. (2012). DNA damage spectra induced by photosensitization. *Photochemical & Photobiological Sciences*, 11, 98–106.

[23] Hanson, K. M., & Clegg, R. M. (2002). Observation and Quantification of Ultraviolet-induced Reactive Oxygen Species in Ex Vivo Human Skin. *Photochemistry and Photobiology*, 76(1), 57–63.

[24] Gibbs, N. K., Tye, J., & Norval, M. (2008). Recent advances in urocanic acid photochemistry, photobiology and photoimmunology. *Photochemical & Photobiological Sciences*, 7(6), 655–667.

[25] Rigel, D. S. (2008). Cutaneous ultraviolet exposure and its relationship to the development of skin cancer. *Journal of the American Academy of Dermatology*, 58(5 Suppl 2), S129–132.

[26] Dessinioti, C., Tzannis, K., Sypsa, V., Nikolaou, V., Kypreou, K., Antoniou, C., et al. (2011). Epidemiologic risk factors of basal cell carcinoma development and age at onset in a Southern European population from Greece. *Experimental Dermatology*, 20(8), 622–626.

[27] Walls, A. C., Han, J., Li, T., & Qureshi, A. A. (2013). Host risk factors, ultraviolet index of residence, and incident malignant melanoma in situ among US women and men. *American Journal of Epidemiology*, 177(9), 997–1005.

[28] Tripp, C. S., Blomme, E. A. G., Chinn, Ã. K. S., Hardy, M. M., Lacelle, P., & Pentland, A. P. (2003). Epidermal COX-2 induction following ultraviolet irradiation: Suggested mechanism for the role of COX-2 inhibition in photoprotection. *The Journal of Investigative Dermatology*, 121(4), 853–861.

[29] Jong, C. T., Finlay, A. Y., Pearse, A. D., Kerr, A. C., Ferguson, J., Benton, E. C., et al. (2008). The quality of life of 790 patients with photodermatoses. *The British Journal of Dermatology*, 159(1), 192–197.

[30] Balogh, T. S., Pedriali, C. A., & Kaneko, T. M. (2011). Ultraviolet radiation protection: current available resources. *Anais Brasileiros de Dermatologia*, 86(4), 732–742.

[31] Dupont, E., Gomez, J., & Bilodeau, D. (2013). Beyond UV radiation: a skin under challenge. *International Journal of Cosmetic Science*, 35(3), 224–232.

[32] Murray, J. C., Burch, J. a, Streilein, R. D., Iannacchione, M. A., Hall, R. P., & Pinnell, S. R. (2008). A topical antioxidant solution containing vitamins C and E stabilized by ferulic acid provides protection for human skin against damage caused by ultraviolet irradiation. *Journal of the American Academy of Dermatology*, 59(3), 418–425.

[33] Nash, J. F., & Tanner, P. R. (2014). Relevance of UV filter/sunscreen product photostability to human safety. *Photodermatology, Photoimmunology & Photomedicine*, 30(2-3), 88–95.

[34] Villalobos-Hernández, J. R., & Müller-Goymann, C. C. (2006). Sun protection enhancement of titanium dioxide crystals by the use of carnauba wax nanoparticles: the synergistic interaction between organic and inorganic sunscreens at nanoscale. *International Journal of Pharmaceutics*, 322(1-2), 161–170.

[35] Gilbert, E., Pirot, F., Bertholle, V., Roussel, L., Falson, F., & Padois, K. (2013). Commonly used UV filter toxicity on biological functions: review of last decade studies. *International Journal of Cosmetic Science*, 35(3), 208–219.

[36] Maier, H., Schauberger, È., Brunnhofer, K., & Ho, H. (2001). Change of Ultraviolet Absorbance of Sunscreens by Exposure to Solar-Simulated Radiation. *The Journal of Investigative Dermatology*, 117, 256–262.

[37] Couteau, C., Faure, A., Fortin, J., Paparis, E., & Coiffard, L. J. M. (2007). Study of the photostability of 18 sunscreens in creams by measuring the SPF in vitro. *Journal of Pharmaceutical and Biomedical Analysis*, 44(1), 270–273.

[38] Manová, E., von Goetz, N., & Hungerbühler, K. (2014). UV filter contact and photocontact allergy: consumer exposure and risk assessment for octocrylene from personal care products and sunscreens. *The British Journal of Dermatology*. 171(6), 1368–1374.

[39] Janjua, N. R., Kongshoj, B., Andersson, A.-M., & Wulf, H. C. (2008). Sunscreens in human plasma and urine after repeated whole-body topical application. *Journal of the European Academy of Dermatology and Venereology : JEADV*, 22(4), 456–461.

[40] Jansen, R., Osterwalder, U., Wang, S. Q., Burnett, M., & Lim, H. W. (2013). Photoprotection: part II. Sunscreen: development, efficacy, and controversies. *Journal of the American Academy of Dermatology*, 69(6), 867.e1–14; quiz 881–882.

[41] Kim, S., & Choi, K. (2014). Occurrences, toxicities, and ecological risks of benzophenone-3, a common component of organic sunscreen products: a mini-review. *Environment International*, 70, 143–157.

[42] US Food and Drug Administration. (2000). Sunscreen Drug Products for Over-the-Counter Human Use. Rockville, MD. Available from: http://www.cfsan.fda.gov/~lrd/fr990521.html

[43] Seixas, V. C., & Serra, O. A. (2014). Stability of sunscreens containing CePO4: proposal for a new inorganic UV filter. *Molecules (Basel, Switzerland)*, 19(7), 9907–9925.

[44] Lewicka, Z., Yu, W.W., Oliva, B.L., Contreras, E.Q., & Colvin, V.L. (2013). Photochemical behavior of nanoscale TiO_2 and ZnO sunscreen ingredients. *Journal of Photochemistry and Photobiology A: Chemistry*, 263, 24–33.

[45] Dunford, R., Salinaro, A., Cai, L., Serpone, N., Horikoshi, S., Hidaka, H., & Knowland, J. (1997). Chemical oxidation and DNA damage catalysed by inorganic sunscreen ingredients. *FEBS Letters*, 418(1-2), 87–90

[46] Byeon, S. W., Pelley, R. P., Ullrich, S. E., Waller, T. A., Bucana, C. D., & Strickland, F. M. (1998). Aloe barbadensis extracts reduce the production of interleukin-10 after exposure to ultraviolet radiation. *The Journal of Investigative Dermatology*, 110(5), 811–817.

[47] Strickland, F. M., Darvil, A., Albersheim, P., Eberhard, S., Pauly, M., & Ronald, P. (1999). Inhibition of UV-induced immune suppression and interleukin-10 production by plant oligosaccharides and polysaccharides. *Photochemistry and Photobiology*, 69(2), 141–147.

[48] Hwang, Y. P., Oh, K. N., Yun, H. J., & Jeong, H. G. (2011). The flavonoids apigenin and luteolin suppress ultraviolet A-induced matrix metalloproteinase-1 expression via MAPKs and AP-1-dependent signaling in HaCaT cells. *Journal of Dermatological Science*, 61(1), 23–31.

[49] Tominaga, K., Hongo, N., Karato, M., & Yamashita, E. (2012). Cosmetic benefits of astaxanthin on humans subjects. *Acta Biochimica Plonica*, 59(1), 43–47.
[50] Stahl, W., & Sies, H. (2012). β-Carotene and other carotenoids in protection from sunlight. *The American Journal of Clinical Nutrition*, 96(5), 1179–1184.
[51] Wertz, K., Hunziker, Ã. P. B., Seifert, Ã. N., Riss, Ã. G., Neeb, Ã. M., Steiner, G., et al. (2005). beta-Carotene interferes with ultraviolet light A-induced gene expression by multiple pathways. *The Journal of Investigative Dermatology*, 124(2), 428–434.
[52] Koone, M.D., & Black, H.S. (1986). A mode of action for butylated hydroxytoluene-mediated photoprotection. *The Journal of Investigative Dermatology*, 87(3), 343–347.
[53] Hanada, K. (2000). Photoprotective role of metallothionein in UV-injury - metallothionein-null mouse exhibits reduced tolerance against ultraviolet-B. *Journal of Dermatological Science*, 23, S51–S56.
[54] Saija, A., Tomaino, A., Trombetta, D., De Pasquale, A., Uccella, N., Barbuzzi, T., et al. (2000). In vitro and in vivo evaluation of caffeic and ferulic acids as topical photoprotective agents. International Journal of Pharmaceutics, 199(1), 39–47.
[55] Koo, S.-W., Hirakawa, S., Fujii, S., Kawasumi, M., & Nghiem, P. (2007). Protection from photodamage by topical application of caffeine after ultraviolet irradiation. *The British Journal of Dermatology*, 156(5), 957–964.
[56] Lee, J., & Il, J. (1998). The photoprotective effect of 1,25-dihydroxyvitamin D3 on ultraviolet light B-induced damage in keratinocyte and its mechanism of action. *Journal of Dermatological Science*, 18(1), 11–18.
[57] Olteanu, E. D., Filip, A., Clichici, S., Daicoviciu, D., Archim, M., Postescu, I. D., et al. (2012). Photochemoprotective effect of Calluna vulgaris extract on skin exposed to multiple doses of ultraviolet B in SKH-1 hairless mice. *Journal of Environmental Pathology, Toxicology and Oncology*, 31, 233–243.
[58] Attaguile, G., Russo, A., Campisi, A., Savoca, F., Acquaviva, R., Ragusa, N., & Vanella, A. (2000). Antioxidant activity and protective effect on DNA cleavage of extracts from Cistus incanus L. and Cistus monspeliensis L. *Cell Biology and toxicology*, 16(2), 83–91.
[59] Katz, D. L., Doughty, K., & Ali, A. (2011). Cocoa and chocolate in human health and disease. *Antioxidants & Redox Signaling*, 15(10), 2779–811.
[60] Yan, H., Sun, X., Sun, S., Wang, S., Zhang, J., Wang, R., et al. (2011). Anti-ultraviolet radiation effects of Coptis chinensis and Phellodendron amurense glycans by immunomodulating and inhibiting oxidative injury. *International Journal of Biological Macromolecules*, 48(5), 720–725.
[61] Tanaka, Y. T., Tanaka, K., Kojima, H., Hamada, T., Masutani, T., Tsuboi, M., & Akao, Y. (2013). Cynaropicrin from Cynara scolymus L. suppresses photoaging of skin by inhibiting the transcription activity of nuclear factor-kappa B. *Bioorganic & Medicinal Chemistry Letters*, 23(2), 518–523
[62] Tee, L.H., Yang, B., Prasad, N., Ramanan, N., Sun, J., Chan, E., et al. (2014). Nutritional compositions and bioactivities of Dacryodes species: a review. *Food Chemistry*, 165, 247–255.
[63] Rostan, E. F., Debuys, H. V, Madey, D. L., & Pinnell, S. R. (2002). Evidence supporting zinc as an important antioxidant for skin. *International Journal of Dermatology*, 41(9), 606-611.

[64] Widyarini, S., Domanski, D., Painter, N., & Reeve, V. E. (2012). Photoimmune protective effect of the phytoestrogenic isoflavonoid equol is partially due to its antioxidant activities. *Photochemical & Photobiological Sciences*, 11(7), 1186–1192.

[65] Rhodes, L. E., Durham, B. H., William, D. F., & Friedmann, P. S. (1995). Dietary fish oil reduces basal and ultraviolet B-generated PGE2 levels in skin and increases the threshold to provocation of polymorphic light eruption. *Journal of Investigative Dermatology*, 105(4), 532–535.

[66] Urikura, I., Sugawara, T., & Hirata, T. (2011). Protective effect of Fucoxanthin against UVB-induced skin photoaging in hairless mice. *Bioscience, Biotechnology, and Biochemistry*, 75(4), 757–760.

[67] Anunciato, T. P., & da Rocha Filho, P. A. (2012). Carotenoids and polyphenols in nutricosmetics, nutraceuticals, and cosmeceuticals. *Journal of Cosmetic Dermatology*, 11(1), 51–54.

[68] Wei, H., Saladi, R., Lu, Y., Wang, Y., Palep, S. R., Moore, J., et al. (2003). Isoflavone genistein: photoprotection and clinical implications in dermatology. *The Journal of Nutrition*, 113(1), 3811–3819.

[69] Li, N., Deng, L., Xiang, L., & Liang, Y. (2014). Photoprotective effect of tea and its extracts against ultraviolet radiation-induced skin disorders. *Tropical Journal of Pharmaceutical Research*, 13(3), 475–483.

[70] Nichols, J., & Katiyar, S. K. (2010). Skin photoprotection by natural polyphenols: anti-inflammatory, antioxidant and DNA repair mechanisms. *Archives of Dermatological Research*, 302(2), 71–83.

[71] Tomaino, A., Cristani, M., Cimino, F., Speciale, A., Trombetta, D., Bonina, F., & Saija, A. (2006). In vitro protective effect of a Jacquez grapes wine extract on UVB-induced skin damage. *Toxicology in Vitro*, 20(8), 1395–1402.

[72] Park, J.E., Pyun, H.B., Woo, S.W., Jeong, J.H., & Hwang, J.K. (2014). The protective effect of Kaempferia parviflora extract on UVB-induced skin photoaging in hairless mice. *Photodermatology, Photoimmunology & Photomedicine*, 30(5), 237–245

[73] Dieamant, G. D. C., Velazquez Pereda, M. D. C., Eberlin, S., Nogueira, C., Werka, R. M., & Queiroz, M. L. D. S. (2008). Neuroimmunomodulatory compound for sensitive skin care: in vitro and clinical assessment. *Journal of Cosmetic Dermatology*, 7(2), 112–119.

[74] Huang, C., Wu, W., Fang, J., Chiang, H., Chen, S., Chen, B., et al. (2007). (-)-Epicatechin-3-gallate, a green tea polyphenol is a potent agent against UVB-induced damage in HaCaT keratinocytes. *Molecules*, 12, 1845–1858.

[75] Vayalil, P. K., Elmets, C. A., & Katiyar, S. K. (2003). Treatment of green tea polyphenols in hydrophilic cream prevents UVB-induced oxidation of lipids and proteins, depletion of antioxidant enzymes and phosphorylation of MAPK proteins in SKH-1 hairless mouse skin. *Carcinogenesis*, 24(5), 927–936.

[76] Andreassi, M., Stanghellini, E., Ettorre, A., Di Stefano, A., & Andreassi, L. (2004). Antioxidant activity of topically applied lycopene. *Journal of the European Academy of Dermatology and Venereology : JEADV*, 18(1), 52–55.

[77] Song, J. H., Bae, E. Y., Choi, G., Hyun, J. W., Lee, M. Y., & Lee, H. W. (2013). Protective effect of mango (*Mangifera indica* L.) against UVB-induced skin aging in hairless mice. *Photodermatology, Photoimmunology & Photomedicine*, 29(2), 84–89.

[78] Chae, S., Piao, M. J., Kang, K. A., Zhang, R., Kim, K. C., Youn, U. J., et al. (2011). Inhibition of matrix metalloproteinase-1 induced by oxidative stress in human keratinocytes by mangiferin isolated from Anemarrhena asphodeloides. *Bioscience, Biotechnology, and Biochemistry*, 75(12), 2321–2325.

[79] Huang, J.H., Huang, C.C., Fang, J.Y., Yang, C., Chan, C.-M., Wu, N.L., et al. (2010). Protective effects of myricetin against ultraviolet-B-induced damage in human keratinocytes. *Toxicology in Vitro*, 24(1), 21–28.

[80] Kang, S., Chung, J. H., Lee, J. H., Fisher, G. J., Wan, Y. S., Duell, E. A., & Voorhees, J. J. (2003). Topical N-acetyl cysteine and genistein prevent ultraviolet-light-induced signaling that leads to photoaging in human skin in vivo. *The Journal of Investigative Dermatology*, 120(5), 835–841.

[81] El-Mahdy, M. A., Zhu, Q., Wang, Q.-E., Wani, G., Patnaik, S., Zhao, Q., et al. (2008). Naringenin protects HaCaT human keratinocytes against UVB-induced apoptosis and enhances the removal of cyclobutane pyrimidine dimers from the genome. *Photochemistry and Photobiology*, 84(2), 307–316.

[82] Sgarbossa, A., Dal Bosco, M., Pressi, G., Cuzzocrea, S., Dal Toso, R., & Menegazzi, M. (2012). Phenylpropanoid glycosides from plant cell cultures induce heme oxygenase 1 gene expression in a human keratinocyte cell line by affecting the balance of NRF2 and BACH1 transcription factors. *Chemico-Biological Interactions*, 199(2), 87–95.

[83] Philips, N., Conte, J., Chen, Y.-J., Natrajan, P., Taw, M., Keller, T., et al. (2009). Beneficial regulation of matrixmetalloproteinases and their inhibitors, fibrillar collagens and transforming growth factor-beta by Polypodium leucotomos, directly or in dermal fibroblasts, ultraviolet radiated fibroblasts, and melanoma cells. *Archives of Dermatological Research*, 301(7), 487–495.

[84] Rodríguez-Yanes, E., Juarranz, Á., Cuevas, J., Gonzalez, S., & Mallol, J. (2012). Polypodium leucotomos decreases UV-induced epidermal cell proliferation and enhances p53 expression and plasma antioxidant capacity in hairless mice. *Experimental Dermatology*, 21(8), 638–640.

[85] Syed, D. N., Malik, A., Hadi, N., Sarfaraz, S., Afaq, F., & Mukhtar, H. (2006). Photochemopreventive effect of pomegranate fruit extract on UVA-mediated activation of cellular pathways in normal human epidermal keratinocytes. *Photochemistry and Photobiology*, 82(2), 398–405.

[86] Mittal, A., Elmets, C. a, & Katiyar, S. K. (2003). Dietary feeding of proanthocyanidins from grape seeds prevents photocarcinogenesis in SKH-1 hairless mice: relationship to decreased fat and lipid peroxidation. *Carcinogenesis*, 24(8), 1379–1388.

[87] Ribeiro, A. B., Chisté, R. C., Freitas, M., da Silva, A. F., Visentainer, J. V., & Fernandes, E. (2014). Psidium cattleianum fruit extracts are efficient in vitro scavengers of physiologically relevant reactive oxygen and nitrogen species. *Food Chemistry*, 165, 140–148.

[88] Alonso, C., Rubio, L., Touriño, S., Martí, M., Barba, C., Fernández-Campos, F., et al. (2014). Antioxidative effects and percutaneous absorption of five polyphenols. *Free Radical Biology & Medicine*, 75, 149–55.

[89] Widyarini, S., Spinks, N., Husband, A. J., & Reeve, V. E. (2001). Isoflavonoid compounds from red clover (Trifolium pratense) protect from inflammation and immune suppression induced by UV radiation. *Photochemistry and Photobiology*, 74(3), 465–470.

[90] Cimino, F., Cristani, M., Saija, A., Bonina, F. P., & Virgili, F. (2007). Protective effects of a red orange extract on UVB-induced damage in human keratinocytes. *BioFactors*, 30(2), 129–138.

[91] Ndiaye, M., Philippe, C., Mukhtar, H., & Ahmad, N. (2011). The grape antioxidant resveratrol for skin disorders: promise, prospects, and challenges. *Archives of Biochemistry and Biophysics*, 508(2), 164–170.

[92] Silveira, J. P. S., Seito, L. N., Eberlin, S., Dieamant, G. C., Nogueira, C., Pereda, M. C. V, & Di Stasi, L. C. (2013). Photoprotective and antioxidant effects of Rhubarb: inhibitory action on tyrosinase and tyrosine kinase activities and TNF-α, IL-1α and α-MSH production in human melanocytes. *BMC Complementary and Alternative Medicine*, 13(2), 49.

[93] Choi, K.S., Kundu, J. K., Chun, K.S., Na, H.K., & Surh, Y.J. (2014). Rutin inhibits UVB radiation-induced expression of COX-2 and iNOS in hairless mouse skin: p38 MAP kinase and JNK as potential targets. *Archives of Biochemistry and Biophysics*, 559, 38–45.

[94] Hwang, I. S., Kim, J. E., Choi, S. Il, Lee, H. R., Lee, Y. J., Jang, M. J., et al. (2012). UV radiation-induced skin aging in hairless mice is effectively prevented by oral intake of sea buckthorn (Hippophae rhamnoides L.) fruit blend for 6 weeks through MMP suppression and increase of SOD activity. *International Journal of Molecular Medicine*, 30(2), 392–400.

[95] Pongcharoen, S., Warnnissorn, P., Lertkajornsin, O., & Limpeanchob, N. (2013). Protective effect of silk lutein on ultraviolet B-irradiated human keratinocytes. *Biological Research*, 46(1), 39–45.

[96] Nichols, J. A., & Katiyar, S. K. (2010). Skin photoprotection by natural polyphenols: anti-inflammatory, antioxidant and DNA repair mechanisms. *Archives of Dermatological Research*, 302(2), 71–83.

[97] Chiu, T.M., Huang, C.C., Lin, T.J., Fang, J.Y., Wu, N.L., & Hung, C.-F. (2009). In vitro and in vivo anti-photoaging effects of an isoflavone extract from soybean cake. *Journal of Ethnopharmacology*, 126(1), 108–113.

[98] Cafardi, J. A., & Elmets, C. A. (2008). T4 endonuclease V: review and application to dermatology. *Expert Opinion on Biological Therapy*, 8(6), 829–838.

[99] Hong, Y.H., Jung, E.Y., Shin, K.S., Kim, T.Y., Yu, K.W., Chang, U. J., & Suh, H. J. (2012). Photoprotective effects of a formulation containing tannase-converted green tea extract against UVB-induced oxidative stress in hairless mice. *Applied Biochemistry and Biotechnology*, 166(1), 165–175.

[100] Kim, S.B., Kang, O.H., Joung, D.K., Mun, S.H., Seo, Y.S., Cha, M.R., et al. (2013). Anti-inflammatory effects of tectroside on UVB-induced HaCaT cells. *International Journal of Molecular Medicine*, 31(6), 1471–1476.

[101] James, A.M., Smith, R.A.J., & Murphy, M.P. (2004). Antioxidant and prooxidant properties of mitochondrial Coenzyme Q. *Archives of Biochemistry and Biophysics*, 423(1), 47–56.

[102] Tanino, Y., Budiyanto, A., Ueda, M., Nakada, A., Nyou, W.T., Yanagisawa, M., et al. (2005). Decrease of antioxidants and the formation of oxidized diacylglycerol in mouse skin caused by UV irradiation. *Journal of Dermatological Sciences*, 2(1), 21–28.

[103] Yue, Y., Zhou, H., Liu, G., Li, Y., Yan, Z., & Duan, M. (2010). The advantages of a novel CoQ10 delivery system in skin photo-protection. *International Journal of Pharmaceutics*, 392(1-2), 57–63.
[104] Haftek, M., Mac-Mary, S., Le Bitoux, M.-A., Creidi, P., Seité, S., Rougier, A., & Humbert, P. (2008). Clinical, biometric and structural evaluation of the long-term effects of a topical treatment with ascorbic acid and madecassoside in photoaged human skin. *Experimental Dermatology*, 17(11), 946–952.
[105] Wu, S., Gao, J., Dinh, Q. T., Chen, C., & Fimmel, S. (2008). IL-8 production and AP-1 transactivation induced by UVA in human keratinocytes: roles of D-alpha-tocopherol. *Molecular Immunology*, 45(8), 2288–2296.
[106] Nassiri-Asl, M., & Hosseinzadeh, H. (2009). Review of the pharmacological effects of Vitis vinifera (Grape) and its bioactive compounds. *Phytotherapy Research*, 23(9), 1197–1204.
[107] Strickland, F. M., Darvil, A., Albersheim, P., Eberhard, S., Pauly, M., & Ronald, P. (1999a). Inhibition of UV-induced immune suppression and interleukin-10 produc- tion by plant oligosaccharides and polysaccharides. *Photochemistry and Photobiology*, 69(2), 141–147.
[108] Gao, S., Qin, T., Liu, Z., Caceres, M. A., Ronchi, C. F., Chen, C. O., et al. (2011). Lutein and zeaxanthin supplementation reduces H2O2-induced oxidative damage in human lens epithelial cells. *Molecular vision*, 17, 3180–3190.
[109] Bissett, D. L., & McBride, J. F. (1996). Synergistic topical photoprotection by a combination of the iron chelator 2-furildioxime and sunscreen. *Journal of the American Academy of Dermatology*, 35(4), 546–549.
[110] Yarosh, D., Bucana, C., Cox, P., Alas, L., Kibitel, J., & Kripke, M. (1994). Localization of liposomes containing a DNA repair enzyme in Murine skin. *Journal of Investigative Dermatology*, 103(4), 461–468.
[111] Gilchrest, B. a, & Eller, M. S. (1999). DNA Photodamage Stimulates Melanogenesis and Other Photoprotective Responses. *Journal of Investigative Dermatology. Symposium Proceedings*, 4(1), 35–40.
[112] Orengo, I. F., Gerguis, J., Phillips, R., Guevara, A., Lewis, A. T., & Black, H. S. (2002). Celecoxib, a cyclooxygenase 2 inhibitor as a potential chemopreventive to UV-induced skin cancer, *Archives of Dermatology*, 138(8), 751–755.
[113] Kitazawa, M., Iwasaki, K., & Sakamoto, K. (2006). Iron chelators may help prevent photoaging. *Journal of Cosmetic Dermatology*, 5(3), 210–217.
[114] Bissett, D. L., & McBride, J. F. (1996b). Synergistic topical photoprotection by a combination of the iron chelator 2-furildioxime and sunscreen. *Journal of the American Academy of Dermatology*, 35(4), 546–549.
[115] Warskulat, U., Reinen, Ã. A., Grether-beck, Ã. S., Krutmann, J., & Ha, D. (2004). The osmolyte strategy of normal human keratinocytes in maintaining cell homeostasis. *Journal of Investigative Dermatology*, 123, 516–521.
[116] Manchester, L.C., Poeggeler, B., Alvares, F.L., Ogden, G.B., & Reiter, R.J. (1995). Melatonin immunoreactivity in the photosyn- thetic prokaryote Rhodospirillum rubrum: implications for an ancient antioxidant system. *Cellular & Molecular Biology Research*, 41(5), 391–395.

[117] Poeggele, B., Balzer, I., Hardeland, R., & Lerchl, A. (1991). Pineal hormone melatonin oscillates also in the dinoflagellate Gonyaulax polyedrae. *Naturwissenschaften*, 78, 268–269.

[118] Sprenger J, Hardeland R, Fuhrberg B, H. S. (1999). Melatonin and other 5-methoxylated indoles in yeast: presence in high concentrations and dependence on tryptophan availability. *Cytologia*, 64, 209–213.

[119] Grace, M. S., Cahill, G. M., & Besharse, J. C. (1991). Melatonin deacetylation: retinal vertebrate class distribution and Xenopus laevis tissue distribution. *Brain Research*, 559(1), 56–63.

[120] Slominski, A., Tobin, D. J., Zmijewski, M. A., Wortsman, J., & Paus, R. (2008). Melatonin in the skin: synthesis, metabolism and functions. *Trends in Endocrinology and Metabolism: TEM*, 19(1), 17–24.

[121] Zhang, H., Squadrito, G. L., & Pryor, W. A. (1998). The reaction of melatonin with peroxynitrite: formation of melatonin radical cation and absence of stable nitrated products. *Biochemical and Biophysical Research Communications*, 251(1), 83–87.

[122] Horstman, J. A., Wrona, M. Z., & Dryhurst, G. (2002). Further insights into the reaction of melatonin with hydroxyl radical. *Bioorganic Chemistry*, 30(5), 371–382.

[123] Dellegar, S. M., Murphy, S. A., Bourne, A. E., DiCesare, J. C., & Purser, G. H. (1999). Identification of the factors affecting the rate of deactivation of hypochlorous acid by melatonin. *Biochemical and Biophysical Research Communications*, 257(2), 431–439.

[124] Semak, I., Naumova, M., Korik, E., Terekhovich, V., Wortsman, J., & Slominski, A. (2005). A novel metabolic pathway of melatonin: oxidation by cytochrome C. *Biochemistry*, 44(26), 9300–9307.

[125] Tan, D.X., Manchester, L. C., Reiter, R. J., Plummer, B. F., Hardies, L. J., Weintraub, S. T., & Shepherd, A. M. M. (1998). A novel melatonin metabolite, cyclic 3-hydroxymelatonin: a biomarker of in vivo hydroxyl radical generation. *Biochemical and Biophysical Research Communications*, 253(3), 614–620.

[126] Peyrot, F., Martin, M.T., Migault, J., & Ducrocq, C. (2003). Reactivity of peroxynitrite with melatonin as a function of pH and CO2 content. *European Journal of Organic Chemistry*, 2003(1), 172–181.

[127] Zhang, H., Squadrito, G. L., Uppu, R., & Pryor, W. A. (1999). Reaction of peroxynitrite with melatonin : a mechanistic study. *Chemical Research in Toxicology*, 12, 526–534.

[128] Hirata, F., Hayaishi, O., Tokuyama, T., & Senoh, S. (1974). In vitro and in vivo formation of two new metabolites of melatonin. *The Journal of Biological Chemistry*, 249(4), 1311–1313.

[129] Hardeland, R., Pandi-Perumal, S. R., & Cardinali, D. P. (2006). Melatonin. *The International Journal of Biochemistry & Cell Biology*, 38(3), 313–316.

[130] Hardeland, R., Poeggeler, B., Niebergall, R., & Zelosko, V. (2003). Oxidation of melatonin by carbonate radicals and chemiluminescence emitted during pyrrole ring cleavage. *Journal of Pineal Research*, 34(1), 17–25.

[131] Almeida, E. A., Martinez, G. R., Klitzke, C. F., Medeiros, M. H. G., & Mascio, P. Di. (2003). Oxidation of melatonin by singlet molecular oxygen (O2(1Deltag)) produces N1-acetyl-N2-formyl-5-methoxykynurenine. *Journal of Pineal Research*, 35(2), 131–137.

[132] Hardeland, R., Balzer, I., Poeggeler, B., Fuhrberg, B., Uría, H., Behrmann, G., et al. (1995). On the primary functions of melatonin in evolution: mediation of photoperiodic

signals in a unicell, photooxidation, and scavenging of free radicals. *Journal of Pineal Research*, 18(2), 104–111.

[133] Fischer, T. W., Sweatman, T. W., Semak, I., Sayre, R. M., Wortsman, J., & Slominski, A. (2006). Constitutive and UV-induced metabolism of melatonin in keratinocytes and cell-free systems. *FASEB Journal*, 20(9), 1564–1566.

[134] Carrillo-Vico, A., Guerrero, J.M., Lardone, P.J., & Reiter, R.J. (2005). A review of the multiple actions of melatonin on the immune system. *Endocrine*, 27(2), 189–200.

[135] Hardeland, R. (2008). Melatonin, hormone of darkness and more: occurrence, control mechanisms, actions and bioactive metabolites. *Cellular and Molecular Life Sciences:CMLS*, 65(13), 2001–2018.

[136] Saija, A., Tomaino, A., Trombetta, D., Pellegrino, M. L., Tita, B., Caruso, S., & Castelli, F. (2002). Interaction of melatonin with model membranes and possible implications in its photoprotective activity. *European Journal of Pharmaceutics and Biopharmaceutics*, 53(2), 209–215.

[137] Maestroni, G.J., Covacci, V., & Conti, A. (1994). Hematopoietic rescue via T-cell-dependent, endogenous granulocyte-macrophage colony-stimulating factor induced by the pineal neurohormone melatonin in tumor-bearing mice. *Cancer Research*, 54, 2429–2432.

[138] Barjavel, M.J., Mamdouh, Z., Raghbate, N., & Bakouche, O. (1998). Differential expression of the melatonin receptor in human monocytes. *Journal of Immunology*, 160(3), 1191–1197.

[139] Kelly, R. W., Amato, F., & Seamark, R. F. (1984). N-acetyl-5-methoxy kynurenamine, a brain metabolite of melatonin, is a potent inhibitor of prostaglandin biosynthesis. *Biochemical and Biophysical Research Communications*, 121(1), 372–379.

[140] Mayo, J. C., Sainz, R. M., Tan, D.-X., Hardeland, R., Leon, J., Rodriguez, C., & Reiter, R. J. (2005). Anti-inflammatory actions of melatonin and its metabolites, N1-acetyl-N2-formyl-5-methoxykynuramine (AFMK) and N1-acetyl-5-methoxykynuramine (AMK), in macrophages. *Journal of Neuroimmunology*, 165(1-2), 139–149.

[141] Tan, D.X., Reiter, R.J., Manchester, L.C., Yan, M.T., El-Sawi, M., Sainz RM, et al. (2002). Chemical and physical properties and potential mechanisms: melatonin as a broad spectrum antioxidant and free radical scavenger. *Current Topics in Medicinal Chemistry*, 2(2), 181–197.

[142] Barlow-Walden, L. R., Reiter, R. J., Abe, M., Pablos, M., Menendez-Pelaez, A., Chen, L.-D., & Poeggeler, B. (1995). Melatonin stimulates brain glutathione peroxidase activity. *Neurochemistry International*, 26(5), 497–502.

[143] Rodriguez, C., Mayo, J. C., Sainz, R. M., Antolin, I., Herrera, F., Martin, V., & Reiter, R. J. (2004). Regulation of antioxidant enzymes: a significant role for melatonin. *Journal of Pineal Research*, 36(1), 1–9.

[144] Ianăş, O., Olinescu, R., & Bădescu, I. (1991). Melatonin involvement in oxidative processes. *Endocrinologie,* 29(3–4), 147–153.

[145] Tan, D.X., Chen, L.D., Poeggeler, B., Manchester, L.C., & Reiter, R.J. (1993) Melatonin: A potent, endogenous hydroxyl radical scavenger. *Endocrine Journal*, 1, 57–60.

[146] Antolin, I., Mayo, J. C., Sainz, R. M., del Brío, M. de los A., Herrera, F., Martín, V., & Rodríguez, C. (2002). Protective effect of melatonin in a chronic experimental model of Parkinson's disease. *Brain Research*, 943(2), 163–173.

[147] Pablos, M. I., Agapito, M. T., Gutierrez, R., Recio, J. M., Reiter, R. J., Barlow-Walden, L., et al. (1995). Melatonin stimulates the activity of the detoxifying enzyme glutathione peroxidase in several tissues of chicks. *Journal of Pineal Research*, 19(3), 111–115.

[148] Martín, M., Macías, M., Escames, G., León, J., & Acuña-Castroviejo D. Melatonin but not vitamins C and E maintains glutathione homeostasis in t-butyl hydroperoxide-induced mitochondrial oxidative stress. *FASEB Journal*, 14(12), 1677–1679.

[149] Urata, Y., Honma, S., Goto, S., Todoroki, S., Iida, T., Cho, S., et al. (1999). Melatonin induces γ-glutamylcysteine synthetase mediated by activator protein-1 in human vascular endothelial cells. *Free Radical Biology and Medicine*, 27(7–8), 838–847.

[150] Pierrefiche G, & Laborit, H. (1995). Oxygen free radicals, melatonin, and aging. *Experimental Gerontology*, 30, 213–227.

[151] Leon, J., Acuña-Castroviejo, D., Sainz, R. M., Mayo, J. C., Tan, D.X., & Reiter, R. J. (2004). Melatonin and mitochondrial function. *Life Sciences*, 75(7), 765–790.

[152] Fuchs, J., Zollner, T., Kaufmann, R., & Podda, M. (2001). Redox-modulated pathways in inflammatory skin diseases. *Free Radical Biology and Medicine*, 30(4), 337–353.

[153] Sainz, R. M., Reiter, R. J., Tan, D.X., Roldan, F., Natarajan, M., Quiros, I., et al. (2008). Critical role of glutathione in melatonin enhancement of tumor necrosis factor and ionizing radiation-induced apoptosis in prostate cancer cells in vitro. *Journal of Pineal Research*, 45(3), 258–270.

[154] Lopez-Burillo, S., Tan, D.X., Rodriguez-Gallego, V., Manchester, L.C., Mayo, J.C., Sainz, R.M., & Reiter, R.J. (2003). Melatonin and its derivatives cyclic 3-hydroxymelatonin, N1- acetyl-N2-formyl-5-methoxykynuramine and 6-hydroxymelatonin reduce oxidative DNA damage induced by Fenton reagents. *Journal of Pineal Research*, 34, 178–184.

[155] Qi, W., Reiter, R. J., Tan, D.-X., Manchester, L. C., Siu, A. W., & Garcia, J. J. (2000). Increased levels of oxidatively damaged DNA induced by chromium(III) and H2O2: protection by melatonin and related molecules. *Journal of Pineal Research*, 29(1), 54–61.

[156] Liu, X., Chen, Z., Chua, C. C., Ma, Y.-S., Youngberg, G. A., Hamdy, R., & Chua, B. H. L. (2002). Melatonin as an effective protector against doxorubicin-induced cardiotoxicity. *American Journal of Physiology. Heart and Circulatory Physiology*, 283(1), H254–263.

[157] Maharaj, D. S., Limson, J. L., & Daya, S. (2003). 6-Hydroxymelatonin converts Fe (III) to Fe (II) and reduces iron-induced lipid peroxidation. *Life Sciences*, 72(12), 1367–1375.

[158] Matuszak, Z., Bilska, M. A., Reszka, K. J., Chignell, C. F., & Bilski, P. (2007). Interaction of singlet molecular oxygen with melatonin and related indoles. *Photochemistry and Photobiology*, 78(5), 449–455.

[159] Burkhardt, S. (2001). DNA oxidatively damaged by chromium(III) and H2O2 is protected by the antioxidants melatonin, N1-acetyl-N2-formyl-5-methoxykynuramine, resveratrol and uric acid. *The International Journal of Biochemistry & Cell Biology*, 33(8), 775–783.

[160] Chen, L., Hu, J. Y., & Wang, S. Q. (2012). The role of antioxidants in photoprotection: a critical review. *Journal of the American Academy of Dermatology*, 67(5), 1013–1024.

[161] Yuan, L., Collins, A. R., Dai, J., Dubocovich, M. L., & Hill, S. M. (2002). MT1 melatonin receptor overexpression enhances the growth suppressive effect of melatonin in human breast cancer cells. *Molecular and Cellular Endocrinology*, 192(1-2), 147–156.

[162] Fischer, T., Zmijewski, M., Zbytek, B., Sweatman, T., Slominski, R., Wortsman, J., & Slominski, A. (2006). Oncostatic effects of the indole melatonin and expression of its cytosolic and nuclear receptors in cultured human melanoma cell lines. *International Journal of Oncology*, 29(3), 665–672.

[163] Kadekaro, A. L., Andrade, L. N. S., Floeter-Winter, L. M., Rollag, M. D., Virador, V., Vieira, W., & Castrucci, A. M. de L. (2004). MT-1 melatonin receptor expression increases the antiproliferative effect of melatonin on S-91 murine melanoma cells. *Journal of Pineal Research*, 36(3), 204–211.

[164] Slominski, A., & Pruski, D. (1993). Melatonin inhibits proliferation and melanogenesis in rodent melanoma cells. *Experimental Cell Research*, 206(2), 189–194.

[165] Lissoni, P., Paolorossi, F., Tancini, G, Ardizzoia, A., Barni, S., Brivio, F., et al. (1996). A phase II study of tamoxifen plus melatonin in metastatic solid tumour patients. *British Journal of Cancer*, 74(9), 1466–1468.

[166] Bangha, E., Elsner, P., & Kistler, G.S. (1997). Suppression of UV-induced erythema by topical treatment with melatonin (N-acetyl-5-methoxytryptamine). Influence of the application time point. *Dermatology*, 195(3), 248–252.

[167] Becker-Andre, M., Wiesenberg, I., Schaeren-Wiemers, N., Andre, E., Missbach, M., Saurat, J., & Carlberg, C. (1994). Pineal gland hormone melatonin binds and activates an orphan of the nuclear receptor superfamily. *The Journal of Biological Chemistry*, 269(46), 28531–28534.

[168] Dreher, F., Denig, N., Gabard, B., Schwindt, D.A., & Maibach, H. I. (1999). Effect of topical antioxidants on UV-induced erythema formation when administered after exposure. *Dermatology*, 198(1), 52–55.

[169] Fischer, T. W., Zbytek, B., Sayre, R. M., Apostolov, E. O., Basnakian, A. G., Sweatman, T. W., et al. (2006). Melatonin increases survival of HaCaT keratinocytes by suppressing UV-induced apoptosis. *Journal of Pineal Research*, 40(1), 18–26.

[170] Fischer, T. W., Scholz, G., Knoll, B., Hipler, U.-C., & Elsner, P. (2001). Melatonin reduces UV-induced reactive oxygen species in a dose-dependent manner in IL-3-stimulated leukocytes. *Journal of Pineal Research*, 31(1), 39–45.

[171] Kleszczyński, K., Tukaj, S., Kruse, N., Zillikens, D., & Fischer, T. W. (2013). Melatonin prevents ultraviolet radiation-induced alterations in plasma membrane potential and intracellular pH in human keratinocytes. *Journal of Pineal Research*, 54(1), 89–99.

[172] Luchetti, F., Betti, M., Canonico, B., Arcangeletti, M., Ferri, P., Galli, F., & Papa, S. (2009). ERK MAPK activation mediates the antiapoptotic signaling of melatonin in UVB-stressed U937 cells. *Free Radical Biology & Medicine*, 46(3), 339–51.

[173] Ryoo, Y. W., Suh, S. I., Mun, K. C., Kim, B. C., & Lee, K. S. (2001). The effects of the melatonin on ultraviolet-B irradiated cultured dermal fibroblasts. *Journal of Dermatological Science*, 27(3), 162–169.

[174] Cho, J., Kim, C., & Lee, K. (2007). Modification of gene expression by melatonin in UVB-irradiated HaCaT keratinocyte cell lines using a cDNA microarray. *Oncology Reports*, 17(3), 573–577.

[175] Fischer, T. W., Scholz, G., Knöll, B., Hipler, U.C., & Elsner, P. (2004). Melatonin suppresses reactive oxygen species induced by UV irradiation in leukocytes. *Journal of Pineal Research*, 37(2), 107–112.

[176] Lee, K.S., Lee, W.S., Suh, S.I., Kim, S.P., Lee, S.R., Ryoo, Y.W., & Kim, B.C. (2003). Melatonin reduces ultraviolet-B induced cell damages and polyamine levels in human skin fibroblasts in culture. *Experimental & Molecular Medicine*, 35, 263–268.

[177] Nickel, A., & Wohlrab, W. (2000). Melatonin protects human keratinocytes from UVB irradiation by light absorption. *Archives of Dermatological Research*, 292(7), 366–368.

[178] Fischer, T. W., Kleszczyński, K., Hardkop, L. H., Kruse, N., & Zillikens, D. (2013). Melatonin enhances antioxidative enzyme gene expression (CAT, GPx, SOD), prevents their UVR-induced depletion, and protects against the formation of DNA damage (8-hydroxy-2'-deoxyguanosine) in ex vivo human skin. *Journal of Pineal Research*, 54(3), 303–312.

[179] Slominski, A., Fischer, T. W., Zmijewski, M. A., Wortsman, J., Semak, I., Zbytek, B., et al. (2005). On the role of melatonin in skin physiology and pathology. *Endocrine*, 27(2), 137–148.

[180] Fischer, T. W., Zmijewski, M. A., Wortsman, J., & Slominski, A. (2008). Melatonin maintains mitochondrial membrane potential and attenuates activation of initiator (casp-9) and effector caspases (casp-3/casp-7) and PARP in UVR-exposed HaCaT keratinocytes. *Journal of Pineal Research*, 44(4), 397–407.

[181] Yamamoto, H., & Mohanan, P. V. (2001). Effects of melatonin on paraquat or ultraviolet light exposure-induced DNA damage. *Journal of Pineal Research*, 31(4), 308–313.

[182] Dreher, F., Gabard, B., Schwindt, D. A., & Maibach, H. I. (1998). Topical melatonin in combination with vitamins E and C protects skin from ultraviolet-induced erythema: a human study in vivo. *British Journal of Dermatology*, 139, 332–339.

[183] Sierra, A. F., Ramírez, M. L., Campmany, A. C., Martínez, A. R., & Naveros, B. C., (2012). In vivo and in vitro evaluation of the use of a newly developed melatonin loaded emulsion combined with UV filters as a protective agent against skin irradiation. *Journal of Dermatological Science*, 69(3), 202–214.

[184] Fischer, T.W., Greif, C., Fluhr, J.W., Wigger-Alberti, W., & Elsner, P. (2004). Percutaneous penetration of topically applied melatonin in a cream and an alcoholic solution. *Skin Pharmacology and Physiology*, 17, 190–194.

In: Sunscreens
Editors: Sean Henry Sharp

ISBN: 978-1-63482-160-5

Chapter 5

UV FILTERS, THEIR DEGRADATION REACTIONS AND ECO-TOXICOLOGICAL EFFECTS

Albano Joel M. Santos and Joaquim C. G. Esteves da Silva*

Centro de Investigação em Química da Universidade do Porto (CIQ-UP),
Departamento de Química e Bioquímica, Faculdade de Ciências,
Universidade do Porto, Porto, Portugal

ABSTRACT

Sunscreens or sunscreen agents are more notoriously known as ultraviolet (UV) filters, and they are the prime components of many personal care products and pharmaceuticals. Most UV filters are organic compounds that absorb UV radiation, therefore protecting us from solar radiation and its nefarious effects on human skin and health. The protective character of UV filters regarding UV radiation, would presuppose a stable nature towards alterations in general. However, the compounds are well known to undergo degradation, and in many cases quite substantially, either by influence of UV radiation itself (by photolysis or photo-isomerization) or through contact with water disinfecting agents, such as chlorine. These degradation reactions might be quite troublesome, since they generate degradation by-products that either do not present the appropriate UV-protective capabilities, as is the case with photo-isomers, or possess toxicological profiles potentially damaging for both the human health and the environment, as is the case with free-radicals or even disinfection by-products (DBP's).

INTRODUCTION

Ultraviolet (UV) radiation constitutes about 6.2% of the total solar radiation that is able to reach the Earth's surface, given the filtration and mitigation capabilities of the protective ozone layer. Out of this specific portion of the solar radiation, mostly is attributed to UVA radiation (320-400 nm) while a very small portion is attributed to UVB radiation (290-320 nm).

* Corresponding author: Joaquim C.G. Esteves da Silva; jcsilva@fc.up.pt.

Table 1. Physical-chemical properties of the UV filters currently approved and regulated in and by the EU (adapted from [3] and [6])

Structure	INCI name	Acronym	Molecular weight	Log K_{OW}§	Log BCF **;§§	Log K_{OC} ††;§§	Solubility /g/L‡‡	λ_{max} /nm
Benzophenones	Benzophenone-3	BZ3	228.24	3.79	1.38	3.10	0.21	290
	Benzophenone-4	BZ4	308.31	0.88	-	-	0.65	240†; 288
PABA and derivatives	*p*-Aminobenzoic acid	PAB	137.14	0.83	-	-	915	282
	PEG-25 PABA	P25	277.41	-	-	-	-	310*
	Ethylhexyl dimethyl PABA	EDP	277.40	6.15	3.74	3.38	2.1×10^{-3}	310
Salicylates	Homosalate	HS	262.35	6.16	-	-	0.02	-
	Ethylhexyl salicylate	ES	250.34	5.77	-	-	0.028	240*
Cinnamates	Ethylhexyl methoxycinnamate	EMC	290.40	5.80	5.80	4.10	0.15	306†
	Isopentyl *p*-methoxycinnamate	IMC	248.32	4.06	-	-	0.06	-
Camphor derivatives	Camphor benzalkonium methosulfate	CBM	409.55	0.28	-	-	-	288*
	Terephtalydene dicamphor sulfonic acid	TDS	562.69	1.35	-	-	0.014	340*
	Benzylidene camphor sulfonic acid	BCS	320.40	2.74	-	-	0.038	297*
	Polyacrylamidomethyl benzylidene camphor[d]	PBC		-	-	-	-	-
	4-Methylbenzylidene camphor	MBC	254.37	4.95	3.51	3.89	5.1×10^{-3}	300†
	3-Benzylidene camphor	3BC	240.34	4.49			9.9×10^{-3}	292*
Triazines	Ethylhexyltriazone	ET	826.10	15.53	-	-	-	310†
	Diethylhexyl butamido triazone	DBT	765.98	11.90	-	-	4.6×10^{-7}	-
	Bis-Ethylhexyloxyphenol methoxyphenyl triazine	EMT	627.81	13.89	-	-	4.9×10^{-8}	340†
Benzotriazoles	Drometrizole trisiloxane	DRT	225.25	9.79	-	-	1.3×10^{-5}	344; 303
	Methylene bis-benzotriazolyl tetramethylbutylphenol	MBT	658.87	14.35	-	-	3.0×10^{-8}	340†
Benzimidazole derivatives	Phenyl benzimidazole sulfonic acid	PBS	274.30	0.01	0.50	2.46	0.26	300†
	Disodium phenyl dibenzimidazole tetrasulfonate	DPD	674.60	-	-	-	-	250
Dibenzoylmethane derivatives	Butyl methoxydibenzoyl methane	BDM	310.39	2.41	4.51	3.23	0.037	358*
	Diethylamino hydroxybenzoyl hexyl benzoate	DHH	397.51	6.93	-	-	9.5×10^{-4}	360†
Others	Octocrylene	OCR	361.49	7.35	-	-	2.0×10^{-4}	300†
	Polysilicone 15	P15		-	-	-	-	313‡

Data is originated from SciFinder, American Chemical Society, 2008.

UV filters shadowed in green colour, represent the most popular and frequently used compounds in commercial formulations of sunscreen products.

* Rastogi, S.C., Jensen, G.H. (1998), Identification of UV filters in sunscreen products by high-performance liquid chromatography–diode-array detection, *J. Chromatogr. A* 828 (1-2), 311-316.

† De Orsi, D., Giannini, G., Gagliardi, L., Porrà, R., Berri, S., Bolasco, A., Carpani, I., Tonelli, D. (2006), Simple extraction and HPLC determination of UV-A and UV-B filters in sunscreen products, *Chromatographia* 64 (9-10), 509-515.

‡ Philippe Maillan Formulation, R&D Cosmetics, DSM Nutritional Products; Measurement of UV Protection in Hair.

§ Octanol-water partition coefficient (K_{OW}); it regards the ratio between the concentration of a substance in octanol and in water, in equilibrium and at a determined temperature.

** Bio-concentration factor (BCF); it regards the concentration of a substance in an organism and in the water body around it.

†† Organic carbon distribution coefficient (K_{OC}); it regards the ratio between the mass of a substance adsorbed into the soil (by unity of mass of organic carbon in the soil) and the concentration of the same substance in equilibrium in solution.

‡‡ In water and at 25°C.

§§ Giokas, D.L., Salvador, A., Chisvert, A. (2007), UV filters: from sunscreens to the human body and the environment, *Trends in Analytical Chemistry* 26 (5), 360-374.

The highly energetic UVC radiation (100-290 nm) is completely blocked by the ozone layer and therefore does not reach the surface of the planet [1]. Despite the beneficial character of UV radiation (it enhances the production of vitamin D, improving the human resistance towards different pathologies; increases the calcium absorption by the organism; etc.), it is also known to enhance the occurrence of skin cancer, as well as other serious but less prominent issues like inflammations, sunburns, and allergic reactions [1]. It is in this context that sunscreens or sunscreen agents play a fundamental role, by preventing or attenuating the damaging effects of UV radiation on the human skin and health [1].

Sunscreen products include complex formulations of different compounds, of which UV filters are of the utmost importance, since these are the compounds that indeed protect us from UV radiation. As Salvador and Chisvert [2] refer, a sunscreen is defined as any product containing UV filters in its formulation, in order to protect the skin from the negative effects of UV radiation, significantly decreasing its impact on human health [2]. The mechanism of protection, however, is based on two processes that are intimately linked to the two existing types of filters in question: essentially absorption of UV radiation in the case of the vastly more numerous organic UV filters; and reflection or scattering in the case of the few existing inorganic UV filters [3].

UV filters generally display either simple or multiple aromatic structures, often conjugated with carbon-carbon double bonds or carbonyl groups, which attributes them the ability to absorb or scatter UV radiation. These compounds will absorb UV radiation, therefore evolving towards a superior energetic state but returning thereafter to the original state by emitting energy through vibrational transitions or photochemical reactions [4]. As it was already mentioned, UV filters are classified as either organic (UV-absorbent) or inorganic (UV-scattering) compounds. The most prominent classes of UV filters are the benzophenones, salicylates, cinnamates, triazines, *p*-aminobenzoic acid derivatives, dibenzoyl methane derivatives and camphor derivatives, and there are globally about 55 filters approved, regulated and controlled worldwide, out of which merely two are inorganic (zinc oxide and titanium dioxide) [1, 4, 5].

Table 1 includes all the UV filters currently approved in the EU, as well as all their relevant physical-chemical properties [3, 6].

As for the nature of UV filters, these compounds present the features common to most priority organic pollutants (POP's), such as the presence of aromatic rings in association with long and unsaturated aliphatic chains. Most of the filters consist of geometrical isomers (*E* and *Z* forms), although the commercial formulations include solely the *E* isomer. As is visible in Table 1, these compounds exhibit commonly increased lipophilicity, enabling their association with particles rich in organic matter content, such as soils and sediments, as well as high resistance towards biotic degradation, which enhances their accumulation, concentration and persistence in the environment and the food chain [3, 6, 7].

UV Filter Degradation Reactions

Regarding their purpose of application, protection of human skin from the effects of UV radiation, there is the assumption that UV filters are quite stable to general degradation.

However, such assumptions are not exactly accurate, in fact, it is well reported and established that UV filters experience degradation from two essential sources: photo-degradation, upon exposure to UV radiation; and degradation induced by disinfecting agents such as chlorine, when in contact with these in aqueous solution [3, 4]. Figure 1 presents the paths of degradation and their consequential by-products.

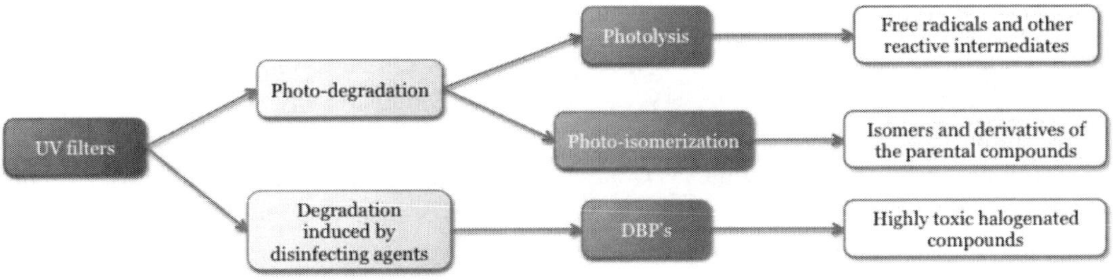

Figure 1. Degradation processes experienced by UV filters.

Photo-Degradation of UV Filters

Photolysis

The direct dissociation of a molecule upon the absorption of a determined amount of energy from a given type of radiation is ever more likely when that amount is equivalent or higher than the bonding energy of that same molecule. When this molecule reaches a higher or excited energy state, it dissociates, and the process is regarded as photolysis [14].

Photolysis is usually a rather complex set of reactions that lead to the formation of reactive species or fragments, and it can be experienced either by direct or indirect paths. Direct photolysis occurs upon the absorption of radiation by specific portions of the UV filters' structure itself, denominated chromophores. Indirect photolysis occurs upon the absorption of radiation by other structures or compounds rather than the UV filter, named photosensitizers, therefore initiating a series of reactions that will induce the transformation or degradation of the filters [3, 8, 9, 14]. Organic compounds will also experience degradation when in contact with reactive species, such as singlet oxygen, hydroxyl radicals, photo-excited organic matter and others [8, 9].

This type of photochemical reactions is one of the most important abiotic processes that control the fate and behaviour of UV filters when in the environment, in particular the aquatic compartments, and in general their prominence is far more significant than the biotic processes of degradation [3, 8], which will be approached in more detail further ahead.

There are numerous studies that have dealt with the subject of photo-degradation, with emphasis on photolysis. The general notion that must be underlined is that as the filters are exposed to UV radiation, they gradually lose their UV-protective features or capabilities [10, 11], which is also accompanied by the formation of several toxic and harmful by-products, as it has been demonstrated with EMC [12]. Sayre [13] stressed the complexity of the photo-degradation issue, since UV filters are used as part of a formulation of several different filters in commercial sunscreen products, and not in singular. In other words, the photochemical profile and behaviour of a matrix of multiple filters is fundamentally different than that displayed by a single UV filter, since the photo-degradation reactions of many filters are known to enhance or even induce the degradation reactions of others, even those supposedly more stable [13]. Serpone has also carried out some interesting studies on the photo-degradation or photo-stability of certain UV filters [10, 11]. His approach [11], delved on the photo-degradation of different UV filters and its extension in aerobic aqueous medium. The study was carried on the basis of the record of any and every alteration to the UV radiation absorbance as a function of irradiation time, with any loss of absorbance being subsequently directly correlated with loss of UV-protective capabilities. Results have shown that, in the case of the filter PAB, for instance, UV radiation absorbance capacity decreased about 35% just within the first hour of irradiation, whereas in the case of a very similar filter, EDP, the UV absorbance decrease was almost complete just after 20 minutes of irradiation. As for TDS, it was defined as the most photo-unstable UV filter of the study, with 90% UV radiation absorbance decrease after just 10 minutes of irradiation, while BZ3 was considered the most photo-stable, with a UV absorbance decrease of 20% and throughout two hours of irradiation.

Photo-degradation studies have always focused on its relation towards photo-protection alterations [10], ability of the filter mixture to enhance photolysis [10, 13], or the toxicological potential of by-products [12], but seldom has it focused on degradation in the environmental context [15]. Sakkas [15] approached simultaneously the disinfection by-product (DBP) formation as well as the photo-degradation by-products. Results have shown that photochemical reaction rates depend, not only on the environmental conditions, but also on the presence of other relevant compounds in solution, in particular dissolved organic matter (DOM). In the case of the filter EDP, degradation decreased significantly with the increase of DOM levels in solution, which is easily explained by the fact that DOM actively competes with any other present organic compound for the incident photons, in regards to photo-degradation. The authors were also able to identify several photo-degradation by-products, namely from dealkylation and hydroxylation, and in all the different sources of water samples studied (distilled water; swimming-pool water; and sea water).

Photo-Isomerization

Contrary to photolysis, photo-isomerization reactions yield new species closely related to the parental structures, but potentially more toxic and harmful than the original compounds. Regarding UV filters in particular, this translates essentially into the production of photo-isomers that may be related but no longer possess the required UV-protective features of the parental molecules, which is prominently evident in several classes of filters: cinnamates; salicylates; camphor derivatives; and dibenzoylmethane derivatives [10, 16-18].

The photo-isomerization of UV filters is both a fast and reversible process, when in aqueous solution, giving origin to a mixture of *E* and *Z* isomers in equilibrium. In the environment, UV filters will always be found in either of these two isomeric forms, given the existence of carbon-carbon exocyclic double bonds in their structure. However, commercial formulations of these compounds contain solely the *E* form of the compounds, despite their immediate photo-isomerization into the *Z* form upon exposure to UV radiation [19].

Another notable disadvantage of these reactions is, as approached earlier, apart from the loss of UV-protective capabilities, the production of potentially more troublesome by-products. For instance, the isomeric forms of UV filters might be chiral and therefore enantiomers, with similar physical-chemical properties, but the compounds will display very distinct environmental fate, behaviour and eco-toxicological profile. Contrary to the biological processes of degradation, that might be stereo-selective or enantio-selective [20], these abiotic processes are apparently not enantio-selective [19]. In light of this, the stereo-isomer composition of UV filters in natural waters seems indeed paramount in order to understand the compounds' fate and behaviour in the environment, but seldom has the theme been the subject of serious and focused investigation [3].

Díaz-Cruz [3] reviews the only existing study focused specifically on the subject: Buser [21] studied the chirality of MBC, showing that the stereo-isomer composition of the filter depended in fact on biological degradation occurring in waste water treatment plants, other water bodies like rivers or lakes, as well as plant or animal life.

There are numerous other studies on the photo-degradation or photo-stability of UV filters in general. One of the most important and popular UV filters, EMC, has been the subject of several interesting studies [10, 22-25]. In a study already mentioned, Sakkas [15] investigated the photochemical behaviour of the filter EDP in different water samples (sea water; swimming pool water; and distilled water) and under natural or artificial solar radiation. Results demonstrate that the filter degrades photo-chemically, originating several by-products; influence of dissolved organic matter (DOM) was also evaluated, showing that its presence decreases the photo-degradation reaction rates, since it competes with the filters for the incident photons; several by-products were also successfully identified. Huong [24] studied the photo-isomerization of EMC under artificial solar radiation and in several different solvents. Results showed significant loss in UV-absorbance capacity after irradiation, occurrence of chemical environmentally-dependent photo-isomerization *E* ➔ *Z* as well as irreversible degradation of the filter structure; *Z* isomer displays considerable lower UV-absorbance capacity; and photo-degradation by-products were also detected and successfully identified. Pattanaargson [22] also approached the photo-isomerization of EMC in different solvents and under natural solar radiation. The relevant results were as follows: photo-isomerization *E* ➔ *Z* resulted in significant loss of UV-absorbance capacity; *E-Z* equilibrium in solution does occur but it depends on solvent polarity. Pattanaargson and Limphong [23] approached the photo-stability of EMC on a chromatographic basis, in order to determine the obtained photo-degradation by-products. The authors have successfully determined one photo-degradation by-product, identified as the *Z* form of the filter, referring that after one day of irradiation, approximately half of the amount of the original *E* form of the filter had been transformed into the by-product. No irreversible compound structure degradation of the filter was detected. Maier [26] carried out a spectroscopically-focused study on the spectral alterations undergone by a set of sunscreen products upon exposure to artificial solar radiation, and its reflection on the UV-absorbance capacity. Results have shown the following: loss in UVB-absorbance capacity never exceeded 5% and considering all the irradiation times; UVA-absorbance capacity loss was generally much more significant and frequent; all products displayed increased spectroscopic photo-instability at increasing wavelengths. Gaspar and Maia Campos [27] evaluated the *in vitro* photo-stability of different combinations of UV filters in sunscreen products, under artificial solar radiation. Results have demonstrated that the interaction between filters within a formulation influences their photo-stability; and formulations containing the filter OCR increased their UVA-absorbance capacity. Huong [28] carried out another study similar to the one mentioned before for EMC [24], but focused now on BDM [28]. As far as the results are concerned, BDM demonstrated photo-instability in non-polar solvents, with significant alterations in its absorption spectra;

these alterations, despite significant, were found to be reversible after protection and storage of the irradiated solutions in the dark, but also found to be inhibited depending on the solvent conditions; the general behaviour of BDM was considered analogous to that of EMC, and it displayed quite significant and irreversible degradation of the filter structure in aqueous solution; several photo-degradation by-products were detected and successfully identified; photo-degradation in general was found to be significantly influenced and dependent on the medium and experimental conditions.

Many other similar studies exist, like Mturi's and Martincigh's [29] that dealt with the photo-stability of BDM in different solvents; or Hojerová's study [30], that ascertained the protective efficiency of several sunscreen products containing different UV filter formulations, and concluded that the sunscreen products' UV-protective efficiency is quite distinct from one another, even between commercial products with the same labeled sun protection factor (SPF); Rodil [25] also evaluated the photo-stability of several UV filters, as well as the eco-toxicological profile of their photo-degradation by-products in aquatic microorganisms; Perugini [31] carried out a very interesting study on the effect of nanoparticle encapsulation of the filter EMC on its photo-stability; and Scalia [32] evaluated the effect of the natural antioxidant quercetin, on the photo-stability of a combination of two of the most popular UV filters used worldwide, EMC and BDM.

Degradation Induced by Disinfecting Agents

The water disinfection process has the fundamental purpose of destroying aquatic microbiological organisms, which represent the ultimate contagion source of disease. This is contrary to the concept of sterilization, which involves complete destruction of every microorganism, something that may not always be achievable or even necessary or beneficial [33].

For more than a century, chlorine has been the most popular disinfecting agent used worldwide, successfully controlling and even eliminating water-borne infectious diseases altogether [8]. Despite this, there are several other types of less popular disinfecting agents, like ozone or even UV radiation, both used in high-scale swimming-pool water disinfection, but also bromide-based water disinfecting agents, used in lower-scale swimming pools [33]. Although the removal of relevant pathogens and microorganisms is rather effective, the removal of DOM is not. Removal of organic pollutants is rather complex and varies significantly [3].

The disinfection process transforms the organic compounds in the water, giving origin to the so-called disinfection by-products (DBP's), or in this particular case, chlorinated DBP's. Over the years, chlorinated DBP's have been directly associated with several and serious potential toxicological effects, which forced authorities to consider the problem of production of these compounds in the context of drinking water disinfection process [3, 8]. Reports indicate that exposure to chlorinated DBP's might be directly associated with the occurrence of several cancers in human vital organs, so Gopal [33] approached predictive models for production and kinetics of DBP formation, their health effects, removal techniques, and guideline implementation.

Given the use of other aforementioned water disinfecting agents, apart from the vastly more popular chlorine, based on either bromide or iodine, important focus is now being given to brominated and iodinated DBP's. These compounds are reported to be significantly toxic, not only in the range of carcinogenicity, but also genotoxicity and cytotoxicity. Such compounds include iodo-acids, like iodo-acetic acid, bromonitromethanes, iodinated-trihalomethanes, 3-Chloro-4-(dichloromethyl)-5-hydroxy-2(5H)-furanone (best known by its historical name, Mutagen X or MX), halogenated-aldehydes, halogenated-amides, bromate, and many others [35]. Also a particular reason for concern is yet another by-product of chlorine disinfection, the production of chloramines, which are originated from the reaction of chlorine with ammonia. Research has indicated that chloramines potentiate the iodo-acids and iodinated-trihalomethane production and accumulation within the water compartments [8].

Researchers have previously approached the general pathways of introduction and movement of synthetic organic pollutants, into and throughout the environment, with emphasis on the aquatic compartments [6, 8]. Generally speaking, the mode of introduction of these compounds into the environmental compartments will very much depend on their pattern of use or application [8]. When in the environment, however, these are transformed, chemically, photo-chemically or biologically. Usually, these processes will lead to the compounds' structure breakdown and subsequent elimination, but at the same time degradation by-products may also be produced, often more persistent and toxic than the original structures [6, 8]. Figure 2 represents the pathways involved in the generic fate and behaviour of UV filters and corresponding by-products in the environment [6].

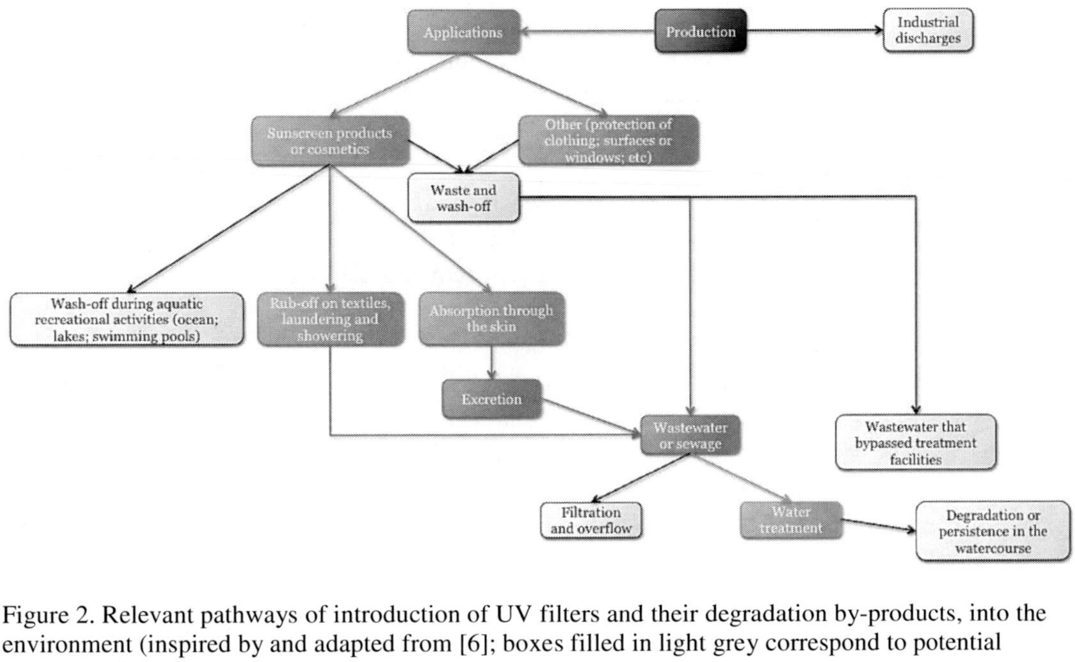

Figure 2. Relevant pathways of introduction of UV filters and their degradation by-products, into the environment (inspired by and adapted from [6]; boxes filled in light grey correspond to potential processes of release into the environment).

An evaluation on the occurrence of DBP's was carried out in Turkish superficial waters with low levels of dissolved organic carbon [36]. Results have shown that, given the susceptibility of the DBP precursors to associate with soils and sediments, events like ground-level run-off or leaching from soils as well as re-suspension into the watercourse from sediments, increased their levels in the superficial aquatic compartments. Upon treatment with chlorine disinfecting agents, it led to the production and increase of DBP's in drinking water.

There isn't any data available on the determination of UV filters DBP's in water treatment facilities [3]. Nonetheless, given the combined action of solar radiation and the presence of disinfecting species in solution, UV filters will be readily halogenated, giving origin to halogenated species of the parental compounds as well as many other DBP's as a result of the degradation of the original structure. Up to this moment, there are only four studies focused on the UV filter degradation reactions in aqueous solution on the presence of chlorine disinfecting agents [1, 37-39], along with a comprehensive review on both the UV filter photo-degradation by-products in aqueous solution, and the UV filters' DBP formation studies until 2012 [40].

Regarding the study of these compounds, very little is still known about the degradation reactions induced by disinfecting agents, and what is indeed known is focused solely on a very limited number of the most popular UV filters [1, 37-39]. More focus should be given towards the disinfection process and its implications on the degradation of UV filters.

Eco-Toxicological Effects of UV Filters and Their Degradation by-Products

The physical-chemical properties of UV filters, presented in Table 1, such as water solubility, vapour pressure and polarity, are crucial in order to determine their behaviour in the environment. As already mentioned, data points to their substantial tendency to concentration and accumulation within the environment and food chain, which, associated with their also reported significant potential for eco-toxicity, is quite problematic [3, 6, 8, 15, 41, 42].

Díaz-Cruz and Barceló [43] have reviewed some of the most important existing eco-toxicological studies, performed both *in vitro* and *in vivo*. What follows, is a brief summary on these and some additional relevant studies and subsequent results and conclusions.

In Vitro Studies

Several UV filters have been reported to display estrogenic activity *in vitro* [7, 44-48]. The *in vitro* models applied or used on these and other studies, often revolve around the highly efficient, sensitive, fast and inexpensive recombinant yeast assay [44, 47, 48], MCF-7 breast cancer cells [45, 48], the human embryonic kidney 293 reporter gene assay (HEK293) [7], the human endometrial Ishikawa cell line [46], or rat and human primary hepatocytes [46].

Regarding the UV filters commonly approached in *in vitro* studies, benzophenones seem to be quite popular in that regard, with Schultz [44] investigating their estrogenic activity in specific, although the compounds have been addressed in many other studies, in particular BZ3 [7, 45, 47].

MBC has also been the subject of some particular studies, regarding its interaction towards estrogenic receptors [46, 48], amongst other more generic *in vitro* eco-toxicological studies [7, 45, 47]. Amidst the most popular UV filters, one must also underline the UV filters EMC, BDM and EDP, also investigated as to their estrogenic activity [7, 45, 47].

As for the relevant eco-toxicological conclusions arisen from these studies, all have emphasized the issues subsequent to this context of investigation. These problems include noncommittal results or the clear inability of the general *in vitro* models to account for the toxico-kinetics and toxico-dynamics of complex whole organisms, which highlights their prominent limitations as to relevant predictive value for a mammalian *in vivo* context. Overall, nearly all filters have demonstrated dose-dependent estrogenic activity, with benzophenones being amongst the most active, as was the case of BZ3 [7, 45], with EMC [7] and BDM [45] being the least active and inactive, respectively, in the same type of studies. The estrogenic activity seems to be directly linked to the presence of benzene rings substituted with polar functional groups, particularly in *para-* position, as well as with the presence of symmetry in the molecule [44]. MBC, one of the filters studied in specific, has demonstrated either estrogenic activity analogous to that of other know weak estrogens [46] or ambiguous results occurring at extremely high levels [48].

Possible effects on thyroid hormonal regulation have also been mentioned [43, 48], but the data on the subject are rather scarce [49]. This study used a new human recombinant thyroid peroxidase stably transfected into a human follicular thyroid carcinoma cell line (FTC-238), in order to assess the possible effects of the filter BZ2.

Very significant disturbance of thyroid hormone homeostasis by inhibition of thyroid peroxidase was reported, making BZ2 the most potent thyroid peroxidase inhibitor found to date [49]. A similar study using human FTC-133 thyroid carcinoma cells [50] showed the opposite results for EMC and MBC.

Evaluation of mere estrogenic activity of UV filters has always been the main focus of hormonal activity studies of these compounds, but multiple combined hormonal effects (estrogenic, anti-estrogenic, androgenic and anti-androgenic effects) have seldom been investigated. Several UV filters have been recently shown to display multiple endocrine-disrupting behaviour like MBC, which displayed estrogenic and anti-estrogenic activities, or BZ3 and HS, which demonstrated estrogenic, anti-estrogenic and anti-androgenic activities [7, 51-53].

In another study [54], out of 19 UV filters and two benzophenone metabolites, all displayed some kind of hormonal effect, merely two (P25 and PAB) did not demonstrate multiple hormonal effects, while the vast majority demonstrated multiple effects. However, as Díaz-Cruz and Barceló argue [43], these effects might be subjective, since individual activities are directly and significantly dependent on the type of tests conducted.

Regarding the *in vitro* studies on UV filters' transformation or degradation by-products, seldom has it been the subject of any studies. The exceptions are a study by Butt and Christensen [12], which dealt with the toxicity of photo-degradation by-products of EMC and BDM in a mouse lymphoma cell line (L5178Y-R), and a more recent study from Nakajima [38], which focused on the mutagenic activity of EMC and EDP using a mutagenic assay on a *Salmonella typhimurium* strain (TA100).

Butt and Christensen [12] demonstrated that exposure to irradiated solutions of UV filter resulted in increased cell mortality, independently of the irradiation time. Regarding Nakajima's study [38], both EMC and EDP were not mutagenic in the referred assay, with the opposite being exhibited after chlorination. EMC's mutagenic by-products of chlorination however, proved to be unstable after 6 hours of completion of the chlorination reactions, since the mutagenicity of the solutions decreased subsequently.

In Vivo Studies

Díaz-Cruz and Barceló [43] mention that benzophenones are the essential focus of study, regarding *in vivo* investigations, and these are mostly centered on evaluation of hormonal effects, effects on reproduction or fertility [54-64].

The usual *in vivo* models of investigation include mostly fish, particularly juvenile or mature fathead minnows (*Pimephales promelas*) [54-58], Japanese rice fish (*Oryzias latipes*) [58, 62] or rainbow trout (*Oncorhynchus mykiss*) [58], with some existing studies also in ovariectomized rats [59, 60, 61], tadpoles [57, 63] or even fetal rats [64]. Benzophenones are indeed a special focus of these studies, particularly BZ2 [56, 59, 60] and BZ3 [58, 60], given the fact that the molecular structure of this class of compounds is quite similar to other known estrogenic chemicals. But camphor derivatives have also been approached often, with particular emphasis on MBC [57, 62-64] and 3BC [55, 57, 63, 64]. There are two existing studies on the extremely popular EMC [61, 62].

Regarding the conclusions of these studies, all have emphasized concerning considerations, and in general, dose-dependent: significant bioaccumulation factors [55, 56], which has also been approached in previous chapters (see Table 1 and corresponding references [3, 6]); quite significant decrease in fecundity or complete cessation of reproductive ability [55-58]; demasculinization of secondary sexual characteristics [55, 57]; significant induction of Vitellogenin [54, 55, 57, 58]; prominent effects in the masculine and feminine gonad histology [55, 56, 57]; and development of both oocytes and spermatocytes, as well as egg production, inhibited [55, 56, 57, 58].

On the other hand, MBC and 3BC displayed no accountable effects on tadpole's hormonal and thyroidal systems during metamorphosis [57], which was described as a critical stage quite susceptible to endocrine disruptions. The filter Ethyl-*p*-aminobenzoate (yet another *p*-aminobenzoic acid derivative) also did not exhibit negative effects on fathead minnows' weight and length development, and mortality was not verified either, upon exposure to the compound [54].

As a counterweight to all the concerning findings, some authors argue that many of the toxicological effects are found and reported at extremely high levels, sometimes as high as 75 fold the levels previously reported for wastewater effluents [58]. At environmental levels, however, MBC and 3BC were both studied as to their effects on the hormonal, thyroidal and sexual systems of tadpoles, during metamorphosis, and after 35 days of exposure, no relevant negative effects were found [63]. Contrary to this fact, studies have also reported that significant toxicological effects may indeed be found at low levels, as was the case with 3BC, which induced prominent histological and reproductive effects in fish and at low concentrations [57].

FUTURE PERSPECTIVES

In light of what was approached in this review, it is important to emphasize that very little is still known about the aqueous degradation reactions of UV filters induced by disinfecting agents. Very few filters have been studied in this context (essentially EMC, BDM and EDP), and considering the findings of these studies, it is imperative to focus even more on this context and extend the investigation towards other filters amongst the most popular.

Special attention should also be given to the determination of their DBP's, which is a field of special concern given their potential hazardous toxicological effects.

Considering the eco-toxicological reviews, it seems clear that additional studies are also required, given the ambiguous results obtained so far. Both the *in vitro* and *in vivo* contexts of toxicological investigation are of paramount importance, and should therefore be used in succession in order to achieve a reliable assessment of the eco-toxicity of UV filters and by-products. However, there are still many issues to consider and solve, particularly regarding the *in vitro* models: the typical models used carry significant unclearness regarding procedures and protocols; many display limited predictive value towards the *in vivo* results; and none reflect or replicate the metabolic processes of complex whole organisms, which is clear from the usually conflicting *in vitro* and *in vivo* results.

Naturally, the *in vitro* models lack the capacity to account for the toxico-kinetics and dynamics of complete organisms, which represents a comprehensive disadvantage. This fact stresses the need to carry out studies *in vivo*, following the investigations made *in vitro*, for these often generate inconclusive results and that do not necessarily reflect what may indeed occur in whole organisms.

ACKNOWLEDGMENTS

A. J. M. Santos wishes to acknowledge Fundação para a Ciência e Tecnologia (FCT) for the Ph.D. Program in Sustainable Chemistry grant PD/BD/52530/2014.

REFERENCES

[1] Chisvert, A., Salvador, A. (2007), *Analysis of Cosmetic Products*, Chapter 3, Elsevier, Amsterdam, The Netherlands.

[2] Salvador, A., Chisvert, A. (2005), Sunscreen analysis – a critical survey on UV filter determination, *Anal. Chim. Acta* 537, 1-14.

[3] Díaz-Cruz, M. S., Llorca, M., Barceló, D. (2008), Organic UV filters and their photodegradates, metabolites and disinfection by-products in the aquatic environment, *Trends in Analytical Chemistry* 27 (10), 873-887.

[4] Shaath, N. A. (2010), Ultraviolet filters, Photochem. *Photobiol.* 9, 464-469.

[5] Shaath, N. A. (2005), The chemistry of UV filters, in: Sunscreens: Regulations and Commercial Development, 3rd Edition, *Taylor and Francis*, New York, USA, pp. 217-238.

[6] Giokas, D. L., Salvador, A., Chisvert, A. (2007), UV filters: from sunscreens to the human body and the environment, *Trends in Analytical Chemistry* 26 (5), 360-374.

[7] Schreurs, R., Lanser, P., Seinen, W., Van der Burg, B. (2002), Estrogenic activity of UV filters determined by an in vitro reporter gene assay and an in vivo transgenic zebrafish assay, *Arch. Toxicol.* 76 (5-6), 257-261.

[8] La Farré, M., Pérez, S., Kantiani, L., Barceló, D. (2008), Fate and toxicity of emerging pollutants, their metabolites and transformation products in the aquatic environment, *Trends in Analytical Chemistry* 27 (11), 991-1007.

[9] Lam, M. W., Tantuco, K., Mabury, S. A. (2003), PhotoFate: a new approach in accounting for the contribution of indirect photolysis of pesticides and pharmaceuticals in surface waters, *Environ. Sci. Technol.* 37 (5), 899-907.

[10] Serpone, N., Salinaro, A., Emeline, A. V., Horikoshi, S., Hidaka, H., Zhao, J. (2002), An in vitro systematic spectroscopic examination of the photostabilities of a random set of commercial sunscreen lotions and their chemical UVB/UVA active agents, *Photochem. Photobiol. Sci.* 1 (12), 970-981.

[11] Serpone, N., Dondi, D., Albini, A. (2007), Inorganic and organic UV filters: their role and efficacy in sunscreens and suncare products, *Inorganica Chim. Acta* 360 (3), 794-802.

[12] Butt, S. T., Christensen, T. (2000), Toxicity and phototoxicity of chemical sun filters, *Radiat. Prot. Dosim.* 91 (1-3), 283-286.

[13] Sayre, R. M., Dowdy, J.C., Gerwig, A.J., Shields, W.J., Lloyd, R.V. (2005), Unexpected photolysis of the sunscreen octinoxate in the presence of the sunscreen avobenzone, *Photochem. Photobiol.* 81 (2), 452-456.

[14] Rohatgi-Mukherjee, K.K. (1978), *Fundamentals of Photochemistry* (Revised Edition), New Age International Limited Publishers.

[15] Sakkas, V.A., Giokas, D.L., Lambropoulou, D.A., Albanis, T.A. (2003), Aqueous photolysis of the sunscreen agent octyl-dimethyl-p-aminobenzoic acid. Formation of disinfection by-products in chlorinated swimming pool water, *J. Chromatogr.* A 1016, 211-222.

[16] Broadbent, J.K., Martincigh, B.S., Raynor, M.W., Salter, L.F., Moulder, R., Sjoberg, P. and Markides, K.E. (1996), Capillary supercritical fluid chromatography combined with atmospheric pressure chemical ionisation mass spectrometry for the investigation of photoproduct formation in the sunscreen absorber 2-ethylhexyl-p-methoxycinnamate, *J. Chromatogr.* A 732 (1), 101-110.

[17] Deflandre, A. and Lang, G. (1988), Photostability assessment of sunscreens. Benzylidene camphor and dibenzoylmethane derivatives, *Int. J. Cosmet. Sci.* 10 (2), 53-62.

[18] Plaguellat, C., Kupper, T., Furrer, R., Alencastro, L., Grandjean, D. and Tarradellas, J. (2006), Concentrations and specific loads of UV filters in sewage sludge originating from a monitoring network in Switzerland, *Chemosphere* 62 (6), 915-925.

[19] Poiger, T., Buser, H.R., Balmer, M.E., Bergqvist, P.A. and Müller, M.D. (2004), Occurrence of UV filter compounds from sunscreens in surface waters: regional mass balance in two Swiss lakes, *Chemosphere* 55 (7), 951-963.

[20] Ariens, E. J. (1989), Stereoselectivity of bioactive agents, general aspects, in: *Stereochemistry and Biological Activity of Drugs*, Ariens, E.J., Soudijn, W., Timmermann, P.B.M.W.M. (Editors), Blackwell, Oxford, UK.

[21] Buser, H.-R., Müller, M.D., Balmer, M.E., Poiger, T., Buerge, I.J. (2005), Stereoisomer Composition of the chiral UV filter 4-Methylbenzylidene camphor in environmental samples, *Environ. Sci. Technol.* 39 (9), 3013-3019.

[22] Pattanaargson, S.T., Munhapol, T., Hirunsupachot, P. and Luangthongaram, P. (2004), Photoisomerization of octyl methoxycinnamate, *J. Photochem. Photobiol.* A 161 (2-3), 269-274.

[23] Pattanaargson, S.T., Limphong, P. (2001), Stability of octyl methoxycinnamate and identification of its photo-degradation product, *Int. J. Cosmet. Sci.* 23 (3), 153-160.

[24] Huong, S.P., Andrieu, V., Reynier, J.-P., Rocher, E., Fourneron, J.-D. (2007), The photoisomerization of the sunscreen ethylhexyl p-methoxy cinnamate and its influence on the sun protection factor, *J. Photochem. Photobiol.* A 186 (1), 65-70.

[25] Rodil, R., Moeder, M., Altenburger, R., Schmitt-Jansen, M. (2009), Photostability and phytotoxicity of selected sunscreen agents and their degradation mixtures in water, *Anal. Bioanal. Chem.* 395 (5), 1513-1524.

[26] Maier, H., Schauberger, G., Brunnhofer, K. and Honigsmann, H. (2001), Change of ultraviolet absorbance of sunscreens by exposure to solar-simulated radiation, *J. Invest. Dermatol.* 117 (2), 256-262.

[27] Gaspar, L.R., Maia Campos, P.M.B.G. (2006), Evaluation of the photostability of different UV filter combinations in a sunscreen, *Int. J. Pharm.* 307 (2), 123-128.

[28] Huong, S.P., Rocher, E., Fourneron, J.-D., Charles, L., Monnier, V., Bun, H., Andrieu, V. (2008), Photoreactivity of the sunscreen butylmethoxydibenzoylmethane (DBM) under various experimental conditions, *J. Photochem. Photobiol. A* 196 (1), 106-112.

[29] Mturi, G.J. and Martincigh, B.S. (2008), Photostability of the sunscreening agent 4-tert-butyl-4′-methoxydibenzoylmethane (avobenzone) in solvents of different polarity and proticity, *J. Photochem. Photobiol. A* 200 (2-3), 410-420.

[30] Hojerová, J., Medovcíková, A., Mikula, M. (2011), Photoprotective efficacy and photostability of fifteen sunscreen products having the same label SPF subjected to natural sunlight, *Int. J. Pharm.* 408 (1-2), 27-39.

[31] Perugini, P., Simeoni, S., Scalia, S., Genta, I., Modena, T., Conti, B., Pavanetto, F. (2002), Effect of nanoparticle encapsulation on the photostability of the sunscreen agent, 2-ethylhexyl-p-methoxycinnamate, *Int. J. Pharm.* 246 (1-2), 37-45.

[32] Scalia, S., Mezzena, M. (2010), Photostabilization effect of quercetin on the UV filter combination, Butyl methoxydibenzoylmethane-Octyl Methoxycinnamate, *Photochem. Photobiol.* 86 (2), 273-278.

[33] Gopal, K., Tripathy, S.S., Bersillon, J.L., Dubey, S.P. (2007), Chlorination by-products, their toxico-dynamics and removal from drinking water, *J. Hazard. Mater.* 140 (1-2), 1-6.

[34] Scholz, M. (2006), *Wetland Systems To Control Urban Runoff*, Chapter 22, Elsevier, Amsterdam, The Netherlands, pp. 155-162.

[35] Richardson, S.D. (2005), New disinfection by-product issues: emerging DBPs and alternative routes of exposure, *Global NEST J.* 7 (1), 43-60.

[36] Ates, N., Kaplan, S.S., Sahinkaya, E., Kitis, M., Dilek, F.B., Yetis, U. (2007), Occurrence of disinfection by-products in low DOC surface waters in Turkey, *J. Hazard. Mater.* 142 (1-2), 526-534.

[37] Negreira, N., Canosa, P., Rodríguez, I., Ramil, M., Rubí, E., Cela, R. (2008), Study of some UV filters stability in chlorinated water and identification of halogenated by-products by gas chromatography–mass spectrometry, *J. Chromatogr. A* 1178 (1-2), 206-214.

[38] Nakajima, M., Kawakami, T., Niino, T., Takahashi, Y., Onodera, S. (2009), Aquatic fate of sunscreen agents Octyl-4-methoxycinnamate and Octyl-4-dimethylaminobenzoate in model swimming pools and the mutagenic assays of their chlorination by-products, *J. Health Sci.* 55 (3), 363-372.

[39] Santos, A.J.M., Crista, D.M.A., Miranda, M.S., Almeida, I.F., Sousa e Silva, J.P., Costa, P.C., Amaral, M.H., Lobão, P.A.L., Sousa Lobo, J.M., Esteves da Silva, J.C.G.

(2013), Degradation of UV filters 2-Ethylhexyl-2-methoxycinnamate and 4-tert-Butyl-4'-methoxydibenzoylmethane in chlorinated water, *Environ. Chem.* 10 (2), 127-134.

[40] Santos, A.J.M., Miranda, M.S., Esteves da Silva, J.C.G. (2012), The degradation products of UV filters in aqueous and chlorinated aqueous solutions, *Water Res.* 46 (10), 3167-3176.

[41] Balmer, M.E., Buser, H.R., Müller, M.D., Poiger, T. (2004), Occurrence of organic UV filter compounds BP-3, 4-MBC, EHMC and OC, in wastewater, surface waters and in fish from Swiss lakes, Agroscope, Swiss Federal Research Station for Horticulture, *Plant Protection Chemistry*, CH-8820 Wädenswill, Switzerland.

[42] Giokas, D.L., Sakkas, V.A., Albanis, T.A. (2004), Determination of residues of UV filters in natural waters by solid-phase extraction coupled to liquid chromatography–photodiode array detection and gas chromatography–mass spectrometry, *J. Chromatogr. A* 1026 (1-2), 289-293.

[43] Díaz-Cruz, M.S., Barceló, D. (2009), Chemical analysis and ecotoxicological effects of organic UV-absorbing compounds in aquatic ecosystems, *Trends in Analytical Chemistry* 28 (6), 708-717.

[44] Schultz, T.W., Seward, J.R., Links, G.D. (2000), Estrogenicity of benzophenones evaluated with a recombinant yeast assay: Comparison of experimental and rules-based predicted activity, *Environ. Toxicol. Chem.* 19 (2), 301-304.

[45] Schlumpf, M., Cotton, B., Consciente, M., Haller, V., Steinmann, B., Linchtesteiger, W. (2001), In vitro and in vivo estrogenicity of UV screens, *Environ. Health Perspect.* 109 (3), 239-244.

[46] Müller, S.O., Kling, M., Firzani, P.A., Mecky, A., Durante, E., Shields-Botella, J., Delansorne, R., Broschard, T., Kramer, P.J. (2003), Activation of estrogen receptor α and β by 4-methylbenzylidene-camphor in human and rat cells: comparison with phyto- and xenoestrogens, *Toxicol. Lett.* 142 (1-2), 89-101.

[47] Kunz, P.Y., Galicia, H.F., Fent, K. (2006), Comparison of In Vitro and In Vivo Estrogenic Activity of UV Filters in Fish, *Toxicol. Sci.* 90 (2), 349-361.

[48] Tinwell, H., Lefevre, P.A., Moffat, G.J., Burns, A., Odum, J., Spurway, T.D., Orphanides, G., Sabih, J. (2002), Confirmation of uterotrophic activity of 3-(4-methylbenzylidine)camphor in the immature rat, Environ. *Health Perspect.* 110 (5), 533-536.

[49] Schmutzler, C., Bacinski, A., Gotthardt, I., Huhne, K., Ambrugger, P., Klammer, H., Schlecht, C., Hoang-Vu, C., Grüters, A., Wuttke, W., Jarry, H., Köhrle, J. (2007), The ultraviolet filter benzophenone-2 interferes with the thyroid hormone axis in rats and is a potent in vitro inhibitor of human recombinant thyroid peroxidase, *Endocrinology* 148 (6), 2835-2844.

[50] Schmutzler, C., Hamann, I., Hofmann, P.J., Kovacs, G., Stemmler, L., Memtrup, B., Schomburg, L., Ambrugger, P., Grüters, A., Seidlova-Wuttke, D., Jarry, H., Wuttke, W., Köhrle, J. (2004), Endocrine active compounds affect thyrotropin and thyroid hormone levels in serum as well as endpoints of thyroid hormone action in liver, heart and kidney, *Toxicology* 205 (1-2), 95-102.

[51] Schreurs, R., Sonneveld, E., Hansen, J.H.J., Seeinen, W., Van der Burg, B. (2005), Interaction of Polycyclic Musks and UV Filters with the Estrogen Receptor (ER), Androgen receptor (AR), and progesterone receptor (PR) in reporter gene bioassays, *Toxicol. Sci.* 83 (2), 264-272.

[52] Ma, R., Cotton, B., Lichtensteiger, W., Schlumpf, M. (2003), UV Filters with antagonistic action at androgen receptors in the MDA-kb2 cell transcriptional-activation assay, *Toxicol. Sci.* 74 (1), 43-50.

[53] Schlumpf, M., Schmid, P., Durres, S., Consciente, M., Maerkel, K., Henseler, E., Gruetter, M., Herzog, I., Reolon, S., Ceccatelli, R., Faass, O., Stutz, O., Jarry, H., Wuttke, W., Lichtensteiger, W. (2004), Endocrine activity and developmental toxicity of cosmetic UV filters—an update, *Toxicol.* 205 (1-2), 113-122.

[54] Kunz, P.Y., Fent, K. (2006), Multiple hormonal activities of UV filters and comparison of in vivo and in vitro estrogenic activity of ethyl-4-aminobenzoate in fish, *Aquatic* Toxicol. *79 (4), 305-324.*

[55] *Kunz, P.Y., Gries, T., Fent, K. (2006), The ultraviolet filter 3-Benzylidene Camphor* adversely affects reproduction in fathead minnow (Pimephales promelas), Toxicol. Sci. 93 (2), 311-321.

[56] Weisbrod, C.J., Kunz, P.Y., Zenker, A.K., Fent, K. (2007), Effects of the UV filter benzophenone-2 on reproduction in fish, *Toxicol. Appl. Pharmacol.* 225, 255-266.

[57] Fent, K., Kunz, P.Y., Gomez, E. (2008), UV filters in the aquatic environment induce hormonal effects and affect fertility and reproduction in fish, *Chimia* 62, 368-375.

[58] Coronado, M., De Haro, H., Deng, X., Rempel, M.A., Lavado, R., Schlenk, D. (2008), UV filters in the aquatic environment induce hormonal effects and affect fertility and reproduction in fish, *Aquatic Toxicol.* 90, 182-187.

[59] Jarry, H., Christofell, J., Rimoldi, G., Koch, L., Wuttke, W. (2004), Multi-organic endocrine disrupting activity of the UV screen benzophenone 2 (BP2) in ovariectomized adult rats after 5 days treatment, *Toxicol.* 205, 87-93.

[60] Schlecht, C., Klammer, H., Jarry, H., Wuttke, W. (2004), Effects of estradiol, benzophenone-2 and benzophenone-3 on the expression pattern of the estrogen receptors (ER) alpha and beta, the estrogen receptor-related receptor 1 (ERR1) and the aryl hydrocarbon receptor (AhR) in adult ovariectomized rats, *Toxicol.* 205, 123-130.

[61] Klammer, H., Schlecht, C., Wuttke, W., Schmutzler, C., Gotthardt, I., Köhrle, J., Jarry, H. (2007), Effects of a 5-day treatment with the UV-filter octyl-methoxycinnamate (OMC) on the function of the hypothalamo-pituitary–thyroid function in rats, *Toxicol.* 238, 192-199.

[62] Inui, M., Adachi, T., Takenaka, S., Inui, H., Nakazawa, M., Ueda, M., Watanabe, H., Mori, C., Iguchi, T., Miyatake, K. (2003), Effect of UV screens and preservatives on vitellogenin and choriogenin production in male medaka (Oryzias latipes), *Toxicol.* 194, 43-50.

[63] Kunz, P.Y., Galicia, H.F., Fent, K. (2004), Assessment of hormonal activity of UV filters in tadpoles of frog Xenopus laevis at environmental concentrations, *Mar. Environ. Res.* 58, 431-435.

[64] Hofkamp, L., Bradley, S., Tresguerres, J., Lichtensteiger, W., Schlumpf, M., Timms, B. (2008), Region-specific growth effects in the developing rat prostate following fetal exposure to estrogenic ultraviolet filters, *Environ. Health. Perspect.* 116 (7), 867-872.

In: Sunscreens
Editors: Sean Henry Sharp

ISBN: 978-1-63482-160-5

Chapter 6

ASSESSMENT OF SUNSCREEN SAFETY BY SKIN PERMEATION STUDIES: AN UPDATE

Lucia Montenegro*
Department of Drug Sciences, University of Catania, Catania, Italy

ABSTRACT

One of the major concerns about the use of sunscreens is their safety. Many investigations performed with different techniques have addressed this issue providing conflicting results. To be safe and effective, sunscreens should remain on the skin surface without penetrating into the underlying living tissue. As these products are normally applied on large skin areas, even small amounts of UV-filters permeating the skin could lead to their systemic absorption, making controversial their safety after topical application. To overcome real or perceived human health concerns arising from the use of sunscreen products, their margin of safety (MoS) can be easily estimated by assessing UV-filters skin permeation using *in vitro* techniques. At present, several *in vitro* and *in vivo* test systems that provide reliable and reproducible results are used by cosmetic and pharmaceutical industries.

In this chapter, physical and chemical parameters affecting UV-filters ability to permeate the skin will be discussed, and *in vitro* and *in vivo* skin permeation studies performed on the most commonly used UV-filters will be reviewed. Estimations of UV-filter MoS from skin permeation studies will highlight the safety of currently used sunscreen formulations.

INTRODUCTION

The increasing incidence of skin cancer has led the international health authorities to recommend protection measures to prevent the harmful effects of skin exposure to UV-radiation. Such measures include avoidance of sun exposure, especially at times when

* Phone: + 39 095 738 4010, Fax: + 39 095 738 4211, E-mail: lmontene@unict.it.

disease-inducing wavelengths are more intense, wearing protective clothing and use of topical sunscreens (González et al., 2008; Lautenschlager et al., 2007).

As sunscreen products have gained the public favor, in the last decades there has been a notable increase of their consumption and of the number and content of UV-filters present in cosmetics and toiletries, thus enhancing the potential human exposure to sun-protecting active ingredients.

To be effective, ideally sunscreens should remain on the skin surface, without penetrating into the deep skin layers. As these products are often applied to large skin areas, even small amounts of UV-filters permeating the skin could lead to their systemic absorption and to adverse reactions.

Reports on the ability of some UV-filters to permeate the skin (Hayden et al., 1997; Janjua et al., 2004) and on their estrogenic effects (Klann et al., 2005; Koda et al., 2005; Kunz and Fent, 2006; Schlumpf and Cotton, 2001; Schlumpf et al., 2004) have given rise to a great concern about the safety of sunscreen products. Therefore, the need to guarantee the safety of sunscreen products has boosted toxicity studies on UV-filters. A recent review (Gilbert et al., 2013), illustrating the available toxicity data on the most commonly used UV-filters, evidenced that their potential estrogenic effects as well as their entrapment into vital organs are still very controversial.

To perform a risk assessment of sunscreen products, reliable information on the toxicological profile of individual sunscreen actives are required as well as data from percutaneous absorption studies designed to mimic actual product use. Therefore, understanding the basic concept of skin penetration/permeation is an essential requisite to conduct a rigorous evaluation of the actual safety of sunscreen agents.

The Process of Percutaneous Absorption

In recent years, a growing attention has been focused on the evaluation of permeation through human skin of exogenous compounds. This evaluation is of significance both in the pharmaceutical and cosmetic fields to assess the efficacy and the safety of products intended for application onto the skin. Predicting skin delivery of active ingredients is still a challenge as many factors are involved in the process of percutaneous absorption. This process relates to the entering of a molecule from the external environment within the skin (penetration) and it can be described as permeation if the molecule reaches the systemic circulation. An exhaustive knowledge of the skin's barrier function is fundamental both in evaluating the (trans)dermal delivery of drugs and in making a risk assessment following dermal exposure to chemicals.

It is well known that the outermost layer of the epidermis, the stratum corneum (SC), limits skin permeation of xenobiotics, acting as the rate-controlling barrier to skin delivery of most drugs (Förster et al., 2009). This thin (15 − 30μm) and highly hydrophobic layer consists of dead keratin cells embedded in a lipid domain and arranged in the so-called bricks and mortar model (Bouwstra et al., 2000; Wertz, 2000). Lipid content and organization within the SC and skin thickness are among the factors affecting drug skin permeation and vary for different anatomical regions in the same individual (intra-subject variability), the same region of different individuals (inter-subject variability) and among species (Akomeah et al., 2007).

The underneath viable epidermis is mostly hydrophilic as its water content is > 50 % while in the dermis the water content reaches 70%, thus favoring the uptake of hydrophilic molecules in these skin layers. Variables such as SC water content, skin extensibility, recovery and elasticity in individuals of different sex and race could play a significant role, as well (Berardesca et al., 1991).

Key factors affecting the process of percutaneous absorption involve physicochemical properties of the applied molecule and type and composition of the vehicle.

As reported in the literature (Guy and Hadgraft 1988; Schaefer and Riedelmayer, 1996), the physicochemical properties that determine the skin permeation of an active ingredient include hydrophilic-lipophilic balance, molar mass, molecular size, dipole moment, vapor pressure and extent of ionization. Molecules showing partition coefficient (log P octanol/water) values in the range 1-3 have been reported to permeate the skin better than very lipophilic compounds as they have a sufficient solubility in the lipid domains of the SC while still having a sufficient hydrophilicity to allow their partitioning into the viable tissue of the epidermis (Beetge et al., 2000; Bunge and Cleek, 1995). Therefore, depending on its lipophilic or hydrophilic properties, an active ingredient will accumulate in the SC (very lipophilic molecules), or remain on the surface (very hydrophilic molecules) or penetrate into the skin (amphiphilic molecules).

The molar mass and the molecular size of a molecule affect mainly its ability to diffuse within the SC. Experiments on drugs with different molecular weights evidenced that the optimal permeability is achieved with molar mass lower than 500 Da (Bos and Meinardi, 2000) while the upper limit for drug ability to penetrate the skin is regarded to be 5000 Da (Schaefer and Riedelmayer, 1996).

In Table 1, calculated partition coefficients (Log P) (www.chemspider.com) and molecular weights of some of the most commonly used UV-filters are reported. All these sunscreen agents show molecular weights lower that 500 Da, suggesting that they would be able to penetrate the skin. However, penetration of the most lipophilic and the most hydrophilic UV-filters is likely to be minor as they should accumulate into the SC or remain on the skin surface, respectively.

The importance of partition coefficients and molecular weights in the structure-skin permeability relationships has been widely reported (Hadgraft and Lane, 2005; Patel et al., 2002). In 1992, Potts and Guy made the first attempt at predicting skin permeability from Log P and molecular weights, calculating the best linear fit for a data set of 93 compounds. The regression coefficient (0.67) obtained from this data set points at a non-linear relationship, with the involvement of other physicochemical features of the permeating molecule.

In the same year, Watkinson et al. (1992) developed a mathematical model to predict the extent of percutaneous absorption of sunscreen agents based on their physicochemical properties. In this model, some of the most common UV-filters such as benzophenone-3 (BP-3), octyl methoxycinnamate (OMC), butyl methoxydibenzoylmethane (BMBM), octyl salicylate (OS), octocrylene (OC), octyl dimethylPABA (OPABA), were analyzed. A rate constant was assigned to each process involved in skin absorption (partitioning of UV-filter from the vehicle to the SC; diffusion across the SC; partitioning from the SC to the viable epidermis; uptake into local circulation and elimination; back partitioning from the viable

Table 1. Physicochemical properties, molecular weight (MW), partition coefficient (Log P), water solubility (S_w), UV absorption, maximum concentration allowed (Max conc.), of commonly used UV-filters

UV-filter	Key	CAS	Max conc.	Physical form	Absorption[a]	MW	Log P[b]	S_w (mg/L)
Octyl methoxycinnamate	OMC	5466-77-3	10	Oily liquid	UVB	290.41	5.66	0.15
Buthyl methoxydi-benzoylmethane	BMBM	70356-09-1	5	Crystalline solid	UVA	310.39	4.81	1.52
Octyl saliclylate	OS	118-60-5	5	Oily liquid	UVB	250.34	5.95	<0.1
Benzophenone-3	BP-3	131-57-7	6	Crystalline solid	UVB-UVAII	228.25	3.64	68.56
Benzophenone-4	BP-4	4065-45-6	5	Crystalline solid	UVB-UVAII	308.31	0.89	$25x10^4$
4-Methylbenzilydene camphor	BC	36861-47-9	4	Crystalline solid	UVB	254.37	4.95	0.57
Octyl dimethyl PABA	OPABA	58817-05-3	8	Oily liquid	UVB	277.41	6.15	0.20
Octocrylene	OC	6197-30-4	10	Oily liquid	UVB	361.48	7.53	<0.1

[a] UVB (290– 320 nm); UVAII (320– 340 nm); UVA (320– 400 nm).

[b] Calculated from www.chemspider.com.

epidermis to the SC and from the SC to the vehicle). Rate constants were calculated considering molecular weight, melting point, and calculated partition coefficients of the UV-filters. Based on this model, sunscreen absorption ranging from 0.0033 to 83 mg/1.4m^2 after a 12-hour application was predicted, indicating a potential significant uptake in the systemic circulation after application to a large surface area for prolonged periods. However, this model did not account for variables such as effect of the vehicle, repeated application, skin metabolism of UV-filters or binding to skin sites, evidencing the need for well-designed *in vivo* and *in vitro* studies to perform an accurate evaluation of UV-filter skin absorption, and of the influence of physiological and formulation factors.

As the main barrier to skin penetration is the non-viable SC, a drug applied in a vehicle on the skin surface penetrates into the skin by a passive mechanism depending on its physicochemical properties and according to Fick's First Law (equation 1).

$$J = -D \frac{\delta C}{\delta x}$$

Equation 1

Equation 1 shows that the flux (rate of transfer per unit area of a chemical at a given time and position) is proportional to the differential concentration change δC over the differential distance δx. Therefore, the driving force of the percutaneous absorption process is the concentration gradient of the active compound between the vehicle and the SC. In Equation 1, D represents the diffusion coefficient and the negative sign indicates that the flow is in the direction of decreasing concentration.

When the flux is constant (steady state), it can be calculated from equation 2:

$$J_{ss} = \frac{D(C_1 - C_2)}{L}$$

Equation 2

J_{ss} represents flux at steady state; C_1 and C_2 represent the concentration of the permeating molecule in the vehicle and in the SC, respectively; L is the length of the diffusion pathway in the SC.

C_1 depends on the partition coefficient of the active ingredient between the SC and vehicle (considered equal to Log P for topical formulations) (Roberts et al., 1996) and on the concentration of the ingredient in the formulation.

Therefore, the extent of skin penetration and/or permeation depends not only on the physicochemical properties of the active ingredient but also on the vehicle in which it is formulated and on the interactions between the vehicle and the skin. After topical application of a pharmaceutical or cosmetic product onto the skin, the first critical step that determines the skin absorption level of an active ingredient is its release from the formulation and partitioning between the vehicle and the SC. The vehicle could alter the partitioning of the compound into the SC lipids and the solubility of the active ingredient in the vehicle will determine the thermodynamic driving force governing release of the chemical from the formulation to the skin. In addition, the vehicle itself could modify skin permeability, thus affecting skin penetration of the active compound.

Additional factors that may affect percutaneous absorption include the way of application of the formulation onto the skin, the presence of penetration modifiers in the vehicle (Trommer and Neubert, 2006), which could alter the barrier properties of the SC, the processes occurring in viable tissues such as metabolism, and biological factors.

Skin Permeation of UV-Filters

Skin permeation can be determined using different methodologies performing a) *in vivo* studies in animals or human volunteers, b) *in vitro* experiments employing excised skin from human or animal sources, or synthetic model membranes (Godin and Touitou, 2007; Rai et al., 2010; Varvaresou, 2006).

Because percutaneous absorption depends on the passive diffusion of the permeating molecule and not on an active transport, the viability of the skin is not a prerequisite for penetration testing, making the results of *in vitro* studies predictive of *in vivo* permeation (Bronaugh et al., 1982a; Franz, 1975).

Although *in vitro* tests are preferable for ethical reasons and feasibility and are well accepted in the European Union, regulatory authorities in the United States and Japan suggest *in vivo* penetration studies in a rodent model (EPA 1992).

Skin from a great variety of animals (e.g., pigs and guinea pigs, rats, rabbits, snakes) has been investigated as a model for human skin (Bartek et al., 1972; Bronaugh et al., 1982b; Chow et al., 1978; Harada et al., 1993; Itoh et al., 1990; Lin et al., 1992). Pigs and rats show the most similar skin barrier to that of human skin and therefore are most commonly used for skin penetration/permeation studies. However, due to the complex nature of the human SC, animal skin provides only an indication of the diffusion characteristics of chemicals, requiring a careful extrapolation to humans. In the following sections, *in vitro* and *in vivo* evaluations of percutaneous absorption through human or animal skin of the most commonly used UV-filters will be illustrated.

Human Studies

The most widely used sunscreen active ingredients such as octylmethoxycinnamate (OMC), benzophenone-3 (BP-3), benzophenone-4 (BP-4), octylsalicylate (OS), octyl dimethylPABA (OPABA), butyl methoxydibenzoylmethane (BMBM), octocrylene (OC), 3-(4-methylbenzylidene) camphor (BC), have been extensively investigated *in vitro* and *in vivo* in humans to assess their retention into the different skin layers and their permeation through the skin into the systemic circulation, applying representative vehicles of cosmetic formulations.

In vivo skin permeation of OMC, BP-3, and BC was evaluated on 32 healthy volunteers (15 men and 17 postmenopausal women) following daily whole-body topical application of a cream (2 mg/cm^2) without (week 1) or with (week 2) the three sunscreens, each at 10% w/w (Janjua et al., 2004). At the end of the study, all the sunscreens were detected in urine. Maximum plasma concentrations were similar for OMC (10 ng/mL in females and 20 ng/mL in males) and BC (20 ng/mL both in females and males) while they were significantly higher for BP-3 (200 ng/mL in females and 300 ng/mL in males). The authors observed minor differences in serum estradiol and inhibin B levels in men only but they concluded that these differences in hormone levels were not related to sunscreen exposure.

An interesting study on the relationship between *in vitro* skin penetration and cytotoxicity of sunscreens was performed to ensure that *in vitro* cytotoxicity studies examined relevant doses of these agents to which viable epidermal cells were realistically exposed. With this aim, *in vitro* percutaneous absorption through human skin of five commonly used sunscreen agents (BMBM, OMC, OC, BP-3 and OPABA) was assessed from mineral oil. After 24 hours, 95-98% of the sunscreen agents was recovered on the surface of the epidermis and detectable amounts of all UV-filters were found in the SC and viable epidermis. BP-3 showed the most evident epidermal penetration. After determining sunscreen concentration-human keratinocyte culture response curves, the authors concluded that the concentrations of each sunscreen found in human viable epidermis after topical application were at least 5-fold lower than those appearing to cause toxicity in cultured human keratinocytes (Hayden et al., 2005).

Due to its high photo-stability, BP-3 is widely used in commercial sunscreen products. However, several studies evidenced a higher skin permeation ability of this UV-filter compared to other commonly used sunscreens. BP-3 percutaneous absorption was evaluated in nine healthy volunteers after topical application (12.4 mg/cm^2) onto the entire surface of their forearms of a commercial available sunscreen lotion containing BP-3 6% (w/v), OMC 7.5% (w/v), OS 5% (w/v) and OC 7% (w/v) (Hayden et al., 1997). BP-3 was recovered in urine for 48 h as unchanged BP-3 and as metabolites and the authors concluded that the actual amount absorbed through the skin over a 10-h period was 1-2% of the applied amount contained in the product. However, in this study, the amount of formulation applied on the skin was about six-fold higher than that recommended to evaluate the sun protection factor of sunscreen products under realistic condition of use (2 mg/cm^2).

An *in vitro* study through excised human skin was performed to assess skin penetration/permeation from six commercial milk/lotion sunscreen products for adults and children of BP-3, along with other UVB-filters (OMC, OS, OC) (Jiang et al., 1999). All these sunscreens were recovered into the skin (14% of the applied dose) but only BP-3 was able to permeate through the skin (10% of the applied dose), thus confirming the results obtained from previous *in vivo* studies.

A further *in vivo* investigation on BP-3 skin permeation was carried out on eleven healthy volunteers who were instructed to apply a commercially available sun-protecting lotion containing 4% BP-3 over the whole body (2 mg/cm^2). Under these experimental conditions, the average total amount excreted in urine was approximately 0.4% of the applied amount of BP-3 (Gustavsson Gonzalez et al., 2002).

In vitro studies through human skin proved that BP-3 skin permeation was enhanced by the concomitant application of the insect repellent N,N-diethyl-m-toluamide (DEET) (Wang and Gu, 2007). DEET permeation was greater than that of BP-3 and a synergistic percutaneous enhancement of both compounds was observed when used simultaneously. The authors reported that the extent of the enhancement effect was dependent on the type of vehicle (lotion or spay) containing the active ingredients.

Synergy effects on *in vitro* absorption through human skin between UV filters and other compounds such as herbicides (Pont et al., 2004) have also been reported.

Vehicle effects on skin permeation of UV-filters have been investigated in many papers. Chatelain et al. (2003) evaluated the skin penetration of five UV- filters (BP-3, OMC,

BMBM, OS, homosalate) from an O/W emulsion gel and a petrolatum jelly both *in vitro* and *in vivo*. The results of *in vitro* experiments showed that after applying the formulations under investigation for 30 min and 6 h, only BP-3 and to a lesser extent OMC were detectable in the dermis while no skin permeation of these UV filters was observed after 6 h application. In addition, the authors reported a greater BP-3 penetration from petrolatum. *In vivo i*nvestigations, performed by tape stripping of the SC, evidenced a clear vehicle effect on penetration of the UV-filters into the SC, being the amount of each UV-filter penetrated greater from the emulsion gel formulation compared to the petrolatum jelly. Treffel and Gabard (1996) reported similar results studying *in vitro* and *in vivo* skin penetration of BP-3 (5%), OMC (7.5%), and OS (3%) from two vehicles (an O/W emulsion-gel and petroleum jelly) applied (2 mg/cm^2) for 2 min to 6 h. The emulsion-gel provided higher epidermal concentrations of all UV-filters than the petroleum jelly both *in vivo* and *in vitro*. However, the authors noticed only for BP-3 a greater skin permeation from the petroleum jelly than from the emulsion gel.

The effects of emulsion composition on *in vitro* skin permeation of different UV-filters (OMC, BMBM) was evaluated evidencing differences in UV filter penetration/permeation among various emulsion-type formulations (Marginean-Lazar et al., 1996; Montenegro et al., 2004).

In vitro percutaneous absorption through human skin of OS was assessed from two representative sunscreen vehicles (an oil-in-water emulsion and a hydro-alcoholic formulation) using both the technique of finite and infinite dosing (Walters et al., 1997). The results of this study evidenced a low skin permeation of OS that was dependent on the amount of formulation applied (finite or infinite dosing) when a hydro-alcoholic vehicle was used.

Animal Studies

Several studies have validated pig skin as a suitable model for human skin to investigate percutaneous absorption of UV-filters.

Benech-Kieffer et al. (2000) performed *in vitro* experiments to compare skin permeation of two UV-filters (OMC and BP-4) through human abdominal skin and pig flank skin. The authors found a good agreement between data obtained from human and pig skin, as after 16 hours the percentage of the applied dose of OMC and BP-4 recovered in the skin was similar for both species. However, due to its lipophilicity, OMC showed a higher affinity for the SC than the hydrophilic BP-4.

Pigskin was used as model to evaluate BP-3 and OMC *in vitro* percutaneous absorption from two vehicles, a hydroaclloholic and a diisopropyl adipate formulation (Gupta et al., 1999). BP-3 permeation was greater than that of OMC while OMC was retained to a greater extent in the SC. It is interesting to note that the authors found that permeation and SC retention were formulation dependent and the ratio of retained to permeated amount of sunscreen from a hydroalcoholic formulation after 10 hours was greater when these UV-filters were present together rather than alone.

Fernandez et al. (2000) evaluated the skin penetration of BP-3 *in vitro* and *in vivo* from six different vehicles, three solvents and three different types of emulsions. *In vitro* experiments were performed using pig skin while *in vivo* data were collected determining BP-3 concentration in the SC by the stripping method after 30-min application on the forearm of volunteers. Pig and human skin provided similar results, highlighting a good correlation between *in vitro* and *in vivo* data and between species. In both experiments, significant differences among the vehicles tested were observed as the highest concentration of BP-3 in the skin was obtained from the hydrophilic solvent (propylene glycol) and O/W submicron emulsion while the two oily solvents, W/O emulsion and O/W coarse emulsion provided lower concentrations of this UV-filter in the skin.

Another *in vitro* study on OMC percutaneous absorption through pig skin evidenced that microencapsulating this UV-filter reduced its absorption in comparison with an emulsion containing free OMC (Jimenez et al., 2004).

The effect two vehicles, an oil-in-water (O/W) emulsion and an alcoholic gel, on *in vitro* permeation of BC was assessed through pig ear skin. The results of this study showed that BC skin penetration was dependent on the vehicle, being more remarkable for alcoholic gel (Sasson et al., 2009).

In the last decade, several studies aimed at entrapping UV-filters in carriers such as cyclodextrins (Shokri et al., 2013), lipid microparticles (Scalia et al., 2007) lipospheres (Mew et al., 2007), lipid microspheres (Mestres et al., 2010; Yener et al., 2003), polymeric nanocapsules (Siqueira et al., 2011; Weiss-Angeli et al., 2010), microemulsions (Montenegro et al., 2011), solid lipid nanoparticles (Gulbake et al., 2010; Wissing and Muller, 2002), polymeric nanoparticles (Vettor et al., 2010) to avoid or at least to reduce skin permeation of sunscreens. Some of these investigations were performed *in vitro* or *in vivo* on rat skin, pointing out a good correlation between this animal model and human skin. In all these studies, incorporating UV-filters in different carriers resulted in a decrease of sunscreen release and penetration into the skin compared to conventional cosmetic formulations.

NOAEL and Risk Assessment of UV-Filters

The risk assessment of sunscreen products requires hazard identification and characterization, exposure assessment, and risk characterization, the last being a basic step that brings together hazard characterization and exposure assessment. For sunscreen products, such evaluations have to be performed taking into account the topical nature of human exposure.

While hazard identification and characterization lead to a qualitative assessment based on the available data of a specific chemical, safety evaluation provides a quantitative estimate of the intake that would not give rise to a significant risk of adverse effects in humans. Therefore, the margin of safety (MoS) is determined comparing the so-called no adverse effect level (NOAEL) to the potential human exposure, expressed as systemic exposure dose (SED).

NOAEL values are obtained from subchronic (90-180 days) or chronic (> 180 days) toxicity studies that are generally performed in animals, using different oral dosing. NOAEL is usually defined as the daily dose that does not elicit any toxic effect and is expressed in mg/kg body weight. However, the definition of NOAEL has been largely debated (Dorato and Engelhardt, 2005). According to the SCCS's notes of guidance for the testing of cosmetic substances and their safety evaluation (2012), the no observed (adverse) effect level is defined as the highest dose or exposure level where no (adverse) treatment-related findings are observed.

After establishing the NOAEL of UV-filters, their percutaneous absorption has to be quantified to determine SED, expressed in mg/kg body weight per single application. As sunscreen products are often applied to large skin areas, SED evaluations are performed considering the worst scenario, i.e., a total body application.

If the steady state flux through the skin (J_{ss}) is used to estimate SED, the weight and the skin surface area of a standard human are needed. According to SCCS's notes of guidance for the testing of cosmetic substances and their safety evaluation (2012), a weight of 60 kg and a skin area of 18.000 cm^2 (Timbrell, 2005) are used to calculate SED.

Therefore, the SED can be determined as follows:

$$SED = J_{ss} \times area_{exp} \times 24\ h\ /body\ weight \qquad \text{Equation 3}$$

where $area_{exp}$ is the exposed area of the skin. In addition, the SED can be estimated from the percentage of a topically applied dose that permeates the skin, according to equation 4:

$$SED = C_{product} \times A_{applied} \times n_{applications} \times area_{exp} \times Perm(\%)/body\ weight \qquad \text{Equation 4}$$

where $C_{product}$ is the concentration of UV-filter in the product (%w/w), $A_{applied}$ is the amount of product applied on the skin (mg/cm^2), $n_{applications}$ is the number of application per day and Perm (%) is the permeation percentage of UV-filter.

As many toxicological studies are carried out on animals, uncertainty factors (UF) have to be applied to convert animal data into an exposure level considered of no toxicological concern for humans; additional UF have to be considered to account for toxico-kinetic variability among healthy adults and in children (SCCS, 2012).

When NOAEL and SED are known, MoS can be calculated as follows:

$$MoS = NOAEL/SED \qquad \text{Equation 5}$$

A MoS < 1 indicates a potential risk associated with a given scenario as the dose considered safe is lower than the SED. In the safety evaluation of cosmetic products in EU, to declare a product safe for use, MoS values greater than 100 are required (SCCS, 2012).

Several authors (Gonzalez 2010; Montenegro et al., 2013; Nohynek and Schaefer, 2001; Walters et al., 1997) have calculated MoS of UV-filters using SED values obtained from percutaneous absorption studies.

As BP-3 shows a greater skin permeation compared to other UV-filters, an extensive assessment of its safety has been carried out (El Dareer et al., 1986; Okereke et al., 1994). Okereke et al., (1995) performed a safety evaluation of BP-3 after topical application in rats and found it nontoxic when applied at a dose of 100 mg/kg body weight for 4 weeks. After evaluating *in vitro* and *in vivo* data on BP-3 skin permeation in animals and humans and the available toxicokinetic data, the Scientific Committee on Consumer Products (SCCP, 2008) concluded that the use of BP-3 up to 6% in cosmetic sunscreen products does not pose a risk to the health of the consumer, apart from its contact allergenic and photoallergenic potential. This conclusion was drawn considering that the mean percentage of the applied dose of BP- 3 permeated was 3.1% plus 2 standard deviations (3.4%). As shown in Table 2, in this condition a MoS value of 112 was obtained.

OMC and BMBM are the most commonly used UV-filters, being contained not only in sunscreen products but also in a great variety of cosmetics and toiletries. Although OMC demonstrated weak estrogenic effects *in vivo* and *in vitro* (Gomez et al., 2005; Klammer et al., 2005), it had no adverse effect on estrus cycle, sperm number, morphology and motility, differential follicle counts, mating, fertility, gestation and parturition (Schneider et al., 2005). The NOAEL for fertility and reproductive performance in rats and for systemic parental and developmental toxicity was determined to be 450 mg/kg/day. The same NOAEL has been reported for BMBM (Montenegro et al., 2013)

In vitro experiments showed that the percentage of the applied dose of OMC that permeated through the skin was 0.2–4.5%, using both human and porcine skin (Benech-Kieffer et al., 2000; Gupta et al., 1999). From *in vivo* studies, lower OMC skin permeation was observed (Chatelain et al., 2003; Janjua et al., 2004; Janjua et al., 2008).

As regards BMBM, *in vitro* studies evidenced that less than 1% of this UV-filter penetrated into the SC and epidermis while no skin permeation occurred (Montenegro et al., 2008; Simeoni et al., 2004; Weigmann et al., 2001).

Recently, Nohynek et al. (2010) have pointed out that *in vitro* experiments tend to overestimate human systemic exposure. According to the authors, this overestimation was supported by the results of a study performed in humans, both *in vivo* and *in vitro*, on the UV-filter Mexoryl SX®. In volunteers, 0.014% of the applied filter was systemically available, while parallel *in vitro* experiments, performed under identical exposure conditions, provided a skin penetration rate of 0.37%, suggesting that *in vitro* results produced a 25-fold overestimation of the human systemic exposure and of the potential human health risk (Benech-Kieffer et al., 2003).

However, as according to SCCS (2012) the worst scenario has to be considered, calculating MoS of OMC and BMBM, the maximum percentage of the applied dose permeated (4.5% and 1%, respectively) was used (see Table 2). Based on a total body application of a formulation containing the maximum percentage of UV-filter allowed, the resulting MoS for OMC and BMBM were 1666 and 15000. A recent investigation on the effects of commercial O/W emulsions on *in vitro* skin permeation of OMC and BMBM evidenced that OMC permeation depended on both its concentration in the formulation and vehicle composition, while BMBM release from the vehicle was the key parameter that determined the permeation rate of this UV-filter (Montenegro et al., 2013). All the commercial products investigated proved safe under normal in use conditions as their MoS values were greater than 100.

Being one of the oldest UV-filters, the human safety of OS has been extensively reviewed, highlighting that this UV-filter is well tolerated (Nash, 2006). Investigating OS skin permeation, Walters et al., (1997) reported that less than 1% of the applied dose of OS penetrates through the human skin. Using these data, the authors demonstrated the safety of this sunscreen agent in cosmetic formulations.

Table 2. Systemic exposure dose (SED) and margin of safety (MoS) of UV-filters in adults

Parameter	UV-filter						
	BP-3[a]	OMC[b]	BC-3[c]	BC-4[d]	OS[e]	BMBM[b]	Mexoryl XL (®)[f]
Typical adult body weight (Kg)	60	60	60	60	60	60	60
Body surface area (cm^2)	18000	18000	18000	18000	18000	18000	18000
Average amount (g) of sunscreen applied per day	18	36	18	36	16	36	18
Maximum allowable concentration in sunscreen products (%)	6	10	2	4	5	5	15
Maximum amount applied ultraviolet filter (g)	1.1	3.6	0.36	1.4	0.8	1.8	1.8
Maximum (*in vitro*) percutaneous absorption of UV filter (%)	9.9	4.5	3.29	2.45	0.65	1	0.8
Systemic Exposure Dose (SED) (mg/kg/day)	1.78	0.27	0.21	0.588	0.087	0.03	0.24
NOAEL of toxicity studies (mg/kg/day)	200	450	7.5	25	250	450	1000
Margin of Safety (MoS=NOAEL/SED)	112	1666	36	42.5	2900	15000	4170

[a] data obtained from Gonzalez (2010).

[b] data calculated from *in vitro* and *in vivo* experiments reported in the literature (see text for details).

[c] data obtained from SCCS/1513/13 (2013).

[d] data obtained from SCCP (2008).

[e] data obtained from Walters et al. (1997).

[f] data obtained from Nohynek and Schaefer (2001).

Nohynek and Schaefer (2001) reported a thorough risk assessment of a new broad UVA filter, drometrizole trisiloxane (Mexoryl XL®), listing all the data needed to calculate its MoS, according to SCCS guidelines.

As illustrated In Table 2, apart from 3-benzilydene camphor (BC-3) and 4-methylbenzilydene camphor (BC-4), all the UV-filters mentioned above show MoS values greater than 100, evidencing their safety of use in sunscreen products at the maximum concentration allowed in EU.

As regards BC-3, Søeborg et al. (2006), studying *in vivo* skin permeation of BC-3 in rats, observed an accumulation of approximately 10% of the applied topical dose in various tissues after 65 days of treatment. Further studies (Søeborg et al., 2007) pointed out that skin permeation of BC-3 was higher than that of BC-4. As both UV-filters affected the endocrine activity, the risk associated with use of BC-3 and BC-4 in sunscreen products was found high. To evaluate the risk of human exposure to BC-3, the SCCP (2013) used a percentage of absorption of 3.29% and a NOAEL value of 7.5 mg/Kg/day obtained from maternal toxicity and embryo-toxicity studies in rats (15 mg/Kg/day), taking into account that BC-3 bioavailability was 50% of the administered dose. Based on the resulting MoS lower than 100, the SCCP declared that the use of BC-3 in cosmetic products in a concentration up 2.0% is not safe. Therefore, BC-3 has been withdrawn from the list of UV-filters approved in EU.

Using a percutaneous absorption rate of 1.9% along with a NOAEL of 25 mg/Kg/day (determined in rats) for human risk assessment of BC-4 (SCCP, 2008), a MoS below 100 was obtained, indicating that BC-4 cannot be considered safe as a UV filter in cosmetic sunscreen products at 4%. However, as detailed toxicokinetic studies in healthy volunteers demonstrated that the actual NOAEL in humans was 100 mg/Kg/day, a MoS value of 25 was considered safe for BC-4. Therefore, as the calculation of the MoS resulted in a value of 42.5, which was higher than the requested threshold of 25, the use of this UV-filter was regarded safe (SCCP, 2008).

CONCLUSION

In recent years, an increasing attention has been paid to the evaluation of UV-filter percutaneous absorption to assess the potential risk of human exposure to these sunscreen agents.

In vitro permeation experiments and animal models, with all their limitations, provide important tools for screening sunscreen products, making possible to estimate the rate and extent of percutaneous absorption of their active ingredients.

The safety evaluation of sunscreen products is based on the two factors that contribute to risk characterization, hazard characterization and potential human exposure and only UV-filters whose MoS are at least 100 times the NOAEL are accepted as safe.

As evidenced in this chapter, when comparing the toxicological properties of the most commonly used UV-A and UV-B filters to the potential human exposure, the human risk caused by exposure to sunscreen products is negligible. Furthermore, modern UV filters are formulated to be retained on or within the upper layers of the horny layer to achieve high protection factors, thus reducing their potential of skin permeation into the underlying living tissue.

Therefore, the benefits of sunscreen products to public health largely outweigh the risk of human topical exposure to such formulations, supporting the recommendation of a proper use of sunscreen products to prevent the deleterious effects of UV-radiation.

REFERENCES

Akomeah FK; Martin GP; Brown MB. Variability in human skin permeability in vitro: comparing penetrants with different physicochemical properties. *J. Pharm. Sci.*, 2007, 96, 824-834.

Bartek M J; LaBudde J A; Maibach HI. Skin permeability in vivo. Comparison in rat, rabbit, pig and man. *J. Invest. Dermatol.*, 1972, 58, 114-123.

Beetge E; Du Plessis J; Muller DG; Goosen C; Van Rensburg FJ. The influence of the physicochemical characteristics and pharmacokinetic properties of selected NSAID's on their transdermal absorption. *Int. J. Pharm.*, 2000, 193, 261-264.

Benech-Kieffer F; Wegrich P; Schwarzenbach R; Klecak G; Weber T; Leclaire J; Schaefer H. Percutaneous absorption of sunscreens in vitro: Interspecies comparison, skin models and reproducibility aspects. *Skin Pharmacol. Appl. Skin Physiol.*, 2000, 13, 324-335.

Benech-Kieffer F; Meuling WJA; Leclerc C; Roza L; Leclaire J; Nohynek G. Percutaneous absorption of Mexoryl SX® in human volunteers: comparison with in vitro data. *Skin Pharmacol. Appl. Skin Physiol.* 2003, 16, 343–355.

Berardesca E; De Rigal J; Leveque JL; Maibach HI. In vivo biophysical characterization of skin physiological differences in races. *Dermatologica*, 1991, 182, 89-93.

Bos JD; Meinardi MMHM. The 500 Dalton rule for the skin penetration of chemical compounds and drugs. *Exp. Dermato*, 2000, 9, 165-9.

Bouwstra JA; Dubbelaar FE; Gooris GS; Ponec M. The lipid organisation in the skin barrier. *Acta Derm Venereol Suppl* 2000, 208, 23–30.

Bronaugh RL; Stewart R F; Congdon ER; Giles AL. Methods for in vitro percutaneous absorption studies. I. Comparison with in vivo results. *Toxicol. Appl. Pharmacol.*, 1982a, 62, 474-480.

Bronaugh RL; Stewart R F; Congdon ER. Methods for in vitro percutaneous absorption studies. II. Animal models for human skin. *Toxicol. Appl. Pharmacol.*, 1982b, 62, 481-488.

Bunge AL; Cleek RL. A new method for estimating dermal absorption from chemical exposure: 2. Effect of molecular weight and octanol-water partitioning. *Pharm Res*, 1995, 12, 88-95.

Chatelain E; Gabarda B; Surber C. Skin penetration and sun protection factor of five UV filters: effect of the vehicle. *Skin Pharmacol. Appl. Skin Physiol.*, 2003, 16, 28–35.

Chow C; Chow AYK; Downie RH; Buttar HS. Percutaneous absorption of hexachlorophene in rats, guinea pigs and pigs. *Toxicology* 1978, 9, 147-154.

Dorato MA; Engelhardt JA. The no-observed-adverse-effect-level in drug safety evaluations: Use, issues, and definition(s). *Regul. Toxicol. Pharmacol.*, 2005, 42, 265–274.

El Dareer SM; Kalin JR; Tillery KF; Hill DL. Disposition of 2-hydroxy-4-methoxybenzophenone in rats dosed orally, intravenously, or topically. *J. Toxicol. Environ. Health* 1986, 19, 491–502.

EPA 1992 Dermal Exposure Assesment: Principles and applications, Interim Report EPA/600/8-91/011B. Exposure Assesment Group, Office of Health and Enviromental Assesment Group, U.S. Enviromental Protection Agency, Washington DC.

Fernández C; Marti-Mestres G; Ramos J; Maillols H. LC analysis of benzophenone-3: II application to determination of 'in vitro' and 'in vivo' skin penetration from solvents, coarse and submicron emulsions. *J. Pharm. Biomed. Anal.*, 2000, 24, 155–165.

Förster M; Bolzinger MA; Fessi H; Briançonet S. Topical delivery of cosmetics and drugs. Molecular aspects of percutaneous absorption and delivery. *Eur. J. Dermatol.*, 2009, 19, 309-23.

Franz TJ. Percutaneous absorption on the relevance of in vitro data. *J. Invest. Dermatol.*, 1975, 64, 190-195.

Gilbert E; Pirot F; Bertholle V; Roussel L; Falson F; Padois K. Commonly used UV filter toxicity on biological functions: review of last decade studies. *Int. J. Cosm. Sci.*, 2013, 35, 208–219.

Godin B; Touitou E. Transdermal skin delivery: Predictions for humans from in vivo, ex vivo and animal models. *Adv Drug Del Rev*, 2007, 59, 1152-61.

Gomez E; Pillon A; Fenet H; Rosain D; Duchesne MJ; Nicolas JC; Balauger P; Casellas C. Estrogenic activity of cosmetic components in reporter cell lines: parabens, UV screens, and musks. *J Toxicol Environ Health*, 2005, 68, 239-251.

Gonzalez H. Percutaneous absorption with emphasis on sunscreens. *Photochem. Photobiol. Sci.,* 2010, 9, 482–488.

González S; Fernández-Lorente M; Gilaberte-Calzada Y. The latest on skin photoprotection. *Clin. Dermatol.*, 2008, 26, 614–626.

Gulbake A; Jain A; Khare P; Jain SK. Solid lipid nanoparticles bearing oxybenzone: in-vitro and in-vivo evaluation. *J. Microencapsul.*, 2010, 27, 226–233.

Gupta VK; Zatz JL; Rerek M. Percutaneous absorption of sunscreens through micro-Yucatan pig skin in vitro. *Pharm. Res.*, 1999, 16, 1602-1607.

Gustavsson Gonzalez H; Farbrot A; Larko O. Percutaneous absorption of benzophenone-3, a common component of topical sunscreens. *Clin. Exp. Dermatol.*, 2002, 27, 691-694.

Guy RH; Hadgraft J. Physicochemical aspects of percutaneous penetration and its enhancement. *Pharm Res*, 1988, 5, 753-8.

Hadgraft J; Lane ME. Skin permeation: The years of enlightenment. *Int. J. Pharm.*, 2005, 305, 2–12.

Harada K; Murakami T; Kawasaki E; Higashi Y; Yamamoto S; Yata N. In-vitro permeability to salicylic acid of human, rodent, and shed snake skin. *J. Pharm Pharmacol.*, 1993, 45, 414-418.

Hayden CG; Roberts MS; Benson HA. Systemic absorption of sunscreen after topical application. *Lancet* 1997, 350, 863-4.

Hayden CGJ; Cross SE; Anderson C; Saunders NA; Roberts MS. Sunscreen penetration of human skin and related keratinocyte toxicity after topical application. *Skin Pharmacol. Physiol.,* 2005, 18, 170-174.

Iannucelli V; Coppi G; Sergi S; Mezzena M; Scalia S. In vivo and in vitro skin permeation of butyl methoxydibenzoylmethane from lipospheres. *Skin Pharmacol. Physiol.*, 2007, 21, 30–38.

Itoh T; Xia J; Magavi R; Nishihata T; Rytting JH. Use of shed snake skin as a model membrane for in vitro percutaneous penetration studies: Comparison with human skin. *Pharm. Res.*, 1990, 7, 1042-1047.

Janjua NR; Mogensen B; Andersson AM; Petersen JH; Henriksen M; Skakkebaek NE; Wulf HC. Systemic absorption of the sunscreens benzophenone-3, octyl-methoxycinnamate, and 3-(4-methyl-benzylidene) camphor after whole-body topical application and reproductive hormone levels in humans. *J. Invest Dermatol.* 2004, 123, 57– 61.

Janjua NR; Kongshoj B; Andersson AM; Wulf, HC. Sunscreens in human plasma and urine after repeated whole-body topical application. *J. Eur. Acad. Dermatol. Venereol*, 2008, 22, 456–61.

Jiang R; Roberts MS; Collins DM; Benson HA. Absorption of sunscreens across human skin: an evaluation of commercial products for children and adults. *Br. J. Clin. Pharmacol.*, 1999, 48, 635–7.

Jimenez MM; Pelletier J; Bobin MF; Martini MC. Influence of encapsulation on the in vitro percutaneous absorptionof octyl methoxycinnamate. *Int. J. Pharm.*, 2004, 272, 45-55.

Klammer H; Schlecht C; Wuttke W; Jarry H. Multi-organic risk assessment of estrogenic properties of octyl-methoxycinnamate in vivo. A 5-day sub-acute pharmacodynamic study with ovariectomized rats. *Toxicology*, 2005, 215, 90-96.

Klann A; Levy G; Lutz I; Müller C; Kloas W; Hildebrandt JP. Estrogen-like effects of ultraviolet screen 3-(4-methylbenzylidene)-camphor (Eusolex 6300) on cell proliferation and gene induction in mammalian and amphibian cells. *Environ Res.* 2005, 97, 274– 81.

Koda T; Umezu T; Kamata R; Morohoshi K; Ohta T; Morita M. Uterotrophic effects of benzophenone derivatives and a p-hydroxybenzoate used in ultraviolet screens. *Environ Res,* 2005, 98, 40 –5.

Kunz PY; Fent K. Estrogenic activity of UV filter mixtures, *Toxicol. Appl. Pharmacol.*, 2006, 217, 86–99.

Lautenschlager S; Wulf HC; Pittelkow MR; Photoprotection. *Lancet* 2007, 370, 528–37.

Lin S Y; Hou S J; Hsu TH; Yeh FL. Comparisons of different animal skins with human skin in drug percutaneous penetration studies. *Methods Find Exp. Clin. Pharmacol.*, 1992, 14, 645-654.

Marginean-Lazar G; Baillet A; Fructus AE; Arnaud-Battandier J; Ferrier D; Marty JP. Evaluation of in vitro percutaneous absorption of UV filters used in sunscreen formulations. *Drug Cosm. Ind*, 1996, 158, 50–62.

Mestres JP; Duracher L; Baux C; Vian L; Marti-Mestres G. Benzophenone-3 entrapped in solid lipid microspheres: formulation and in vitro skin evaluation. *Int. J. Pharm.*, 2010, 400, 1-7.

Montenegro L; Paolino D; Puglisi G. (2004). Effects of silicone emulsifiers on in vitro skin permeation of sunscreens from cosmetic emulsions. *J. Cosmet Sci*, 2004, 55, 509–518.

Montenegro L.; Carbone C.; Paolino D.; Drago R.; Stancampiano A.H.; Puglisi G. *In vitro* skin permeation of sunscreen agents from O/W emulsions. *Int. J. Cosmet. Sci.*, 2008, 30, 57-65.

Montenegro L; Carbone C; Puglisi G. Vehicle effects on in vitro release and skin permeation of octylmethoxycinnamate from microemulsions. *Int. J. Pharm.*, 2011, 405, 162-8.

Montenegro L; Puglisi G. Evaluation of sunscreen safety by in vitro skin permeation studies: effects of vehicle composition. *Pharmazie,* 2013, 68, 34-40.

Nash JF. Human safety and efficacy of ultraviolet filters and sunscreen products. *Dermatol. Clin.*, 2006, 24, 35 – 51.

Nohynek GJ; Schaefer H. Benefit and Risk of Organic Ultraviolet Filters. *Regul. Toxicol. Pharmacol.,* 2001, 33, 285–299.

Nohynek GJ; Antignac E; Re T; Toutain H. Safety assessment of personal care products/cosmetics and their ingredients. *Toxicol. Appl. Pharmacol.*, 2010, 243, 239–259.

Okereke CS, Abdel-Rhaman MS, Friedman MA. Disposition of benzophenone-3 after dermal administration in male rats. *Toxicol. Lett.* 1994, 73, 113– 22.

Okereke CS; Barat SA; Abdel-Rahman MS. Safety evaluation of benzophenone-3 after dermal administration in rats. *Toxicol. Lett.* 1995, 80, 61–7.

Patel H; Berge W; Cronin MTD. Quantitative structure-activity relationships (QSARs) for the prediction of skin permeation of exogenous chemicals. *Chemosphere,* 2002, 48, 603-613.

Pont AR; Charron AR; Brand RM. Active ingredients in sunscreens act as topical penetration enhancers for the herbicide 2,4-dichlorophenoxyacetic acid. *Toxicology Appl. Pharmacol.,* 2004, 195, 348–354.

Potts RO; Guy RH. Predicting skin permeability. *Pharm. Res.*, 1992, 9, 663- 669.

Rai V;, Ghosh I; Bose S; Silva SMC; Chandra P; Michniak-Kohn B. A transdermal review on permeation of drug formulations, modifier compounds and delivery methods. *J. Drug Del. Sci. Tech.*, 2010, 20, 75-87.

Roberts MS; Pugh WJ; Hadgraft J. Epidermal permeability: Penetrant structure relationships. 2. The effect of h-bonding groups in penetrants on their diffusion through the stratum corneum. *Int. J. Pharm.*, 1996, 132, 23-32.

Sasson CS; Sato ME; da Silva Beletti K; Cunha Mota F; Dakiw Piaceski A. Influence of cosmetics vehicles on 4-methylbenzylidene-camphor's skin penetration, in vitro. *Braz. Arch. Biol. Technol.*, 2009, 52, 299-303.

Scalia S; Mezzena M; Iannuccelli V. Influence of solid lipid microparticle carriers on skin penetration of the sunscreen agent, 4-methylbenzylidene camphor. *J. Pharm. Pharmacol.,* 2007, 59, 1621–1627.

SCCP Opinion on 4-Methylbenzylidene camphor (4-MBC) COLIPA n° S60, 24 June 2008.

SCCS's notes of guidance for the testing of cosmetic substances and their safety evaluation SCCS/1501/12, 8th Revision, 11 December 2012.

SCCS/1513/13 Opinion ion 3-Benzylidene camphor COLIPA n° S61, 18 June 2013.

Schaefer H; Riedelmayer TE. Skin Barrier: Principles of Percutaneous Absorption. Karger, Basel, 1996, pp. 118–28.

Schlumpf M, Schmid P, Durrer S, Conscience M; Maerkel K; Henseler M; Gruetter M; Herzog I; Reolon S; Ceccatelli R; Faass O; Stutz E; Jarry H; Wuttke W; Lichtensteiger W. Endocrine activity and developmental toxicity of cosmetic UV filters—an update. *Toxicology,* 2004, 205,113–22.

Schlumpf M; Cotton B; Conscience M; Haller V; Steinmann B; Lichtensteiger W. In vitro and in vivo estrogenicity of UV screens. *Environ Health Perspect*, 2001, 109, 239– 44.

Schneider S; Deckardt K; Hellwig J; Kuttler K; Mellert W; Schulte S; van Ravenzwaay B. Octyl methoxycinnamate: Two-generation reproduction toxicity in Wistar rats by dietary administration. *Food Chem. Toxicol.*, 2005, 43, 1083-1092.

Shokri J; Hasanzadeh D; Ghanbarzadeh S; Dizadji-Ilkhchi M; Adibkia K. The effect of Beta-cyclodextrin on percutaneous absorption of commonly used Eusolex® sunscreens. *Drug Res*, 2013, 63, 591-6.

Siqueira NM; Contri RV; Paese K; Beck RCR; Pohlmann AR; Guterres SS. Innovative sunscreen formulation based on benzophenone-3-loaded chitosan-coated polymeric nanocapsules. *Skin Pharmacol. Physiol.*, 2011, 24, 166–174.

Simeoni S; Scalia S; Benson HA. Influence of cyclodextrins on in vitro human skin absorption of the sunscreen, butylmethoxydibenzoylmethane. *Int. J. Pharm.*, 2004, 280, 163–71.

Søeborg T; Ganderup NC; Kristensen JH; Bjerregaard P; Pedersen KL; Bollen P; Hansen SH; Halling-Sørensen B. Distribution of the UV filter 3-benzylidene camphor in rat following topical application. *J. Chromatogr B,* 2006, 834, 117–121.

Søeborg T; Hollesen Basse L; Halling-Sørensen B. Risk assessment of topically applied products. *Toxicology,* 2007, 236, 140–148.

Timbrell, J. Principles of Biochemical Toxicology, 3rd ed. Taylor & Francis, New York, 2005.

Treffel P; Gabard B. Skin penetration and sun protection factor of ultra- violet filters from two vehicles. *Pharm. Res.,* 1996, 13, 770–774.

Trommer H; Neubert RHH. Overcoming the stratum corneum: the modulation of skin penetration. *Skin Pharmacol. Physiol.* 2006, 19, 106–121.

Varvaresou A. Percutaneous absorption of organic sunscreens. *Journal of Cosmetic Dermatology,* 2006, 5, 53–57.

Vettor M; Bourgeois S; Fessi H; Pelletier J; Perugini P; Pavanetto F; Bolzinger MA. Skin absorption studies of octyl-methoxycinnamate loaded poly(D,L-lactide) nanoparticles: estimation of the UV filter distribution and release behaviour in skin layers. *J. Microencapsul*, 2010, 27, 253–262.

Walters KA; Brain KR; Howes D; James VJ; Kraus AL; Teetsel NM; Toulon M; Watkinson AC; Gettings SD. Percutaneous penetration of octyl salicylate from representative sunscreen formulations through human skin in vitro. *Food Chem. Toxicol.*, 1997, 35, 1219-25.

Wang T; Gu X. In vitro percutaneous permeation of the repellent DEET and the sunscreen oxybenzone across human skin. *J. Pharm. Pharm. Sci.*, 2007, 10, 17-25.

Watkinson AC; Brain KR; Walters KA; Hadgraft J. Prediction of the percutaneous penetration of ultraviolet filters used in sunscreen formulations. *Int. J. Cosmet Sci.* 1992, 14, 265–75.

Weigmann HJ; Lademann J; Schanzer S; Lindemann U; von Pelchrzim R; Schaefer H; Sterry W; Shah V. Correlation of the local distribution of topically applied substances inside the stratum corneum determined by tape-stripping to differences in bioavailability. *Skin Pharmacol. Appl. Skin Physiol.*, 2001, 14 (Suppl 1), 98–102.

Weiss-Angeli V; Bourgeois S; Pelletier J; Guterres SS; Fessi H; Bolzinger MA. Development of an original method to study drug release from polymeric nanocapsules in the skin. *J. Pharm. Pharmacol.*, 2010, 62, 35–45.

Wertz PW. Lipids and barrier function of the skin. *Acta Derm Venereol Suppl* (Stockh) 2000, 208, 7-11.

Wissing S A; Muller RH. Solid lipid nanoparticles as carrier for sunscreens: in vitro release and in vivo skin penetration. *J. Control Rel.*, 2002, 81, 225–233.

Yener G; Incegül T; Yener N. Importance of using solid lipid microspheres as carriers for UV filters on the example octyl methoxy cinnamate. *Int. J. Pharm.*, 2003, 258, 203–207.

In: Sunscreens
Editors: Sean Henry Sharp

ISBN: 978-1-63482-160-5

Chapter 7

UV PROTECTION BY WOOLEN FABRIC DYED WITH NATURAL DYESTUFF

Ana Sutlović, Anita Tarbuk*, Ana Marija Grancarić and Đurđica Parac-Osterman
University of Zagreb, Faculty of Textile Technology,
Department of Textile Chemistry and Ecology, Zagreb, Croatia

ABSTRACT

The UV protection by textiles highly depends on large number of factors such are type of fiber, fabric surface, construction, porosity, density, moisture content, type and concentration of dyestuff, fluorescent whitening agents (FWA), UV-B protective agents (UV absorbers), as well as nanoparticles, if applied. The dyes are selective absorbers. They all absorb visible light, but some absorb light in the near ultraviolet region, as well. Even though synthetic dyes are cheaper, their usage led to such consequences as carcinogenicity and some of them are toxic to the environment. Due to increased awareness of the environmental and health hazards associated with the synthesis, processing and use of synthetic dyes, most of the commercial dyers have started to re-looking to the maximum possibilities of using natural dyes for dyeing and printing of different textiles for targeting niche market. Natural dyes are usually derived from the plants, animal and mineral sources. The shades produced by natural dyes are usually soft, lustrous and soothing to the human eye, can be produced a wide range of colors by mix and match system and are usually renewable and biodegradable. However, it needs longer dyeing time and excess cost for mordants and mordanting. Applied on textiles, provide some UV blocking which depends on the structure of dye molecules, type of dye or pigment, present absorptive groups, depth of dyeing and the uniformity. According to colour physic principles, darker colors (e.g., black, navy blue and dark red) absorb UV-R much more strongly than light pastel colors. For that reason, in this chapter the UV protection by woolen fabric dyed with natural dyestuff extracted from European Ash bark (*Fraxinus excelsior)* and European black elderberry berries (*Sambucus nigra)* was researched. Since these natural dyes, as most of the natural dyes, are non-substantive and must be applied on textiles in the combination with mordants i.e., metallic salts, 4

* Corresponding address: Prilaz baruna Filipovića 28a, HR-10000 Zagreb, Croatia; E-mail: anita.tarbuk@ttf.hr.

different mordants were applied. The color parameters were measured on remission spectrophotometer. The fabric UV protection was determined according to AS/NZS 4399:1996 *Sun Protective Clothing: evaluation and classification*, by UV-A and UV-B transmission measurement on transmission spectrophotometer and calculation of Ultraviolet protection factor (UPF).

Keywords: Wool, UV protection, natural dyestuff, *Sambucus nigra, Fraxinus excelsior*

INTRODUCTION

The application of a number of synthetic dyes is associated with allergies, toxic and carcinogenic effect as well as impact on the environment. Due to increased awareness of the environmental and health hazards associated with the synthesis, processing and use of synthetic dyes, most of the commercial dyers have started to re-looking to the maximum possibilities of using natural dyes for dyeing and printing of different textiles for targeting niche market [1-6]. Natural dyes are usually derived from the plants, animal/insects and mineral sources, and can be classified according to dyeing properties, chemical structure, origin, hue or application area [1-6]. In regards to dyeing properties, most natural dyes can be sorted into group of mordant dyes; some can be classified as vat, while a small number of natural dyes belong to groups of direct and basic dyes [6-13].

Table 1. Review of main groups of natural dyes according hues [6, 12, 13, 26, 27]

Name	Colour Index	Source	Mordant	Main colouring matters
Red colour hues				
Alkanet root *(Anchusa tinctoria L.)*	Natural Red 20	roots	Al	alkannin
Henna *(Lawsonia inrmis L.)*	Natural Orange 6	leaves	Al	lawsone
Kermes *(Coccus ilicis L.)*	Natrual Red 3	insect	Al, Sn, Cu, Fe	kermesic and flavokermesic acid
Cochineal *(Coccus cacti L.)*	Natural Red 4	insect	Al, Sn, Cu, Fe	carminic acid
Madder *(Rubia tinctorum L.)*	Natural Red 8	root	Al, Fe, Sn	alizarin, pseudopurpurin, purpurin, xanthopurpurin
Brazilwood *(Caesalpinia sappan L.)*	Natural Red 24	wood	Al, Fe, Sn	brazilin, brazilein
Yellow colour hues				
Tree of Sorrow *(Nyctanthes arbor-tristis L.)*	Natural Yellow 19	flower	Al	crocetin
Chamomile *(Chamaemelum recutica L.)*	Natural Yellow 1	flowers and leaves	Sn, Al	luteolin, palulitrin, rutin
Jasmine *(Gardenia jasminoides L.)*	Natural Yellow 6	fruit	Sn, Al	crocetin

Name	Colour Index	Source	Mordant	Main colouring matters
Saffron *(Crocus sativus)*	Natural Yellow 6	stigmas	Al	crocetin
Pomegranate *(Punica granatum)*	Natural Yellow 3	fruit	Al	gallotannins, anthocyanins, betalains
Curcuma *(Curcuma longa)*	Natural Yellow 3	root	Al, Cu	curcumin
Marygold (Calendula officinalis L.)	Natural Yellow 27	flower	Al	rubixanthin
Ashtree *(Fraxinus excelsior)*	Natural Yellow 10	bark	Sn, Al	quercitrin, isoquercitrin
Spanish broom *(Spartium junceum L.)*	Natural Yellow 2	flower	Al, Cu	isoflavon, genistin
Blue colour hues				
Logwood *(Haematoxylum campenhianum L.)*	Natural Black 1	heartwood	Al, Sn, Cu, Fe	haematoxylin, haematein
Indigo *(Indigofera tinctoria L.)*	Natural Blue 1	leaves	-	indigotin, indirubin
Purple colour hues				
Tyrian purple *(Murex brandraris L. and Murex trunculus L.)*	Natural Violet 1	shellfish	-	6,6′-dibromoindigotin, 6,6′-dibromoindirubin, 6-bromoindigotin
Brown colour hues				
Walnut-tree *(Junglans regia)*	Natural Brown 7	green scale or leaves	Fe	juglone
Sicilian Sumac *(Ruhus coriaria L.)*	Natural Brown 6	leaves	Fe	chebulinic acid - eutannin

Complexing with metal salts, mordant dyes give different colorations. Aluminum, copper, iron and tin salts are most usually used mordants. Mordants are usually applied in protein fiber dyeing as mordant pre-treatment of fibres (prior to dyeing); during the process of dyeing, or mordant after-treatment. The most common source of these dyestuffs are madder (*Rubia tinctorum*), cochenil bug (*Dactylopius coccus*), as well as herbs from which most widely used mordant dyes are obtained – flavonoid dyes [14-19]. Second important group of natural textile dyes are in water insoluble vat dyes, which have to be transformed into soluble form with the addition of reduction agent and alkali. Most commonly known representatives of this group are indigo and purple 6,6'-dibromindigo dye obtained from murex sea snail (*Murex brandaris and Murex trunculus*) [7, 20-23]. Among most important natural direct dyes are turmeric or yellow root (*Curcuma longa*) and powderd bark or roots of common barberry (*Berberis vulgaris*) [7, 24, 25]. Review of main groups of natural dyes [6,12,13,26,27] is shown in Table 1. Some other plants commonly used as natural dyes are: Dyer's woad (*Isatis tinctoria L.),* Lipsticktree (*Bixa orellana L.*), Brasilwood (*Caesalpina brasiliensis L.*), Weld (*Reseda luteola L.*), Juniper (*Juniperus Communis*); Elder (*Sambucus Nigra*), Oak (Quercus Aegilops), Bramble (*Rubus fruticosus*), Nettle (*Urtica dioica*), St. John

Wart (*Hypericum perforatum*), Hibiscus (*Hibiscus L.*), Oak (*Quercus Aegilops*), Bottlebrush (*Callistemon citrinus*), Eucalyptus (*E. Camaldulensis),* etc. [1-37].

When classifying natural dyes according to color hue, the type and process of mordant should be regarded. Only a few natural dyes are substantive (direct and vat dyes), whilst all other require inorganic oxides or salts – metal salts (mordant dyes). Division of natural dyes according to chemical constitution is in accordance to botanical nomenclature. Most important chemical groups of natural dyes are: carationoide, diaril-methane, benzoquinone, anthraquinone, indigoide, flavonoide, anthociane, betalaine, neoflavonoide, basic, alcaloide, benzofenon, galotannine, tannins, chlorophyll, natural pigments, etc. [7,8]. Flavonoids and flavonoid derivatives are most represented compounds in watery herbal extracts [38-42]. In regards to dyeing properties flavonoids belong to a group of mordant dyes. Most commonly used dyeing method uses a pretreatment process in which wool is mordanted in watery solution of metal salts, followed by a process of dyeing in the solution of watery extracted natural dyes [7, 10-13, 38-41]. The combination dye-metal salt has a strong infuence on the color hue and color fastness properties [10]. Depending on the structure of flavonoid derivative metal complexes 1:1 or 1:2 may be formed [38] (Figure 1).

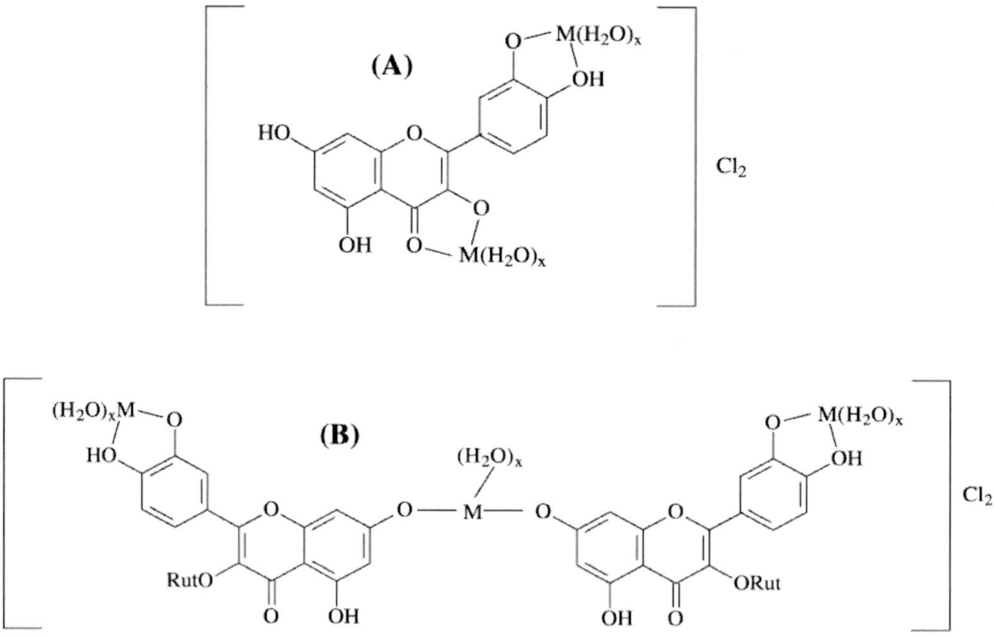

Figure 1. Tentative structures of the complexes: (A) quercetin complexes (1:1); (B) rutin complexes (1:1 and 1:2). x =2 for M = Cu (II); x = 4 for M = Fe(II) [42].

Natural dyes represent renewable and sustainable bioresource products with minimum environmental impact and as such are a potential 'Green chemistry' option as an alternative/co-partner to some extent to synthetic dyes [43-45]. The shades produced by natural dyes are usually soft, lustrous and soothing to the human eye, can be produced a wide range of colors by mix and match system and are usually renewable and biodegradable. However, it needs longer dyeing time and excess cost for mordants and mordanting. There are some issues yet to be solved regard optimization of the amount and contents of natural extracts, increase of dye exhaustion to material, increase in colour fastness, selection and optimization of mordants used. Although, water is the most usual solvent used to prepare natural extract it is being substituted with another solvent (ethanol, methanol) in the aim of increasing the overall amount of the extract, isolation of certain extract components or simply to remove unwanted impurities such as waxes and lipids from watery extracts [46-49].

During the last few decades, increasing attention has been paid by researchers to various aspects of natural dye applications. A large number of plant and animal/insect sources have been identified for extraction of color [2,3] and their diversified use in textile dyeing [9, 29] and functional finishing [30, 31, 50-56], food coloration, cosmetics, and other application disciplines [5]. Natural dyes in functional finishing of textiles has become as a result of a careful balance between compatibility of different finishing products and treatments and the application processes used to provide eco-friendly textiles with desirable properties, such as antimicrobial [30, 31, 43, 49-56], insect repellent, deodorizing and UV-protective [54-64] properties. Several new techniques of modern innovative finishing have been added to dyeing technologies: CO_2, chitosan treatment [65], enzymatic treatment [66, 67], plasma treatment [68, 69], cationization [70-72], microencapsulation and cross-linking [73], etc. for enhancement of protective properties of naturally dyed textile materials, e.g., antimicrobial and UV protection.

The primary cause of skin cancer is believed to be a long exposure to solar ultraviolet (UV) radiation crossed with the amount of skin pigmentation in the population [74-76]. Intermittent sun exposure in childhood and adolescence is considered to be a stronger risk factor for melanoma than continuous exposure. In addition to some beneficial effects of UV radiation it may cause skin and eye damage, especially during the summer time. The proper and early photoprotection may reduce the risk of subsequent occurrence of skin cancer [76]. Therefore, photoprotection is based on protection from UV-B (from 280 nm to 320 nm) and UV-A (from 320 nm to 400 nm) radiation, which are reaching the Earth due to diminishing of the ozone layer.

Textile and clothing show some UV protection, but in the most cases it does not provide full sun screening properties. A good fabric UV protection depends on a large number of factors, such as, the type of fiber, fabric surface and construction, porosity, density, moisture content, type and concentration of dyestuff, fluorescent whitening agent (FWA), UV-B protective agents, as well as nanoparticles, if applied [57,77-91].

The dyestuffs are selective absorbers. They all absorb visible light, but some absorb light in the near ultraviolet region, as well. Applied on textiles, provide some UV blocking which depends on the structure of dye molecules, type of dye or pigment, present absorptive groups, depth of dyeing and the uniformity. According to colour physic principles, darker colors (e.g., black, navy blue and dark red) absorb UV-R much more strongly than light pastel colors. Therefore, dyed fabrics protect more than undyed ones and their protection levels rise with the increase in dye concentration [57-60, 64, 77]. However, most of these results concern synthetic dyes.

There are only few studies that focused on the UV protection properties of natural dyes. Sarkar [57] characterized UV protection of plain, twill or sateen weave cotton fabrics dyed with colorants of plant (madder and indigo) and insect (cochineal) origins. Feng et al. [58] in an experiment conducted to evaluate UV protection properties of two natural dyes (Rheum and Lithospermum erythrorhizon) applied on cotton and silk found that these natural dyes exhibit a comparable UV-absorption performance to benzophenone. Results demonstrated that UV-protective effect was strongly dependent on absorption characteristics of natural dyes for UVR. Grifoni et al. [59, 60] studied the effect of color on UVR transmission of cotton, flax, hemp and ramie fabrics with different construction parameters dyed with some common natural dyes: dyer's woad, madder, logwood, lipsticktree, brasilwood, weld and cochineal by in vitro and outdoor assessments. Metallic salt mordants have been reported to enhance UV-protective properties of naturally dyed cotton [55], wool and silk [61-63] fabrics to a substantial account depending on nature of fibre, mordant and natural dye used. Recently, Hou et al. [75] used natural dyes extracted from orange peel, an abundant, cheap and readily available agricultural byproduct, for producing highly durable UV protective wool fabrics. The authors could not found any research considering UV protection of fabric dyed with European Ash bark *(Fraxinus excelsior)*. On the other hand, there has been ne report regarding European black elderberry berries (*Sambucus nigra)* in photoprotective UVA and UVB; photostability in cosmetic emulsions [92].

For that reason, in this chapter the UV protection by woolen fabric dyed with natural dyestuff extracted from European Ash bark (*Fraxinus excelsior)* and European black elderberry berries (*Sambucus nigra)* was researched. Since these natural dyes are non-substantive and must be applied on textiles in the combination with mordants i.e., metallic salts, 4 different mordants were applied. Additionally, color parameters were measured.

EXPERIMENTAL

Materials

Fabric

Twill woven fabric of 100 % wool fibers, having mass per unit area of 162 g/m^2 was used for this research. Warp in the fabric was 30 tex, of density 33 yarns/cm; and weft 25 tex, of density 28 yarns/cm.

Plant Selection

Natural dyestuff was extracted from European Ash bark (*Fraxinus excelsior)* and European black elderberry berries (*Sambucus nigra)* from Croatia.

Mordants

The chemicals (from Kemika, Zagreb) used as mordants in this research were: $KAl(SO_4)_2$ $12H_2O$, $CuSO_4 \cdot 5H_2O$, $FeSO_4 \cdot 7H_2O$ and $SnCl_2 \cdot 2H_2O$.

Procedure

The dyeing of the wool fabric was done in 3 stages: extraction of dyes from the plant, mordanting in pre-treatment or after-treatment, and dyeing.

Extraction of Dyestuff

Air-dryed and powered plants were dried 6 hours at 105 °C and cooled. Water extract of European Ash bark (*Fraxinus excelsior)* and European black elderberry berries (*Sambucus nigra*) was performed in deionized water for 1 hour at the 100 °C, in bath ratio (BR) 1:20. The solution was cooled down and filtered.

Mordanting

The woolen fabrics were treated with metal salts – mordants:

$KAl(SO_4)_2 \cdot 12H_2O$, $CuSO_4 \cdot 5H_2O$, $FeSO_4 \cdot 7H_2O$ and $SnCl_2 \cdot 2H_2O$ as pre-treatment or after-treatment for wool fabric dyed with water extract of European Ash bark (Fraxinus excelsior); and as pre-treatment for wool fabric dyes with water extract of European black elderberry berries (*Sambucus nigra*) due to it is more effective. In pre-treatment, woolen fabrics were treated with metal salts, followed by dyeing in a water extract of natural dyes. In after-treatment mordants were applied after the dyeing process.

Procedure of mordating

Mordant was dissolved in deionized water to make the liquor. pH 4.5 was set by adding 2 % oxalic acid and 2 % tartaric acid. Wool fabrics were mordanted for 60 min at 100 °C using laboratory dyeing machine (Polycolor, Mathis) at a material to BR 1:20. Mordanting was carried out with 4 different mordants: Pottasium alum dodecahydrate ($KAl(SO_4)_3 \cdot 12\ H_2O$), Copper (II) sulfate pentahydrate ($CuSO_4 \cdot 5H_2O$), Iron (II) sulfate heptahydrate ($FeSO_4 \cdot 7\ H_2O$) and Tin(II) chloride dihydrate ($SnCl_2 \cdot 2H_2O$)in wide concentration range (0.1 % - 5 % owf – over weigth of fabric). The mordant material was than rinsed and dried.

Dyeing

Untereated and woolen fabric treated with mordants were dyed with plant extract solution of pH value 6.5. Dyeing process was done in laboratory dyeing machine (Polycolor, Mathis) at a material to liquor ratio of 1:20. The dye bath temperature was raised at a rate of 3 °C/min to 100 °C, maintained at this temperature for 60 min and cooled down to room temperature. Dyed fabrics were rinsed in cold and hot water and allowed to air-dry.

Measurements

The electrokinetic (zeta) potential is part of the total potential drop occurring in the intermediate surface layer at the boundary of the solid/liquid phases as a consequence of the ions distribution from the solid surface to the liquid mass. It was measured by streaming potential/current method using Brookhaven-Paar Electrokinetic Analyzer with a stamp cell and calculated according to Helmholtz-Smoluchowsky equation [93]. Isoelectric Point (IEP) is a numeric value of pH where electrokinetic surface potential equals zero and indicate the nature of solid surface. Therefore, the zeta potential (ZP) was investigated versus pH, and the Isoelectric Point (IEP) of woolen fabric was determined.

HPLC of plant water extract using Shimadzu HPLC system of LC-10 series was performed to determine composition of primary dyeing agent in natural dyestuffs. Based on the best selectivity of flavonoides that should contain these plant extracts, measurement was performed at 300 nm, bandwidths of 10 nm, in time of 15 min. Column C18 Shodex RSpak DS-613 were used. Analysis was performed by binary system where the mobiles phase included water (pH 2 adjusted with phosphoric acid) and acetonitrile in a ratio of 77,5:22,5; at a flow rate 1 ml/min.

Color parameters of woolen fabrics after dyeing were measured using remission spectrophotometer SF 600 PLUS CT (Datacolor) under illuminant D65, 8° standard observer with the specular component excluded and the UV component included. The coordinates used to determine color values are "L*" for lightness, "a*" for redness (positive value) and greenness (negative value), "b*" for yellowness (positive value) and blueness (negative value), "C*" for chroma and "h°" for hue angle in the range of 0° to 360°.

Colour strength (K/S) was calculated by the Kubelka-Munk equation:

$$K/S = (1-R)^2/2R \quad (1)$$

where R is the remission value (reflectance of the dyed fabric) at λ_{max}, K is the absorption coefficient.

The fabric UV protection was determined according to AS/NZS 4399:1996 *Sun Protective Clothing: evaluation and classification.* UVA and UVB transmission through fabric were measured on Varian Cary 50 Spectrophotometer. The *ultraviolet protection factor* (*UPF*) was calculated automatically. Fabrics UV protection was rated accordingly (Table 2).

Table 2. UV protection rating according to AS/NZS 4399:1996

UPF range	UPF rating	UV-R protection category	UV-R blocking [%]
< 14	0, 5, 10	non-rateable	<93,3
15-24	15, 20	good	93,3-95,8
25-39	25, 30, 35	very good	95,9-97,4
> 40	40, 45, 50, 50+	excellent	> 97,5

RESULTS AND DISCUSSION

In this chapter the UV protection by woolen fabric dyed with natural dyestuff extracted from European Ash bark (*Fraxinus excelsior)* and European black elderberry berries (*Sambucus nigra)* was researched. Prior to dyeing with these natural dyes, the zeta potential and Isoelectric Point (IEP), a numeric value of pH where electrokinetic surface potential equals zero, were determined by streaming potential/current method using Brookhaven-Paar Electrokinetic Analyzer with a stamp cell. The results are shown in Figure 2.

The wool fibre has an anionic character at pH 10 due to the presence of numerous carboxylate groups. The is also a large number of other chargeable groups, including nitrogen containing groups, that will protonate and give rise to positive charge at lower pH values. All these groups result in a high ZP of wool fabric (-48 mV) and IEP = 4.3. The net charge is due to the balance of these different groups and is the reason for positive zeta potential of wool at low pH. Isoelectric point, IEP, depends on molecular and supramolecular structure of fibres in textile fabric. It is important parameter for fabric dyeability and finishing process. Therefore, mordating was performed near the isoelectric point, at pH 4.5, what resulted in yellow shade; whilst in alkali medium it would be brown.

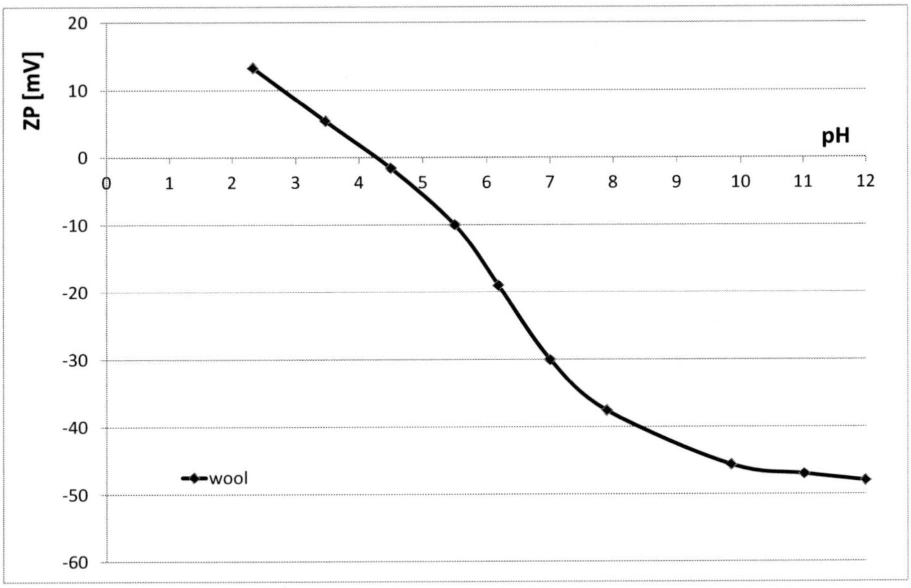

Figure 2. Zeta potential (ZP, ζ) of the wool fabrics vs. pH of 0.001 M KCl (IEP=4.3).

Based on the retention times of occurrence of peaks of standard solutions of flavonoids proved to be in alcocholic extract of European Ash bark obtained the strongest signal in the retention time of 2.61 min, which corresponds to the rutine and less intensity at retention times 3.44 and 4.40 min corresponding isoquercitrin and quercetin. In the alcoholic extract of European black elderberry berries resulted in two spades and at retention time 2.61 min (characteristic of rutin) and 1.85 min which corresponds to anthocyanines. Based on literature data and HPLC measurement in European Ash bark (*Fraxinus excelsior)* extract primary dyeing agents are rutin, quercetin and isoquercitrin [6, 30, 94], and in European black elderberry berries (*Sambucus nigra)* rutine and anthocyanin, especially Cyanidin 3-glucoside and Cyanidin 3-sambubioside [6, 94-96]. The chemical structures of primary dyeing agents are listed in the Table 3. These compounds were taken account when applied to textiles in the combination with 4 different mordants.

Natural dyes derived from plants are usually acid mordant dyes which create metal-flavonoid complexes with metal ions. Depending on the chosen metal the different tones of the coloration can be obtained. Since all these flavonoid pigments belong to the group of mordant dyes, 4 different mordants were used in pre-treatment or after-treatment. The woolen fabrics were pre-treated with metal salts, followed by dyeing in an aqueous extract of natural dyes. In after-treatment mordants (metal salts) were applied after the dyeing process. In both cases, it was essential that the flavonoid component from the extract creates colored metal complex where, depending on the structure of flavonoid derivatives, metal complexes 1:1 or 1:2 may arise.

Table 3. The primary dyeing agents in European Ash bark (*Fraxinus excelsior)* and European black elderberry berries (*Sambucus nigra)*

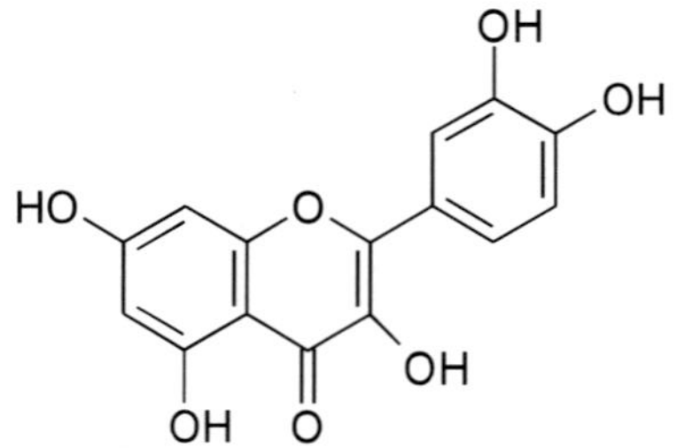 quercetin dihydrate *3,3',4',5,7-pentahydroxyflavon*	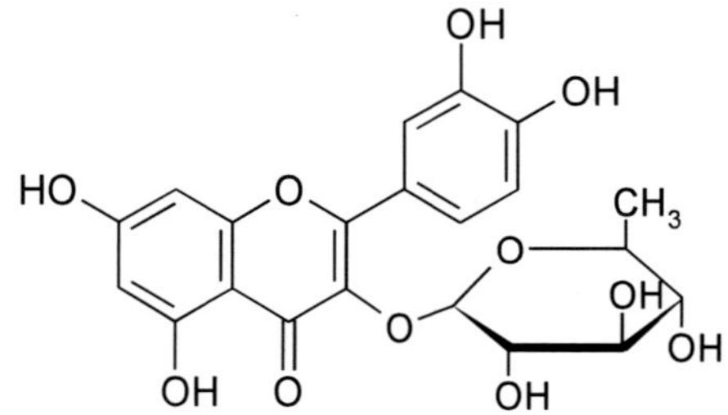 isoquercitrin *quercetin* 3-glucoside
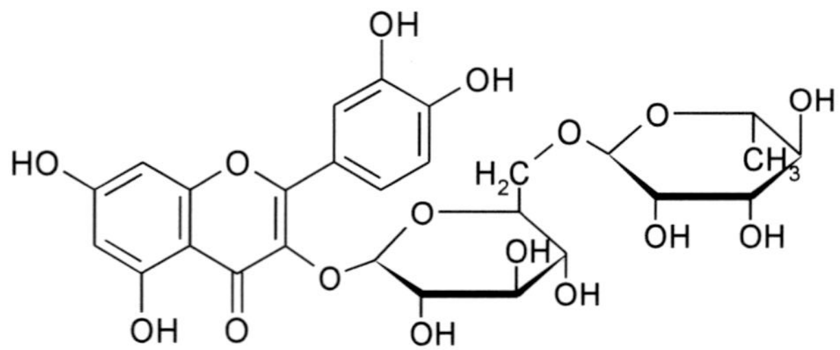 rutin trihydrate *quercetin -3-rutinoside*	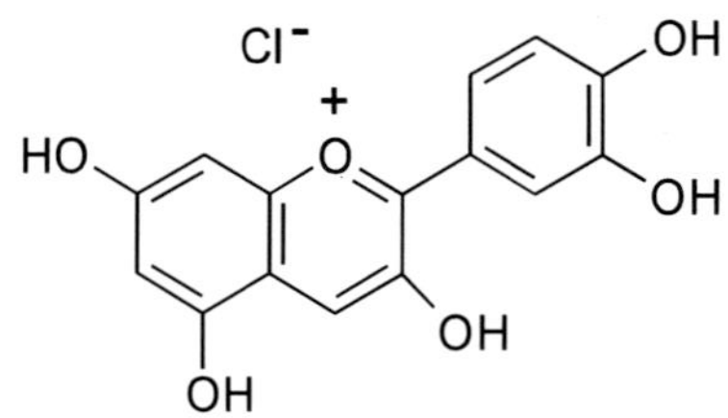 Anthocyanin *Cyanidin*

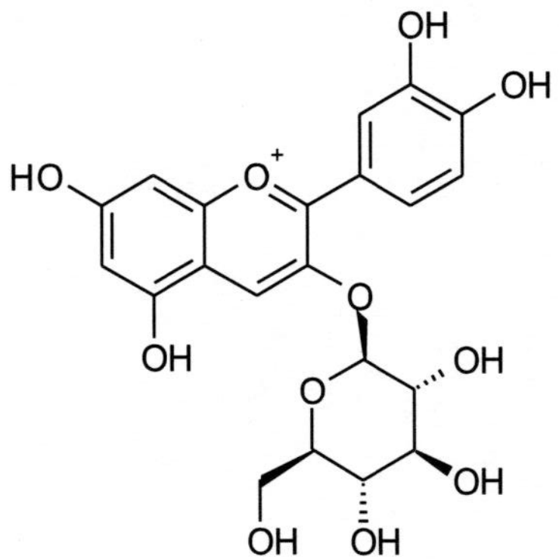

Cyanidin 3-glucoside
(796 mg/100 g)

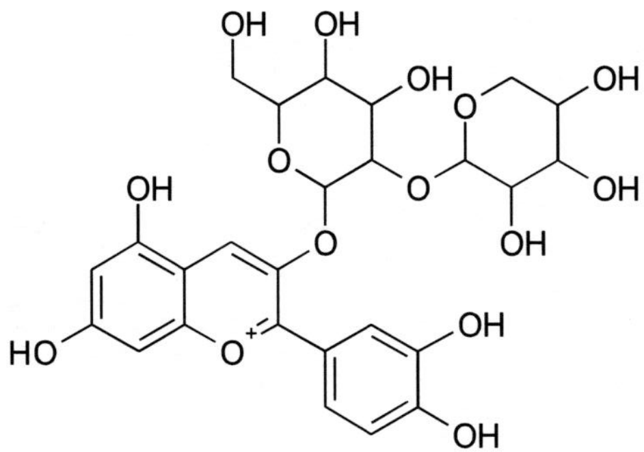

Cyanidin 3-sambubioside
(463 mg/100 g)

Possible copper complexes with quercetin and rutin are shown in Figures 3 and 4. In neutral aglycone quercetin dihydrate reactivity is [94]: $Sn^{2+} > Al^{3+} > Fe^{2+} > Cu^{2+}$. On the other hand, glycoside rutin trihydrate and isoquercetin showed oposite reactivity: $Cu^{2+} > Fe^{2+} > Al^{3+} > Sn^{2+}$. The resulting inverse selectivity of aglycone and glycosides in favor of "natural series" H. Irving and R.J.P. Williams who proved that the stability of metal complexes is growing in a number of divalent central ions: $Mn^{2+}<Fe^{2+}<Co^{2+}<Ni^{2+}<Cu^{2+}$.

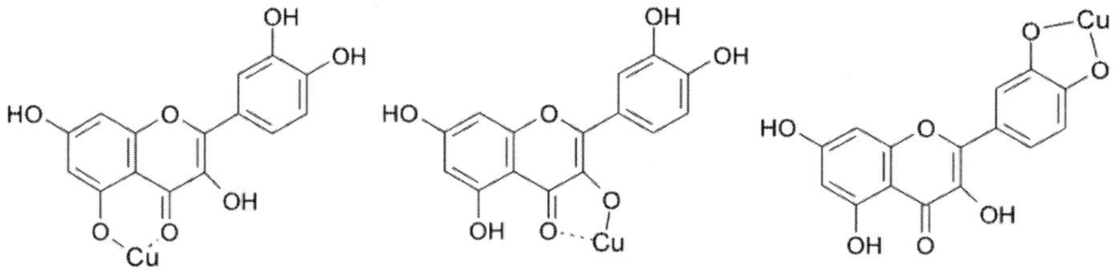

Figure 3. Possible quercetin:copper complex (1:1).

In order to confirm the formation of the colored complex on the dyed woolen fabric, samples were analyzed with a remission spectrophotometer SF 600 PLUS CT (Datacolor). The coloristic parameters are given in Tables 4-6. Color depth (K/S) of all dyed woolen fabrics is presented in Figures 5-9.

From the Tables 4 and 5 can be seen that woolen fabrics dyed in water extract of European Ash bark (*Fraxinus excelsior*) resulted with tones in yellow-orange region, a range of values tons h* = 77 – 87 regardless of mordant or procedure of its application. The effect of mordant concentration and its application procedure to saturation (C*) can be observed. The maximum differences are observed for the metal salts of iron and copper which is in correlation with their ionic potential.

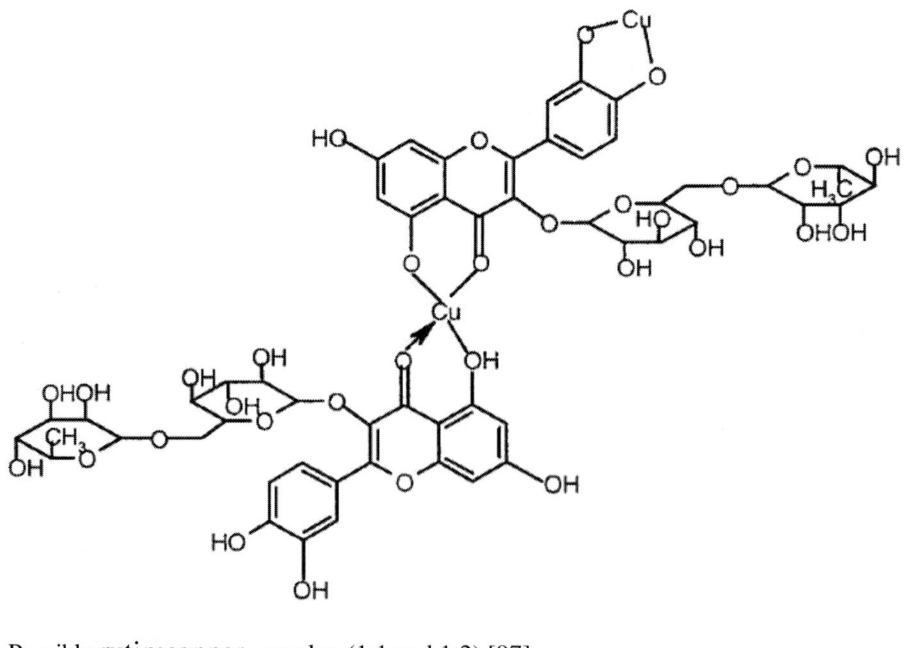

Figure 4. Possible rutin:copper complex (1:1 and 1:2) [97].

Table 4. Color parameters of woolen fabrics dyed in water extract of European Ash bark (*Fraxinus excelsior)* with $KAl(SO_4)_2 \cdot 12H_2O$ and $CuSO_4 \cdot 5H_2O$ as mordants

Mordant	a*	b*	L*	C*	h*	X	Y	Z	x	y
No mordant	4.42	24.38	61.29	24.78	79.72	30.44	29.58	13.42	0.41	0.40
Pre-treatment $KAl(SO_4)_2 \cdot 12H_2O$										
0.1%	5.61	25.77	53.41	26.37	77.71	22.40	21.42	8.61	0.43	0.41
0.5%	5.87	26.36	52.61	27.01	77.44	21.71	20.69	8.08	0.43	0.41
1.0%	5.77	26.41	53.48	27.04	77.68	22.51	21.49	8.47	0.43	0.41
1.5%	5.49	26.23	53.27	26.80	78.17	22.25	21.29	8.42	0.43	0.41
2.0%	5.62	26.28	53.20	26.88	77.94	22.21	21.23	8.38	0.43	0.41
3.0%	5.75	26.25	52.42	26.87	77.65	21.51	20.52	8.02	0.43	0.41
4.0%	5.63	25.99	51.86	26.59	77.79	20.96	20.02	7.84	0.43	0.41
5.0%	5.90	26.27	50.89	26.92	77.35	20.16	19.18	7.35	0.43	0.41
After-treatment $KAl(SO_4)_2 \cdot 12H_2O$										
0.1%	4.66	24.07	67.84	24.52	79.05	38.81	37.76	18.19	0.41	0.40
0.5%	4.88	23.74	67.92	24.24	78.39	38.99	37.86	18.40	0.41	0.40
1.0%	5.05	24.02	67.24	24.55	78.13	38.11	36.95	17.75	0.41	0.40
1.5%	4.77	25.03	63.98	25.48	79.21	33.79	32.78	14.96	0.41	0.40
2.0%	5.13	25.03	63.55	25.55	78.41	33.35	32.25	14.66	0.42	0.40
3.0%	4.61	25.43	61.51	25.84	79.72	30.75	29.83	13.18	0.42	0.40
4.0%	4.84	25.68	62.03	26.13	79.32	31.42	30.43	13.42	0.42	0.40
5.0%	4.85	24.31	63.45	24.79	78.73	33.15	32.12	14.87	0.41	0.40
Pre-treatment $CuSO_4 \cdot 5H_2O$										
0.1%	4.27	23.99	54.54	24.37	79.90	23.20	22.49	9.68	0.42	0.41
0.5%	4.60	24.38	54.30	24.81	79.31	23.04	22.26	9.45	0.42	0.41
1.0%	3.85	24.10	54.45	24.40	80.92	23.01	22.40	9.60	0.42	0.41
1.5%	4.10	24.85	53.30	25.18	80.62	21.97	21.32	8.82	0.42	0.41
2.0%	3.84	24.61	53.97	24.91	81.13	22.55	21.95	9.21	0.42	0.41
3.0%	4.23	24.62	54.48	24.99	80.25	23.13	22.43	9.46	0.42	0.41
4.0%	4.58	24.95	55.20	25.37	79.61	23.91	23.12	9.73	0.42	0.41
5.0%	4.54	25.93	54.45	26.32	80.07	23.17	22.40	9.07	0.42	0.41
After-treatment $CuSO_4 \cdot 5H_2O$										
0.1%	3.77	24.20	62.06	24.49	81.16	31.17	30.48	13.99	0.41	0.40
0.5%	3.16	22.63	65.05	22.85	82.06	34.66	34.10	16.70	0.41	0.40
1.0%	2.08	23.00	61.45	23.09	84.82	30.00	29.77	14.05	0.41	0.40
1.5%	1.20	21.37	61.35	21.40	86.79	29.64	29.64	14.61	0.40	0.40
2.0%	1.78	22.56	58.60	22.63	85.50	26.75	26.60	12.41	0.41	0.40
3.0%	2.47	23.24	59.30	23.38	83.94	27.68	27.35	12.59	0.41	0.40
4.0%	1.56	22.48	63.53	22.53	86.04	32.31	32.22	15.67	0.40	0.40
5.0%	2.37	23.36	61.64	23.48	84.22	30.29	29.98	14.03	0.41	0.40

Table 5. Color parametres of woolen fabrics dyed in water extract of European Ash bark (*Fraxinus excelsior)* with $FeSO_4 \cdot 7H_2O$ and $SnCl_2 \cdot 2H_2O$ as mordants

MORDANT	a*	b*	L*	C*	h*	X	Y	Z	x	y
Pre-treatment $FeSO_4 \cdot 7H_2O$										
0.1%	2.33	15.71	45.23	15.89	81.58	14.93	14.70	7.54	0.40	0.40
0.5%	1.04	12.75	41.77	12.80	85.32	12.37	12.35	6.81	0.39	0.39
1.0%	0.58	10.66	37.55	10.67	86.91	9.80	9.84	5.67	0.39	0.39
1.5%	0.59	9.99	36.98	10.00	86.63	9.50	9.53	5.60	0.39	0.39
2.0%	0.42	10.31	37.54	10.31	87.65	9.78	9.83	5.74	0.39	0.39
3.0%	0.80	10.97	37.04	11.00	85.81	9.55	9.56	5.42	0.39	0.39
4.0%	0.89	12.03	38.52	12.07	85.78	10.39	10.38	5.73	0.39	0.39
5.0%	0.99	12.53	38.20	12.56	85.46	10.22	10.20	5.51	0.39	0.39

Table 5. (Continued)

MORDANT	a*	b*	L*	C*	h*	X	Y	Z	x	y
After-treatment $FeSO_4 \cdot 7H_2O$										
0.1%	2.02	16.47	54.91	16.59	83.01	23.05	22.84	12.31	0.40	0.39
0.5%	1.29	13.90	53.72	13.96	84.70	21.76	21.71	12.50	0.39	0.39
1.0%	1.39	14.92	51.12	14.98	84.66	19.44	19.38	10.66	0.39	0.39
1.5%	1.22	16.43	46.74	16.47	85.76	15.86	15.82	8.03	0.40	0.40
2.0%	1.07	16.21	49.21	16.25	86.23	17.77	17.76	9.26	0.40	0.40
3.0%	1.50	17.02	46.50	17.09	84.96	15.73	15.64	7.77	0.40	0.40
4.0%	1.47	18.29	47.34	18.35	85.39	16.37	16.28	7.82	0.40	0.40
5.0%	1.96	18.53	45.32	18.63	83.96	14.94	14.77	6.90	0.41	0.40
Pre-treatment $SnCl_2 \cdot 2H_2O$										
0.1%	6.13	30.06	59.18	30.67	78.48	28.49	27.23	10.27	0.43	0.41
0.5%	5.94	30.46	60.05	31.03	78.97	29.42	28.18	10.61	0.43	0.41
1.0%	5.99	30.86	61.56	31.44	79.01	31.18	29.89	11.32	0.43	0.41
1.5%	6.18	31.49	62.20	32.09	78.90	32.01	30.64	11.48	0.43	0.41
2.0%	6.44	32.62	62.29	33.25	78.83	32.18	30.74	11.15	0.43	0.42
3.0%	6.45	32.42	62.43	33.05	78.74	32.36	30.90	11.30	0.43	0.41
4.0%	6.53	31.59	60.98	32.25	78.33	30.65	29.22	10.76	0.43	0.41
5.0%	7.00	31.75	59.60	32.51	77.57	29.18	27.68	9.97	0.44	0.41
After-treatment $SnCl_2 \cdot 2H_2O$										
0.1%	5.10	24.81	66.92	25.33	78.38	37.70	36.53	17.16	0.41	0.40
0.5%	4.99	26.23	65.64	26.70	79.22	35.98	34.86	15.63	0.42	0.40
1.0%	4.88	26.41	66.08	26.86	79.54	36.52	35.43	15.87	0.42	0.40
1.5%	4.27	25.70	71.05	26.05	80.58	43.25	42.27	20.02	0.41	0.40
2.0%	5.53	26.84	66.99	27.41	78.36	37.93	36.62	16.34	0.42	0.40
3.0%	5.39	26.64	62.12	27.18	78.56	31.69	30.54	13.12	0.42	0.41
4.0%	4.93	26.12	62.40	26.58	79.32	31.89	30.87	13.49	0.42	0.40
5.0%	5.26	26.71	68.00	27.22	78.86	39.22	37.97	17.14	0.42	0.40

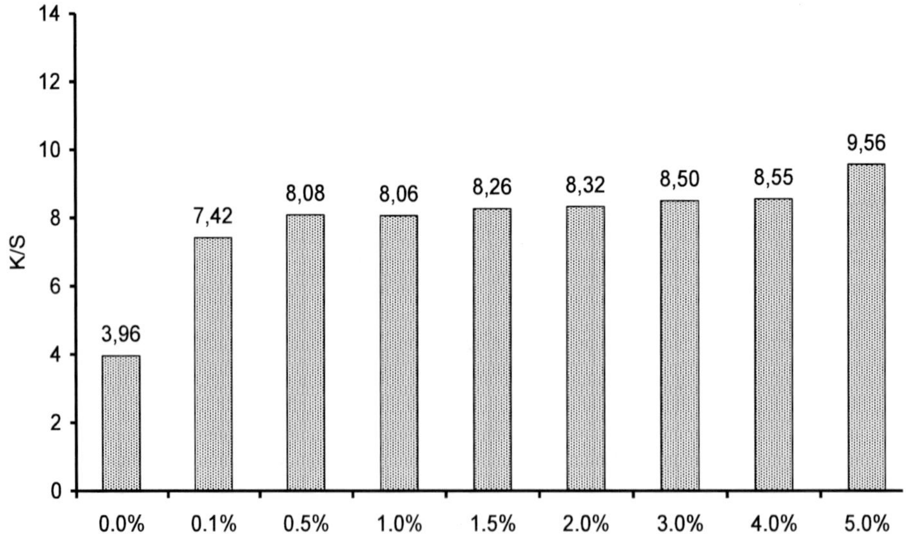

a

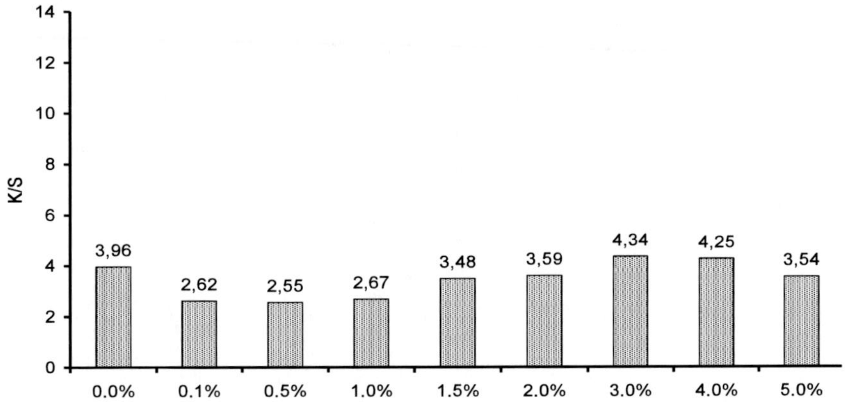

b

Figure 5. K/S values of woolen fabrics dyed in water extract of European Ash bark (*Fraxinus excelsior)* mordanted with $KAl(SO_4)_2{\cdot}12H_2O$ (0.1 % - 5 % owf) in a. pre-treatment and b. after-treatment.

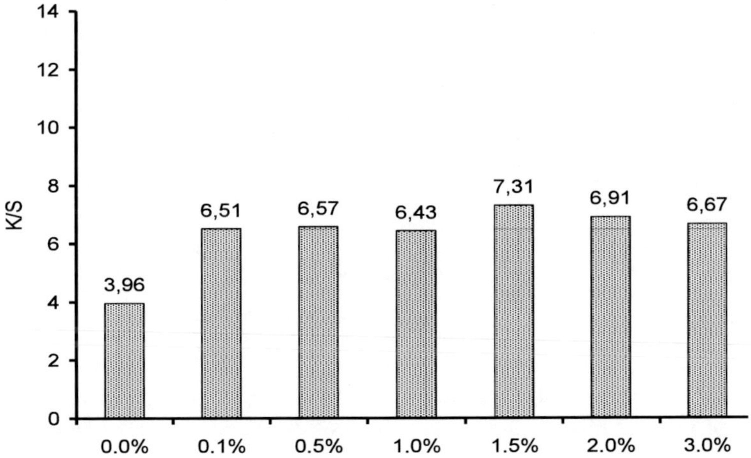

a

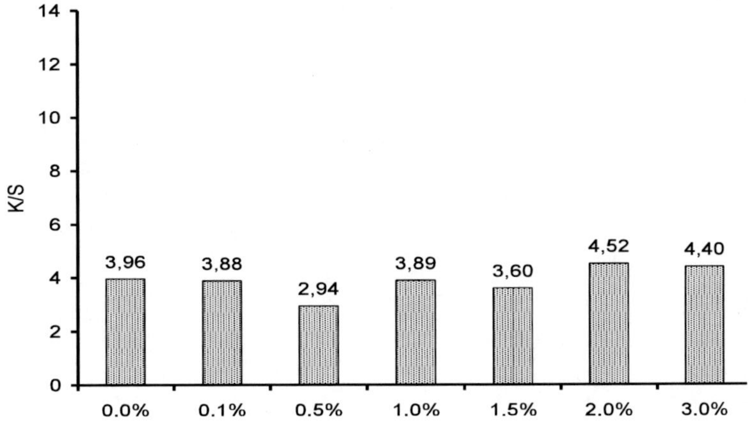

b

Figure 6. K/S values of woolen fabrics dyed in water extract of European Ash bark (*Fraxinus excelsior)* mordanted with $CuSO_4{\cdot}5H_2O$ (0.1 % - 5 % owf) in a. pre-treatment and b. after-treatment.

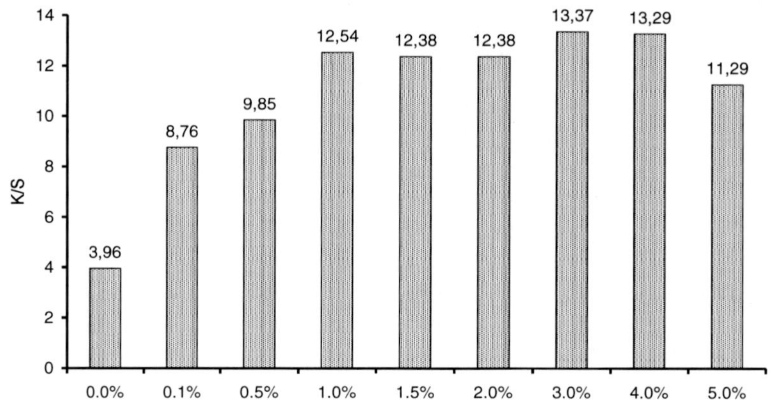

a

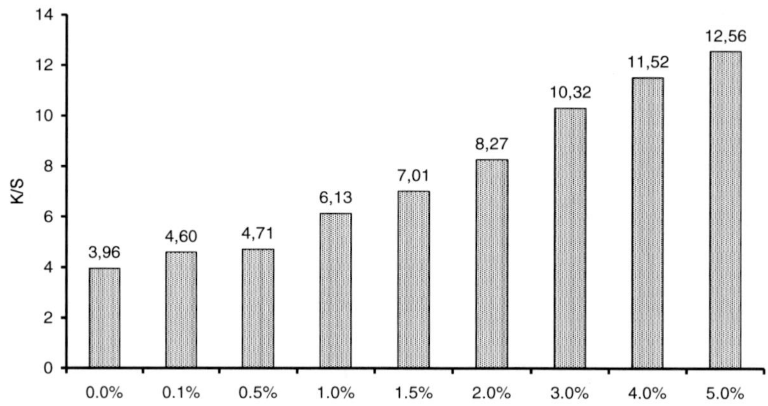

b

Figure 7. K/S values of woolen fabrics dyed in water extract of European Ash bark (*Fraxinus excelsior)* mordanted with $FeSO_4 \cdot 7H_2O$ (0.1 % - 5 % owf) in a. pre-treatment and b. after-treatment.

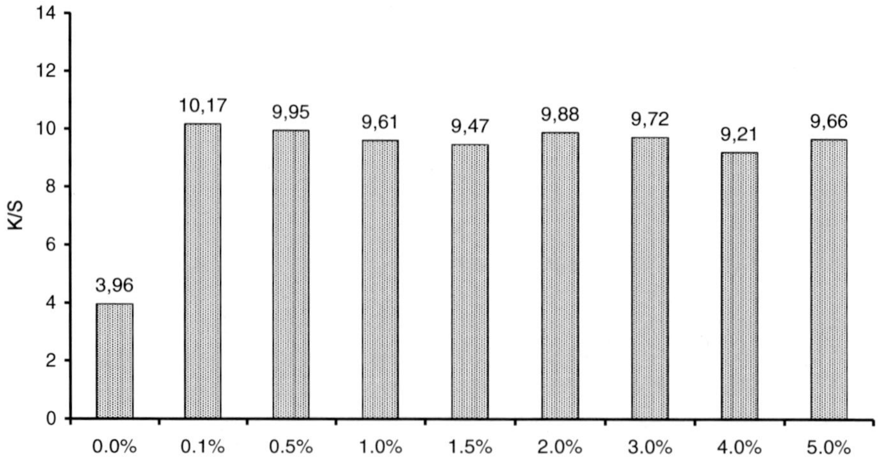

a

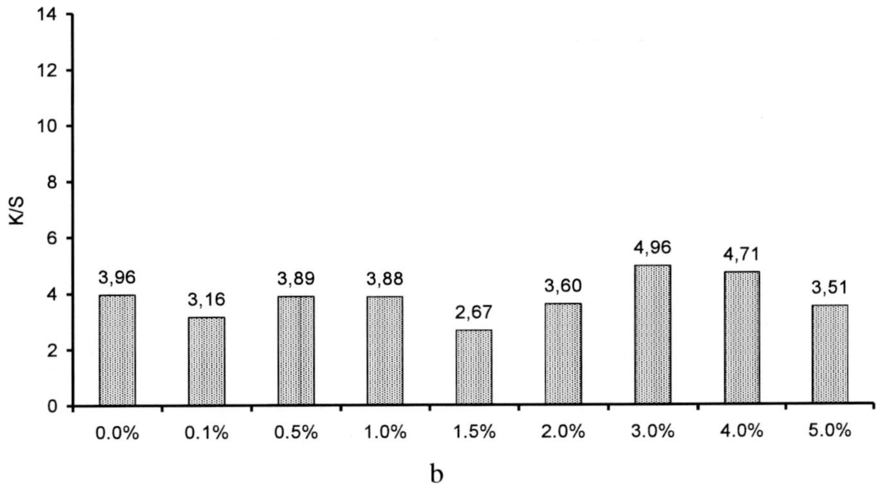

Figure 8. K/S values of woolen fabrics dyed in water extract of European Ash bark (*Fraxinus excelsior)* mordanted with $SnCl_2 \cdot 2H_2O$ (0.1 % - 5 % owf) in a. pre-treatment and b. after-treatment.

However, two-dimensional relationship between hue and saturation, can not make conclusive experience of color without the third dimension - the ligthness (L*). In general, on the basis of the coloristic parameters for all samples the $L^* > 60$, except for samples processed with salt $FeSO_4 \cdot 7H_2O$, $L^* < 40$. It is recognized, based on the x and y, these color samples are closer to achromatic point, resulting in olive shade. This pheomenon is more evident if the mordant was applied in pre-treatment. Comparing the procedures of applying mordants it is evident that pre-treatment results in better saturation than if applied in after-treatment.

This can be considered from two aspects: 1st supstantivity of plant extract to the wool substrate and 2nd stability of resulting metal complexes. In the complexing was done in solution of quercetin dihydrate, and isoquercitrin, rutin trihydrate, the highest reactivity was obtained with the copper salt [94]. However, according to the color measurement, these results are not the best ones. This confirms that all components in plant extract, as well as the textile substrate, participate in creating of colored complex on the fiber/textile material. Mechanism of dyeing with flavonoid dyes is similar to the mechanism of antiradical behaviour of flavonoids in biological system and chelat bonding of metal ions. In biological systems the mechanism has not yet been completely explained on molecular level since there are great differences in chemical properties and significant structural heterogenity. However, the relationship between the structure and activity of the flavonoid and certain structural components and properties of bonding free radicals, formation of chelate complexes and anti oxidation activities have been proofed.

Depending on chemical structure and chemico-morphological characteristics of the fibres being dyed by flavonoid dyes, following chemical bond are formed: hydrogen bonds are formed among poliphenol hydroxyl groups with free amino and amid groups of the protein fibre; ionic bonds are formed among free and available anionic groups in poliphenols and cationic groups of protein fibre [41, 97-100].

Table 6. Color parameters of woolen fabrics dyed in water extract of European black elderberry berries (*Sambucus nigra)*

MORDANT	a*	b*	L*	C*	h*	X	Y	Z	x	y
No mordant	7.29	21.07	52.10	22.30	70.91	20.65	20.23	11.99	0.39	0.38
Pre-treatment $KAl(SO_4)_2{\cdot}12H_2O$										
0.1%	6.67	18.57	45.65	19.74	70.24	12.60	12.28	7.08	0.39	0.38
0.5%	7.58	19.83	44.17	21.23	69.09	14.43	13.96	7.92	0.40	0.38
2.0%	6.45	18.97	42.91	20.04	71.23	13.39	13.10	7.56	0.39	0.38
Pre-treatment $CuSO_4{\cdot}5H_2O$										
0.1%	7.51	18.60	43.17	20.06	68.00	13.73	13.27	7.78	0.39	0.38
0.5%	7.25	18.45	42.73	19.83	68.56	13.39	12.98	7.62	0.39	0.38
2.0%	7.46	19.11	40.58	20.51	68.68	12.05	11.61	6.48	0.40	0.39
Pre-treatment $FeSO_4{\cdot}7H_2O$										
0.1%	6.67	18.57	41.65	19.74	70.24	12.60	12.28	7.08	0.39	0.38
0.5%	5.46	15.62	38.37	16.54	70.72	10.46	10.30	6.40	0.39	0.38
2.0%	4.00	12.88	33.96	13.48	72.75	8.01	7.99	5.28	0.38	0.38
Pre-treatment $SnCl_2{\cdot}2H_2O$										
0.1%	6.67	18.57	41.65	19.74	70.24	12.60	12.28	7.08	0.39	0.38
0.5%	5.61	17.64	42.20	18.51	72.36	12.80	12.63	7.59	0.39	0.38
2.0%	4.82	17.38	40.56	18.04	74.49	11.66	11.59	6.90	0.39	0.38

Considering the mordant concentration, it is evident that optimal color was obtained for samples pre-treated with 2 % of metal salts. By increasing the concentration of mordant, no significant change in color depth (K/S) occured. If mordant applied in wide concentration range in after-treatment, the significant change in color parameters occurred if salt $FeSO_4{\cdot}7H_2O$ was applied. The obtained K/S values can be used as an indicator of water plant extract supstantivity. Approximately the same color depth (K/S) of woolen fabric achieved by pre-treated with 2 %, and after-treated with 5 % of $FeSO_4{\cdot}7H_2O$, can be attributed to the reactivity of the whole system. If pre-treated with 2% $FeSO_4{\cdot}7H_2O$ whole system is more reactive, because in the chelating participate both, the textile substrate and the plant extract. Considering these observations, mordating was performed only in pre-treatment prior to dyeing with European black elderberry berries (*Sambucus nigra)* water extract. Color parameters are collected in Table 6, and color depth (K/S) is shown in Figure 9.

Considering the color parameters of woolen fabrics dyed with European black elderberry berries (*Sambucus nigra)* it can be seen that fabrics have yellow-orange to yellow coloration (h* = 68 – 75). Samples with the highest lightness values were obtained using aluminum salts as mordant (L = 45) and the darkest samples were obtained using copper and iron salts, e.g., L = 34, respectively.

Considering color depth (K/S) of woolen fabrics dyed in water extract of European black elderberry berries (*Sambucus nigra)* mordanted in pre-treatment with $KAl(SO_4)_2{\cdot}12H_2O$, $CuSO_4{\cdot}5H_2O$; $FeSO_4{\cdot}7H_2O$ and $SnCl_2{\cdot}2H_2O$ it can be seen that the highest K/S value has fabric mordaned with iron salt.

However, these samples showed lower chromaticity and the subjective visual assessment noted that the samples have more pronounced grey shade. It is to point out mordating with $SnCl_2{\cdot}2H_2O$ as well, which resulted in high K/S value of 13.33. Other properties and observations are similar to the ones dyes with water extract of European Ash bark (*Fraxinus excelsior).*

It is to notice lower reactivity of water extract of European black elderberry berries (*Sambucus nigra)* than European Ash bark (*Fraxinus excelsior).*

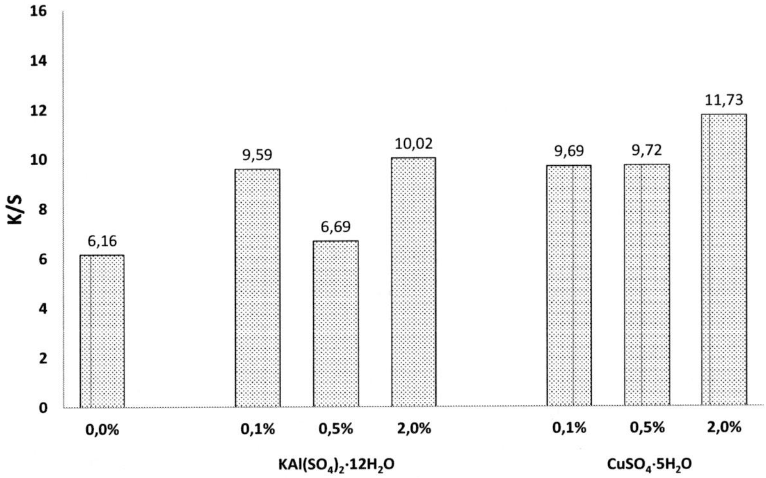

a

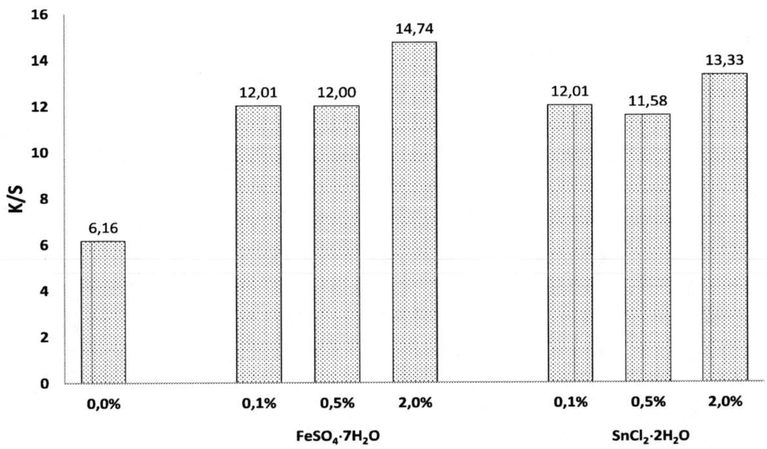

b

Figure 9. K/S values of woolen fabrics dyed in water extract of European black elderberry berries (*Sambucus nigra)* mordanted in pre-treatment with: a. $KAl(SO_4)_2 \cdot 12H_2O$ and $CuSO_4 \cdot 5H_2O$; b. $FeSO_4 \cdot 7H_2O$ and $SnCl_2 \cdot 2H_2O$ (0.1 %, 0.5 %, 2 % owf).

On the basis of the literature, this lower reactivity of isoquercitrin and rutin trihydrate is a result of flavonoid glycosidation. Additionally, the berries in a greater proportion contain anthocyanosides and betalaines, which are considerably more reactive towards metal ions [6, 94-96].

The most of results of the UV protective fabrics concern application of synthetic dyes, whilst only few studies reports of natural dyes. Since it was found that European black elderberry berries (*Sambucus nigra)* helps in cosmetic emulsions giving of photoprotection to UV-A and UV-B irradiation, its application and European Ash (*Fraxinus excelsior)* bark were choosen for the application on light woollen fabric which could protect from harmful UV radiation.

The fabric UV protection was determined according to AS/NZS 4399:1996 *Sun Protective Clothing: evaluation and classification*, by UV-A and UV-B transmission measurement on transmission spectrophotometer and calculation of Ultraviolet protection factor (UPF). The results are presented in Tables 7-9.

Table 7. UV protection of woolen fabrics dyed in water extract of European Ash bark (*Fraxinus excelsior)* with $KAl(SO_4)_2{\cdot}12H_2O$ and $CuSO_4{\cdot}5H_2O$ as mordants

MORDANT	Mean UPF	τ UVA	τ UVB	Stand. Dev.	Stand. Err.	Calc. UPF	UV protection
Wool	32.070	7.634	2.194	1.069	1.326	30.744	30
No mordant	54.800	5.043	1.103	1.481	2.444	52.356	50
Pre-treatment $KAl(SO_4)_2{\cdot}12H_2O$							
0.1%	210.273	0.574	0.455	64.604	80.109	130.163	50+
0.5%	188.651	0.651	0.509	47.362	58.728	129.922	50+
1.0%	188.513	0.615	0.481	15.142	18.776	169.737	50+
1.5%	96.801	1.031	0.981	3.529	4.376	92.425	50+
2.0%	134.488	0.812	0.700	12.303	15.256	119.232	50+
3.0%	77.371	1.300	1.237	6.584	8.164	69.207	50+
4.0%	147.360	0.124	0.634	7.927	9.829	137.531	50+
5.0%	70.494	1.449	1.367	7.667	9.507	60.987	50+
After-treatment $KAl(SO_4)_2{\cdot}12H_2O$							
0.1%	344.562	0.630	0.206	1.160	54.465	290.097	50+
0.5%	427.916	0.527	0.193	43.923	189.108	238.808	50+
1.0%	265.127	0.771	0.336	152.506	130.034	135.093	50+
1.5%	197.291	0.910	0.418	104.866	64.764	132.528	50+
2.0%	197.056	0.855	0.391	52.229	15.342	181.714	50+
3.0%	364.845	0.567	0.209	12.373	124.600	240.245	50+
4.0%	308.848	0.698	0.299	144.756	179.498	129.350	50+
5.0%	158.789	1.027	0.496	12.907	16.005	142.785	50+
Pre-treatment $CuSO_4{\cdot}5H_2O$							
0.1%	204.600	0.600	0.440	34.831	43.191	161.409	50+
0.5%	147.816	0.759	0.616	10.199	12.647	135.168	50+
1.0%	105.849	1.008	0.890	13.102	16.246	89.648	50+
1.5%	119.909	0.924	0.787	19.677	24.400	95.509	50+
2.0%	150.996	0.752	0.601	12.028	14.915	136.081	50+
3.0%	147.508	0.787	0.642	31.394	38.928	108.579	50+
4.0%	103.013	1.057	0.909	7.773	9.639	93.374	50+
5.0%	140.480	0.786	0.656	10.790	13.379	127.101	50+
After-treatment $CuSO_4{\cdot}5H_2O$							
0.1%	456.846	0.446	0.239	250.687	310.852	145.993	50+
0.5%	408.100	0.529	0.206	152.717	189.369	218.731	50+
1.0%	335.774	0.600	0.303	166.050	205.902	129.872	50+
1.5%	546.108	0.416	0.138	111.925	138.787	407.321	50+
2.0%	488.220	0.398	0.154	58.708	72.798	415.422	50+
3.0%	772.257	0.230	0.116	184.463	228.734	543.523	50+
4.0%	347.056	0.573	0.229	93.859	116.385	230.671	50+
5.0%	939.780	0.163	0.100	15.416	19.115	920.665	50+

Table 8. UV protection of woolen fabrics dyed in water extract of European Ash bark (*Fraxinus excelsior)* with $FeSO_4 \cdot 7H_2O$ and $SnCl_2 \cdot 2H_2O$ as mordants

MORDANT	Mean UPF	τ UVA	τ UVB	Stand. Dev.	Stand. Err.	Calc. UPF	UV protection
Pre-treatment $FeSO_4 \cdot 7H_2O$							
0.1%	156.575	0.699	0.604	28.632	35.504	121.071	50+
0.5%	288.053	0.395	0.306	30.565	37.901	250.153	50+
1.0%	102.195	0.972	0.935	8.843	10.966	91.230	50+
1.5%	125.637	0.786	0.760	2.921	3.622	122.051	50+
2.0%	167.955	0.599	0.570	20.070	24.887	143.068	50+
3.0%	146.659	0.681	0.645	3.414	4.234	142.426	50+
4.0%	168.330	0.593	0.576	18.537	22.986	145.344	50+
5.0%	99.988	0.945	0.970	5.214	6.465	93.523	50+
After-treatment $FeSO_4 \cdot 7H_2O$							
0.1%	665.082	0.275	0.125	83.611	103.677	561.404	50+
0.5%	982.979	0.116	0.100	19.794	24.544	958.435	50+
1.0%	734.727	0.249	0.116	86.981	107.857	626.870	50+
1.5%	967.769	0.119	0.101	41.580	51.559	916.210	50+
2.0%	953.918	0.127	0.101	71.234	60.330	893.588	50+
3.0%	999.824	0.100	0.100	0.497	0.616	999.209	50+
4.0%	949.955	0.119	0.104	66.391	82.325	867.630	50+
5.0%	987.772	0.105	0.101	16.573	20.551	967.222	50+
Pre-treatment $SnCl_2 \cdot 2H_2O$							
0.1%	221.733	0.468	0.419	46.565	57.741	163.991	50+
0.5%	167.333	0.581	0.560	13.917	17.257	150.076	50+
1.0%	136.940	0.700	0.689	12.894	15.989	120.951	50+
1.5%	696.052	0.194	0.128	61.790	76.619	619.433	50+
2.0%	791.720	0.160	0.117	124.593	154.495	637.225	50+
3.0%	305.541	0.345	0.309	66.323	82.241	223.300	50+
4.0%	660.171	0.204	0.138	107.995	133.913	526.258	50+
5.0%	254.974	0.432	0.397	62.367	77.335	168.639	50+
After-treatment $SnCl_2 \cdot 2H_2O$							
0.1%	594.845	0.344	0.128	41.231	514.127	543.719	50+
0.5%	218.308	0.657	0.384	33.397	41.413	176.896	50+
1.0%	317.715	0.512	0.235	27.706	34.355	283.360	50+
1.5%	681.892	0.412	0.106	50.341	62.423	619.469	50+
2.0%	612.764	0.357	0.125	90.445	112.152	500.612	50+
3.0%	443.513	0.384	0.168	15.942	19.769	423.745	50+
4.0%	257.243	0.549	0.325	54.372	67.422	189.821	50+
5.0%	756.154	0.279	0.107	40.552	50.284	821.869	50+

Table 9. UV protection of woolen fabrics dyed in water extract of European black elderberry berries (*Sambucus nigra)*

MORDANT	Mean UPF	τ UVA	τ UVB	Stand. Dev.	Stand. Err.	Calc. UPF	UV protection
Wool	32.070	7.634	2.194	1.069	1.326	30.744	30
No mordant	59.489	4.949	0.826	2.371	1.460	58.029	50+
Pre-treatment $KAl(SO_4)_2 \cdot 12H_2O$							
0.1%	856.997	0.167	0.107	76.302	94.689	762.307	50+
0.5%	743.963	0.193	0.124	185.664	230.223	513.739	50+
2.0%	482.273	0.275	0.189	96.842	120.084	362.181	50+
Pre-treatment $CuSO_4 \cdot 5H_2O$							
0.1%	399.652	0.366	0.314	245.563	304.498	95.154	50+
0.5%	164.585	0.616	0.567	10.381	12.872	151.677	50+
2.0%	439.309	0.349	0.309	289.529	359.016	80.293	50+

Table 9. (Continued)

MORDANT	Mean UPF	τ UVA	τ UVB	Stand. Dev.	Stand. Err.	Calc. UPF	UV protection
Pre-treatment $FeSO_4 \cdot 7H_2O$							
0.1%	847.995	0.143	0.112	161.190	199.876	648.119	50+
0.5%	279.710	0.394	0.347	60.479	74.994	204.717	50+
2.0%	952.089	0.119	0.102	49.075	60.853	891.236	50+
Pre-treatment $SnCl_2 \cdot 2H_2O$							
0.1%	740.017	0.179	0.139	247.636	307.068	432.949	50+
0.5%	735.046	0.181	0.140	245.511	304.433	430.613	50+
2.0%	996.544	0.102	0.100	3.978	4.933	991.612	50+

Since no UV-C radiation reaches the earth's surface due to absorption by oxygen and ozone in the upper atmosphere, the transmittance of ultraviolet including UV-A and UV-B through the fabrics was measured on transmission spectrometer Cary 50 (Varian). The ultraviolet transmittance spectra of the woolen fabric without dyeing and after mordating and dyeing with European black elderberry berries (*Sambucus nigra)* and European Ash bark (*Fraxinus excelsior)* was compared. As can be seen from Tables 7-9, there was a significant difference between the dyed fabrics and un-dyed one. Even thoug woolen fabric is the only one that absorbs radiation throughout the entire UV spectrum even when completely untreated due to its chemocal composition, it transmit 7.6 % of UV-A nad 2.2 % UV-B radiation, resulting in very good UV protection (UPF=32.070).

Dyeing with water extract of European Ash bark (*Fraxinus excelsior)* without mordant, results already in excellent UV protection (UPF=54.8). It is to point out that UV-B transmission is lower 50 %, whilst UV-A transmission only 30 %. As proved in cosmetics, dyeing with European black elderberry berries (*Sambucus nigra),* improve UV-B absorption for 63 %, and UV-A for 35 %, resulting in excellent UV protection (Highest class 50+).

From the Tables 7-9 it can be clearly seen that the values of spectral transmittance decrease with all mordants applied, resulting in excellent UV protection. However, it is possible to evaluate the influence of mordants to UV protection considering the mean UPF values. Considering mordant concentration, similar behaviour was noticed as for the color parameters. The concentration of 2 % of mordant was selected as optimal one. Therefore, these results are presented in Figure 10.

The best UV protection has been achieved applying $FeSO_4 \cdot 7H_2O$ as mordant resulting in UPF almost 1000. The reason for that is the lowest ligthness, suggesting darkest shade with the highest absorption of UV radiation what results in the lowest UV transmittion. The results of color parameters confirm that.

For the difference of color depth which was achieved if mordant was applied in pre-treatment; the significantly better UV protection was achieved if mordant was applied in after-treatment. Ibrahim et al. [101] research of UV-protective finishing of cotton knits by addition of the metal-oxide into the finishing bath. It resulted in better UV protection probably because of ligth scattering [89, 90, 102]. Considering the metal-oxides applied, UV protection was the next: Cu > Zr > Zn ≫ Al ≈ none. For that reason, if the metal salts were applied as mordants in after-treatment, it is to assume that ligth scattering form the fabric surface was higher, what led to better UV protection. In the case of mordating in after treatment dyed fabrics with water extract of Fraxinus excelsior, UV protection was next: Fe > Sn > Cu > Al, and significantly higher than if applied as pre-treatment. Again, the difference in chelating played an important role. It is to point out mordating with $SnCl_2 \cdot 2H_2O$ as well, which resulted in higher K/S values, and the highest UV protection as well.

Comparing the influence of European Ash bark (*Fraxinus excelsior)* and European black elderberry berries (*Sambucus nigra),* it can be seen that *Sambuctus nigra* gave off better UV protection.

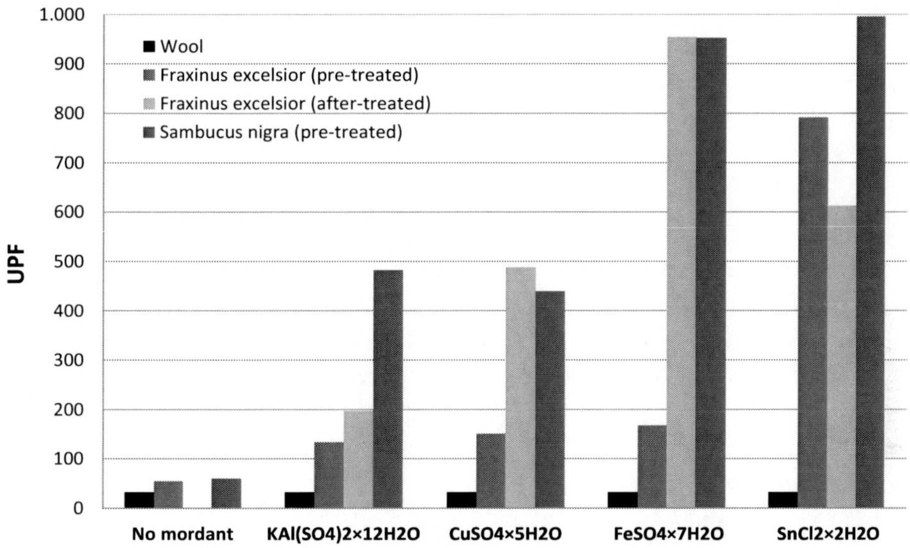

Figure 10. Mean UPF of woollen fabrics dyed with 2 % water extracts of *Fraxinus excelsior* and *Sambuctus nigra* pre-treated or after-treated with 4 different mordants.

CONCLUSION

In this chapter the UV protection by woolen fabric dyed with natural dyestuff extracted from European Ash bark (*Fraxinus excelsior)* and European black elderberry berries (*Sambucus nigra)* was researched. As most of natural dyes water extracts were applied on textiles in the combination with mordants - $KAl(SO_4)_2 \cdot 12H_2O$, $FeSO_4 \cdot 7H_2O$, $CuSO_4 \cdot 5H_2O$ and $SnCl_2 \cdot 2H_2O$. The woolen fabric was characetrized by its zeta potential and isoelectric point; therefore mordants were applied at pH 4.5. The active components, which are the most responsible for achieved colour hue, respectively for the forming of coloured chelates, were determined for the *Fraxinus excelsior* and *Sambucus nigra* by HPLC. Analyzed extracts contained flavonoids substances: quercetin dihydrate, isoquercitrin and rutin trihydrate. It was confirmed that the water based herbal extracts has got certain substantivity towards woolen substrates. The influence of a sort of the metal on a hue of a coloured complexes was confirmed by the color parameters on remission spectrophotometer determination. For $KAl(SO_4)_2 \cdot 12H_2O$ and $SnCl_2 \cdot 2H_2O$ as mordants, the yellow – orange hues were obtained, for $CuSO_4 \cdot 5H_2O$ orange – brown, and for the $FeSO_4 \cdot 7H_2O$ achromatic – chromatic olive green hues. In dependence to reactivity and property of forming the coloured chelates, the largest colour depth (K/S) was achieved using Fe^{2+} ions.

Since flavonoids and anthocyanosides have an important role in protecting against harmful effects of UV radiation the fabric UV protection was determined according to AS/NZS 4399:1996 *Sun Protective Clothing: evaluation and classification*, by UV-A and UV-B transmission measurement on transmission spectrophotometer and calculation of Ultraviolet protection factor (UPF). It was confirmed that woolen fabrics dyed with natural dyes, extracted from *Fraxinus excelsior* and *Sambucus nigra, ensure* excellent UV protection (UPF > 50). It is to point out that it offers protection against UVB radiation as well, and therefore it may reduce the risk of subsequent occurrence of skin cancer. In the case of application, it is to suggest European black elderberry berries (*Sambucus nigra),* which gave maximum UV protection (UPF=1000).

REFERENCES

[1] Taylor G. W. 1986. Natural dyes in textile applications, *Rev. Prog. Coloration,* 16: 53-61.

[2] Kumar, J.K., Sinha, A.K., 2004. Resurgence of natural colourants: a holistic view. *Nat. Prod. Res.* 18: 59-84

[3] Samanta, A.K., Agarwal, P., 2009. Application of natural dyes on textiles. *Indian J. Fibre Text. Res.* 34: 384-399.

[4] Islam, S. U.; M. Shahid, F. Mohammad. 2013. Perspectives for natural product based agents derived from industrial plants in textile applications – a review. *Journal of Cleaner Production* 57: 2-18.

[5] Shahid, M.; S. U. Islam, F. Mohammad. 2013. Recent advancements in natural dye applications: a review. *Journal of Cleaner Production* 53: 310-331.

[6] Schweppe H. 1992. Handbuch der Naturfarbstoffe. Vorkommen, Verwendung, Nachweis, ecomed, *Landsberg/Lech.*

[7] Sekar, N. 1999. Application of natural colourants to textiles – principles and limitations. *Colourage* 46(7): 33-34.

[8] Teli, M. D.; Paul, R.; Pardeshi, P. D. 2000. Natural Dyes: Classification, chemistry and extraction methods, Part – I: Chemical classes, extraction methods and future prospects. *Colourage.* 47 (12): 43-48.

[9] Guinot, P., Roge, A., Gargadennec, A., Garcia, M., Dupont, D., Lecoeur, E., Candelier, L., Andary, C. 2006. Dyeing plants screening: an approach to combine past heritage and present development. Color. Technol. 122: 93-101.

[10] Tušek, L., Golob, V. 1998. Natural Dyes in textile in history and today (Naravna barvila v tekstilstvu včasih in danes). *Tekstilec* 41(3-4): 75-83.

[11] Fakin D., D. Tepeš, A. Majcen le Marechal, A. Ojstršek, M. Božič. 2010. Dyeing of Wool with Plant Dyes and Sample Evaluation with CIE Colour System, *Tekstilec* 53(7–9): 179–193.

[12] Parac-Osterman, Đ.; Karaman, B.; Horvat, A.; Pervan, M. 2001. Dyeing Wool with Natural Dyes in the Ligth of Ethnological Heritage of Lika (Bojadisanje vune prirodnim bojilima u svjetlu etnografske baštine Like). *Tekstil* 50: 339-344.

[13] Sutlović, A.; Đ. Parac-Osterman, V. Đurašević. 2011. Croatian Traditional Herbal Dyes for Textile Dyeing; TEDI 1:65-69. Available at: http://www.ttf.unizg.hr/tedi/pdf/TEDI-1-1-65.pdf; accesed: 2014-12-12.

[14] Bird, C. L., Boston W. S. 1975. The Theory of coloration of textiles. *Dyers Company Publications Trust,* Bradford.

[15] Zollinger, H. Color Chemistry. 1987. Syntheses, Properties and Applications of Organic Dyes and Pigments. VCH, New York.

[16] Goodwin, J. 1990. A Dyer's Manual. Pelham books, *Stephen Greene Press,* Middlesex

[17] Doran, A. 1993. Latest developments in the low-temperature dyeing of wool with 1:2 matal-complex and milling acid dyes. *JSDC* 109 (1): 15-20.

[18] Engeler, E. 1997. Wollfarbstoff – Gammen und ihr ökologisches Umfeld. *Texilveredlung* 32 (7-8): 156-161.

[19] Imming, P.; Zentgraf, M.; Imhof, I. 2000. Welche Farbe hatte der antike Purpur?. *Texilveredlung* 35 (9-10): 22-24.

[20] Grdenić, D. 2002. Purpur i grimiz. *Priroda,* 6-8.

[21] Pötsch, W. R. 2002. Naturfarbstoffherstellung aus Waidpflanzen: Gesank als Qualitätsmerkmal. *Melliand Textilberichte* 83 (3): 170-171.

[22] Lokhande, H. T.; Dorugade, V. A.; Sandeep R. N. 1998. Applicaton of Natural Dyes on Polyester. *American Dyestuff Reporter* 87 (9): 40-50.

[23] Samanta, A. K.; Singhee, D.; Sethia, M. 2003. Application of single and mixture of selected natural dyes on cotton fabric: A scientific approach. *Colourage* 50(10): 29-42.

[24] Ansari, A. A.; Thakur, B. D. 2000. Extraction, characterisation and application of a natural dye: The eco-friendly textile colorant. *Colourage* 47(7): 15-20.

[25] Grotewold, E. 2006. The Science of Flavonoids. *Springer.*

[26] Hofenk de Graaff, J.H. 2004. The Colourful Past: Origins, Chemistry, and identification of Natural Dyestuffs, Archetype Publications, Ltd., London, *Abegg-Stiftung,* Riggisberg.

[27] Nemeth E. Colouring (Dye) Plants. In Cultivated Plants, Primarly as Food Sources – Vol. II. EOLSS (Encyclopedia of Life Support Systems), available at: http://www.eolss.net/Sample-Chapters/C10/E5-02-05-08.pdf; accesed: 2014-11-12.

[28] Bechtold, T., Mussak, R. 2009. Handbook of Natural Colorants, *John Wiley and Sons,* Ltd. UK.

[29] Samanta, A. K., Konar, A. 2011. Dyeing of Textiles with Natural Dyes. In Natural Dyes, InTech, pp. 29-56. Available at: http://www.intechopen.com /books/natural-dyes/dyeing-of-textiles-with-natural-dyes, accessed: 2014-06-19.

[30] Bechtold T., A. Mahmud-Ali, R.A. M. Mussak. 2007. Reuse of ash-tree (Fraxinus excelsior L.) bark as natural dyes for textile dyeing: process conditions and process. *Coloration Technology* 123 (4): 271-279.

[31] Đorđević, D., Šmelcerović, M.; Tarbuk, A. 2009. Environmental-Friendly Cotton Fabric Finishing by Alcohol Extract of Hibiscus Flowers. *Proceedings of VIIIth Symposium, Tehnološki fakultet, Leskovac;* 226-232.

[32] Kovačević, Z; A. Sutlović, S. Bischof. 2014. Spartium Junceum L. as a Natural Dyestuff for Wool Dyeing. Book of *Proceedings 7th International Textile, Clothing & Design Conference – Magic World of Textiles, University of Zagreb, Faculty of Textile Technology, Zagreb;* 220-225.

[33] Kechi, A. R.B. Chavan, R. Moeckel. 2013. Dye Yield, Color Strength and Dyeing Properties of Natural Dyes Extracted from Ethiopian Dye Plants. *Textiles and Light Industrial Science and Technology* 2(3): 137-145.

[34] Baishya, D., J. Talukdar, S. Sandhya S. 2012. Cotton Dyeing with Natural Dye Extracted from Flower of Bottlebrush (Callistemon citrinus), Universal Journal of Environmental Research and Technology 2(5): 377-382.

[35] Deo H. T, Desai B. K. 1999. Dyeing cotton and jute with tea as a natural dye, *J. Soc. Dyers Color.* 115(7-8): 224-227.

[36] Bhattacharya N, Doshi B. A., Sahasrabudhe A. S. 1998. Dyeing jute with natural dyes, *Am. Dyst. Rep.,* 87(4): 26-29.

[37] Nishida K, Kobayashi K. 1992. Dyeing properties of natural dyes from vegetable sources, Part II, *Am. Days. Rep.* 81(9): 26-30.

[38] Kazaić, S. 2004. Antioxydative and antiradical activity of flavonoids. *Archives. of Industrial Hygiene and Toxicology* 55(4): 279-290.

[39] Malešev, D.; Kuntić, V. 2007. Investigation of metal-falvonoid chelates and the determination of flavonoids via matel-falvonoid complexing reactions *Serbian Soc. Chem. Ind. Jour.* 72(10): 921-939.

[40] Cornard, J. P.; Boudet, A. C.; Merlin, J. C. 2001. Complexes of Al(III) with 3′4′-dihydroxy-flavone: characterization, theoretical and spectroscopic study. *Spectrochemica Acta Part A* 57(3): 591-602.

[41] Raj Narayana, K.; Sripal Reddy, M.; Chaluvadi, M. R.; Krishna D. R. Bioflavonoids classification, pharmacological, biochemical effects and therapeutic potential. *Indian Journal of Pharmacology*, 2001, 33 (1), 2-16

[42] R.F. V. de Souza, E.M. Sussuchi, W. F. De Giovani. 2003. Synthesis, Electrochemical, Spectral, and Antioxidant Properties of Complexes of Flavonoids with Metal Ions. *Synthesis and Reactivity in Inorganic and Metal-Organic Chemistry* 33(7): 1125-1144.

[43] Kasiri, M.B., S. Safapour. 2014. Natural dyes and antimicrobials for green treatment of textiles, *Environ Chem Lett* 12: 1-13.

[44] Mirjalili, M., Nazarpoor, K., Karimi, L., 2011. Eco-friendly dyeing of wool using natural dye from weld as co-partner with synthetic dye. *J. Clean. Prod.* 19: 1045-1051.

[45] Yusuf, M., Shahid, M., Khan, M.I., Khan, S.A., Khan, M.A., Mohammad, F. 2011. Dyeing studies with henna and madder: a research on effect of tin (II) chloride mordant. *J. Saudi Chem. Soc.,* available at: http://dx.doi.org/10.1016/j.jscs.2011.12.020, accesed: 2014-12-12.

[46] Robinson, T.; Chandran, B.; Nigam, P. 2002. Removal of dyes from a synthetic textile dye effluent by biosorption on apple pomace and wheat straw. *Water Res.* 36(11): 2824-2830.

[47] Talreja, D.; Talreja, P.; Mathur, M. 2003. Eco-friendliness of natural dyes. *Colourage* 50(7): 35-44.

[48] Singh, R.; Jain, A.; Panwar, S.; Gupta, D.; Khare, S. K. 2005. Antimicrobial activity of some natural dyes. *Dyes and Pigments* 66(2): 99-102.

[49] Kosalec, I.; Pepeljnjak, S.; Bakmaz, M.; Vladimir-Knežević, S. 2005. Flavonoid analysis and antimicrobial activity of commercially available propolis products. *Acta Pharm.* 55(4): 423-430.

[50] Yusuf M., M. Shahid, S.A. Khan, M.I. Khan, S.U. Islam, F. Mohammad, M.A. Khan. 2013. Eco-Dyeing of Wool Using Aqueous Extract of the Roots of Indian Madder (Rubia cordifolia) as Natural Dye. *Journal of Natural Fibers* 10(1): 14-28.

[51] Yusuf, M., Ahmad, A., Shahid, M., Khan, M.I., Khan, S.A., Manzoor, N., Mohammad, F. 2012. Assessment of colorimetric, antibacterial and antifungal properties of woollen yarn dyed with the extract of the leaves of henna (Lawsonia inermis). *J. Clean. Prod.* 27: 42-50.

[52] Šmelcerović M., Mizdraković M., Đorđević D. 2007. Environmental-friendly wool fabric finishing by some water plant extracts. *Serbian Soc. Chem. Ind. Jour.* 61(5): 251-256.

[53] Šmelcerović M., D. Đorđević, A. M. Grancarić. 2009. Spectral properties of cotton fabric treated with marigold flowers water extract. *Zbornik radova Tehnološkog fakulteta u Leskovcu* 19: 315-321.

[54] Šmelcerović, M.; Đorđević, D.; Grancarić, A. M.; Tarbuk, A. 2009. Ecological Finishing of Woolen Fabric with Extracts of Marigold, St.-John's-Wart and Hibiscus Plants. *Book of Proceedings of 2nd Scientific-Professional Symposium Textile Science & Economy. University of Zagreb, Faculty of Textile Technology,* Zagreb, 163-166.

[55] Gupta, D., Jain, A., Panwar, S., 2005. Anti-UV and anti-microbial properties of some natural dyes on cotton. Indian J. Fibre Text. Res. 30: 190-195.

[56] Ibrahim N. A., S. Zhang, M. R. El-Zairy, H. A. Ghazal. 2013. Enhancing the UV-protection and Antibacterial Properties of Polyamide-6 Fabric by Natural Dyeing. *Textiles and Light Industrial Science and Technology* (TLIST) 2(1): 36-41.

[57] Sarkar, A.K., 2004. An evaluation of UV protection imparted by cotton fabrics dyed with natural colorant. *BMC Dermatol.* 4: 15.

[58] Feng, X.X., Zhang, L.L., Chen, J.Y., Zhang, J.C., 2007. New insights into solar UVprotective properties of natural dye. *J. Clean. Prod.* 15: 366-372.

[59] Grifoni, D., Bacci, L., Zipoli, G., Carreras, G., Baronti, S., Sabatini, F. 2009. Laboratory and outdoor assessment of UV protection offered by flax and hemp fabrics dyed with natural dyes. *Photochem. Photobiol.* 85: 313-320.

[60] Grifoni, D., Bacci, L., Zipoli, G., Albanese, L., Sabatini, F. 2011. The role of natural dyes in the UV protection of fabrics made of vegetable fibres. *Dyes Pigm.* 91: 279-285

[61] Mongkholrattanasit, R., Krystufek, J., Wiener, J. 2010. Dyeing and fastness properties of natural dyes extracted from eucalyptus leaves using padding techniques. *Fiber. Polym.* 11: 346-350.

[62] Mongkholrattanasit, R., Krystufek, J., Wiener, J., Vikova, M. 2011. Dyeing, fastness, and UV protection properties of silk and wool fabrics dyed with eucalyptus leaf extract by the exhaustion process. *Fibres Text. East. Eur.* 19(3): 94-99.

[63] Mongkholrattanasit, R., Krystufek, J., Wiener, J., Vikova, M. 2011. UV protection properties silk fabric dyed with eucalyptus leaf extract. *J. Text. Inst.* 102(3): 272-279.

[64] Hustvedt G., P. Cox Crews. 2005. The Ultraviolet Protection Factor of Naturally-pigmented Cotton. *The Journal of Cotton Science* 9: 47–55.

[65] Hou, X., Chen, X., Cheng, Y., Xu, H., Chen, L., Yang, Y. 2013. Dyeing and UV protection properties of water extracts from orange peel. *J. Clean. Prod.* 52: 410-419.

[66] Dev, V.R.G., Venugopal, J., Sudha, S., Deepika, G., Ramakrishna, S., 2009. Dyeing and antimicrobial characteristics of chitosan treated wool fabrics with henna dye. *Carbohydr. Polym.* 75, 646-650.

[67] Raja, A.S.M., Thilagavathi, G. 2011. Influence of enzyme and mordant treatments on the antimicrobial efficacy of natural dyes on wool materials. *Asian J. Text* 1: 138-144.

[68] Popescu A., L. Chirila; C. P. Ghituleasa; C. Hulea; M. Vamesu. 2014. Influence of enzyme pre-treatments on natural dyeing of proteinic substrates. *Annals of the University of Oradea, Fascicle of Textiles, Leatherwork* 15(1): 83-88.

[69] Ghoranneviss, M., Shahidi, S., Anvari, A., Motaghi, Z., Wiener, J., Slamborova, I., 2011. Influence of plasma sputtering treatment on natural dyeing and antibacterial activity of wool fabrics. *Prog. Org. Coat* 70: 388-393.

[70] Chen, C., Chang, W.Y., 2007. Antimicrobial activity of cotton fabric pretreated by microwave plasma and dyed with onion skin and onion pulp extractions. *Indian J. Fibre Text. Res.* 32: 122-125.

[71] Tarbuk, A., A. M. Grancarić, D. Đorđević, M. Šmelcerović. 2009. Adsorption of Plant Extracts on Cationized Cotton. *Zbornik radova Tehnološkog fakulteta u Leskovcu* 19: 257-264.

[72] Đorđević, D., Tarbuk, A., Grancarić, A. M., Šmelcerović, M. 2009. Ecological Finishing of Cationized Cotton Fabric with Extracts of Marigold, St.-John's- Wart and Hibiscus Plants, *Proceedings of 9th AUTEX Conference, Ege Univresity, Izmir,* 1441-1446.

[73] Hong, K.H., Bae, J.H., Jin, S.R., Yang, J.S., 2012. Preparation and properties of multifunctionalized cotton fabrics treated by extracts of gromwell and gallnut. *Cellulose* 19: 507-515.

[74] Sathiyanarayanan, M.P., Bhat, N.V., Kokate, S.S., Walnuj, V.E., 2010. Antibacterial finish for cotton fabric from herbal products. *Indian J. Fibre Text. Res.* 35: 50-58.

[75] Armstrong, B. K., Kricker, A. 1993. How much melanoma is caused by sun exposure? *Melanoma Res* 3(6): 395-401.

[76] Šitum M. 2012. Melanoma. Chapter 57 in Guidliness in common dermatoses and skin cancers diagnostics and treatments (in Croatian: Smjernice u dijagnostici i liječenju najčešćih dermatoza i tumora kože). *Naklada Slap, Jastrebarsko.*

[77] Tarbuk, A., Grancarić A. M., Šitum, M., Martinis M. 2010. UV Clothing and Skin Cancer. *Collegium Antropologicum.* 34(Suppl. 2): 179-183.

[78] Hoffmann, K., Laperre, J., Avermaete, A., Altmeyer, P., Gambichler, T. 2001. Defined UV protection by apparel textiles. *Arch Dermatol.* 137(8): 1089-1094.

[79] Reinert, G., Fuso, F., Hilfiker, R., Schmidt, E. 1997. UV-protecting properties of textile fabrics and their improvement. *Textile Chemist and Colorist* 29(12): 36-43.

[80] Gies, P. H., Roy, C. R., Toomey, S., Mclennan, A. 1998. Protection against solar ultraviolet radiation. *Mutation Research* 422: 15-22.

[81] Grancarić, A. M., Tarbuk, A., Dumitrescu, I., Bišćan J. 2006. UV Protection of Pretreated Cotton – Influence of FWA's Fluorescence. *AATCC Review* 6(4): 44-48.

[82] Tarbuk, A., Grancarić, A.M., Jančijev, I., Sharma, S. 2006. Protection against UV radiation using a modified polyester fabric. *Tekstil* 55(8): 383-394.

[83] Hilfiker, R., Kaufmann, W., Reinert, G., Schmidt, E. 1996. Improving sun protection factors of fabrics by applying UV- absorbers. *Text. Res. J.* 66(2): 61-70.

[84] Algaba, I., Riva, A., Cox Crews, P. 2004. Influence of Fiber Type and Fabric Porosity on the UPF of Summer Fabrics. *AATCC Review* 4(2):26-31.

[85] Grancarić, A.M., Penava, Ž., Tarbuk, A. 2005. UV Protection of Cotton – the Influence of Weaving Structure. *Serbian Soc. Chem. Ind. Jour.* 59(9-10): 230-234.

[86] Saravanan, D. 2007. UV protection textile materials. *AUTEX Research Journal* 7(1): 53-62.

[87] Zhou Y., Cox Crews P. 1998. Effect of OBAs and repeated launderings on UVR transmission through fabrics. *Textile Chemist and Colorist* 30(11): 19-24.

[88] Dekanić, T., Pušić, T., Soljačić I. 2014. Impact of artificial light on optical and protective effects of cotton after washing with detergent containing fluorescent compounds, *Tenside Surf. Det.* 51(5): 451-459.

[89] Farouk, A., Textor, T. Schollmeyer, E. Tarbuk, A. Grancarić, A. M. 2010. Sol-gel Derived Inorganic-organic Hybrid Polymers Filled with ZnO Nanoparticles as Ultraviolet Protection Finish for Textiles, *AUTEX research journal* 10(8): 58-63.

[90] Grancarić, A. M., Tarbuk, A., Kovaček, I. 2009. Nanoparticles of Activated Natural Zeolite on Textiles for Protection and Therapy, *Chem. Ind. & Chem. Engineering Quarterly*. 15(4): 203-210.

[91] Sundaresan, K., Sivakumar A., Vigneswaran, C., Ramachandran, T. 2012. Influence of nano titanium dioxide finish, prepared by sol-gel technique, on the ultraviolet protection, antimicrobial, and self-cleaning characteristics of cotton fabrics. *Journal of Industrial Textiles* 41(3): 259-277.

[92] Jarzycka A., Lewińska A., Gancarz R., Wilk K.A. 2013. Assessment of extracts of Helichrysum arenarium, Crataegus monogyna, Sambucus nigra in photoprotective UVA and UVB; photostability in cosmetic emulsions. *J Photochem Photobiol B.* 128: 50-7.

[93] Grancarić, A. M., Tarbuk, A., Pušić, T. 2005. Electrokinetic Potential of Some of the Most Important Textile Fabrics; *Coloration Technology* 121(4): 221-227.

[94] Sutlović, A. Study of Natural Dyestuff – Contribution to Human Ecology, Doctoral dissertation.University of Zagreb, Faculty of Textile Technology, Zagreb, July 2008.

[95] Häkkinen, S. Flavonols and Phenolic Acids in Berries and Berry Products. Doctoral dissertation, University of Kuopio, Kuopio, 2000

[96] Kananykhina, E. N.; Pilipenko I.V. 2000. Characteristics of the pigments from anthocyan-containing food plants, raw material for production of bioflavonoid dyes, *Chemistry of Natural Compounds* 36(2): 148-151.

[97] Bai Y, Song F, Chen M, Xing J, Liu Z, Liu S. 2004. Characterization of the rutin-metal complex by electrospray ionization tandem mass spectrometry. *Anal Sci.* 20(8): 1147-1151.

[98] Amić, D.; Davidović-Amić, D.; Bešlo, D.; Trinajstić, N. 2003. Structure-Radical Scavenging Activity Relationships of Flavonoids. *Croatica Chem. Acta* 76(1): 55-61.

[99] Dalby, G. 1993. Greener mordants for natural coloration. JSDC 109(1): 8-9.

[100] Glover, B.; Pierce, J. H. 1993. Are natural colorants good for your health? *JSDC* 109(1): 5-7.

[101] Ibrahim N. A., M. Gouda, Sh. M. Husseiny, A. R. El-Gamal, F. Mahrous. 2009. UV-protecting and antibacterial finishing of cotton knits. *Journal of Applied Polymer Science* 112(6): 3589-3596.

[102] Grancarić, A. M., A. Tarbuk, L. Botteri. 2014. Light Conversion and Scattering in UV Protective Textiles. *AUTEX research journal.* 14(4): 247-258.

In: Sunscreens
Editors: Sean Henry Sharp

ISBN: 978-1-63482-160-5

Chapter 8

LIGHT CONVERSION FOR UV PROTECTION BY TEXTILE FINISHING AND CARE

Tihana Dekanić, Anita Tarbuk*, Tanja Pušić, Ana Marija Grancarić and Ivo Soljačić
University of Zagreb, Faculty of Textile Technology,
Department of Textile Chemistry and Ecology, Zagreb, Croatia

ABSTRACT

The incidence of skin cancer is increasing by epidemic proportions. Its primary cause is a long exposure to solar ultraviolet (UV) radiation crossed with the amount of skin pigmentation in the population. It is believed that in childhood and adolescence 80 % of UV-R gets absorbed, whilst in the remaining 20 % gets absorbed later in the lifetime. This suggests that proper and early photoprotection may reduce the risk of subsequent occurrence of skin cancer. Textile and clothing can show UV protection, but in the most cases it does not provide full sun screening properties. UV protection highly depends on large number of factors such are type of fiber, fabric surface and construction, type and concentration of dyestuff, fluorescent whitening agent (FWA), UV-B protective agents, as well as nanoparticles, if applied. Based on electronically-excited state by energy of UV-R (usually 340-370 nm) the molecules of FWAs show the phenomenon of fluorescence giving to white textiles high whiteness of outstanding brightness by reemitting the energy at the blue region (typically 420-470 nm) of the spectrum, what leads to better UV protection. Molecules of UV absorbers are able to absorb the damaging UV-R range of 290 nm to 360 nm, and convert it into harmless heat energy. Latest research declares that FWA's and UV absorbers can be applied in textile care – washing process as well. Therefore, the UV protective properties of cotton and cotton/polyester blend fabrics achieved by light conversion in textile finishing and care was researched in this chapter. For that purpose, three stilbene derivative fluorescent compounds were selected – fluorescent whitening agent commonly used in textile finishing, the other one used in detergent formulations, and UV absorber. In textile finishing process fluorescent compounds were applied by exhaustion procedure in wide

* Corresponding address: Prilaz baruna Filipovića 28a, HR-10000 Zagreb, Croatia. E-mail: anita.tarbuk@ttf.hr, tpusic@ttf.hr.

concentration range. In textile care fluorescent compounds were applied through 9 washing cycles at 60°C with standard ECE reference detergent and commercial detergent. UV protection was determined *in vitro* through Ultraviolet protection factor, UPF. Additionally the influence to fabric whiteness was researched. Since the fabric properties change in wet state, the discrepancy in whiteness and UV protection was research in distilled water as well as Adriatic Sea water.

Keywords: UV protection, Cotton, polyester/cotton blend, FWA, UV absorber, Wet state

INTRODUCTION

The incidence of skin cancer is increasing by epidemic proportions. Basal cell cancer remains the most common skin neoplasm, and simple excision is generally curative. On the other hand, aggressive local growth and metastasis are common features of malignant melanoma, which accounts for 75 percent of all deaths associated with skin cancer [1]. The reason for that is most likely that in the most cases melanoma was diagnosed in an advanced stage. The back sides in men and women, as well as the lower limbs in women, are the most common site for melanomas [2, 3]. The primary cause of skin cancer is believed to be a long exposure to solar ultraviolet (UV) radiation crossed with the amount of skin pigmentation in the population [1-6]. Melanoma incidence rates in white populations increase with proximity to the Equator, and vary across Europe, with the highest rates for both sexes in Switzerland, Denmark, Norway, Sweden and the Netherlands and the lowest rates in Central and Southeastern Europe [1].

UV as a whole does not exceed 5% of the total energy emitted by the sun, but their impact on the organic molecules is very important and it induces significant physiological responses in all areas of life. In addition to some beneficial effects of UV radiation (UV-R; wavelengths from 100 nm to 400 nm) on skin it may cause skin and eye damage, especially during the summer time (UV-C). The UV-C radiation (from 100 nm to 280 nm) is absorbed by atmosphere. However, diminishing of the Earth´s atmospheric ozone layer raised the UV exposure health risk, since both, UV-B (from 280 nm to 320 nm) and UV-A (from 320 nm to 400 nm) radiation, are reaching the Earth. Dangerous UV-B rays can cause acute and chronic reactions and damages such as erythema (sunburn), sun tanning, "photoaging", DNA and eye damage, photokeratitis and cataract, and photocarcinogenesis; increase risk factor for melanoma, or cause various skin cancers [3,6-33]. Experts estimate about 90 % of melanomas are associated with severe UV exposure and sunburns over a lifetime. Intermittent sun exposure, especially in childhood and adolescence is considered to be a stronger risk factor for melanoma than continuous exposure [1]. It is believed that in that period of life 80 % of UV-R gets absorbed, whilst in the remaining 20 % gets absorbed later in the lifetime. This suggests that proper and early photoprotection may reduce the risk of subsequent occurrence of skin cancer [2].

Textile and clothing are the most suitable interface between environment and human body. It can show UV protection, but in the most cases it does not provide full sun screening properties. Literature sources claim that only 1/3 of the spring and summer collections tested give off proper UV protection [11]. In contact with textile fabric, UV radiation can be reflected and/or scattered from fabric surface, or get absorbed or transmitted (Figure 1).

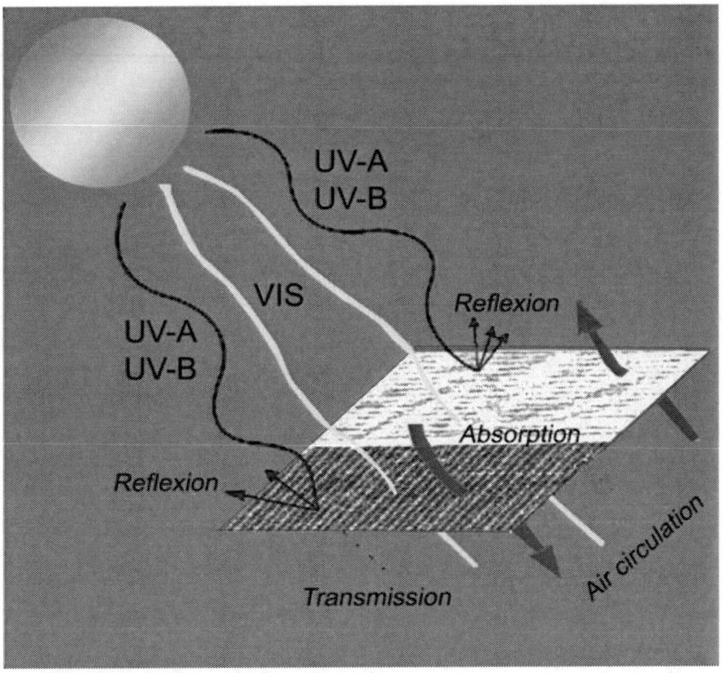

Figure 1. UV radiation in contact with textile fabric [28].

A good fabric UV protection depends on a large number of factors, such as, the type of fiber, fabric surface and construction, porosity, density, moisture content, type and concentration of dyestuff, fluorescent whitening agent (FWA), UV-B protective agents, as well as nanoparticles, if applied [13-37]. For example, polyester fabric gives off better UV protection than cellulose one, due to the polyester benzene rings [17, 30].

Fluorescent whitening agents (FWAs), commonly used for reaching higher whiteness degrees, are chemical compounds that absorb UV-R (usually 340-370 nm), show the phenomenon of fluorescence, and re-emit in the blue region (typically 420-470 nm) of the spectrum.

When P. Krais in 1929 discovered fluorescent compound *Aesculin* by water extraction from wild chestnut, he wrote “About the new white ...“. It was the new white indeed, never seen before such high whiteness degree. However, he could never assume that this UV-A absorption of FWA’s would result in better UV protection as well [6, 15-17, 26, 30, 32]. The phenomenon of fluorescence can be explained by modified diagram according Jablonski (Figure 2) [38].

The molecules of FWAs go to electronically-excited state by absorbing energy of UV-R. An electronically-excited molecule can lose its energy by emission of radiation which is known as “luminescence”. In this case, the emission is fluorescence, which is, according to Figure 2, an emission process occurring from lowest excited state (S_1) to the ground state (S_0). The frequency of fluorescence radiation is lower than that of excitation light (which is known Stokes Law). For the same compound an ideal emission should be the mirror image of the absorption band system [39].

Textile finishing agents for UV protection can be incorporated into the fiber matrix, or it can be applied to the surface of the fabric [3]. Usually sun protection effect is achieved through the use of UV absorbers [6, 16-18].

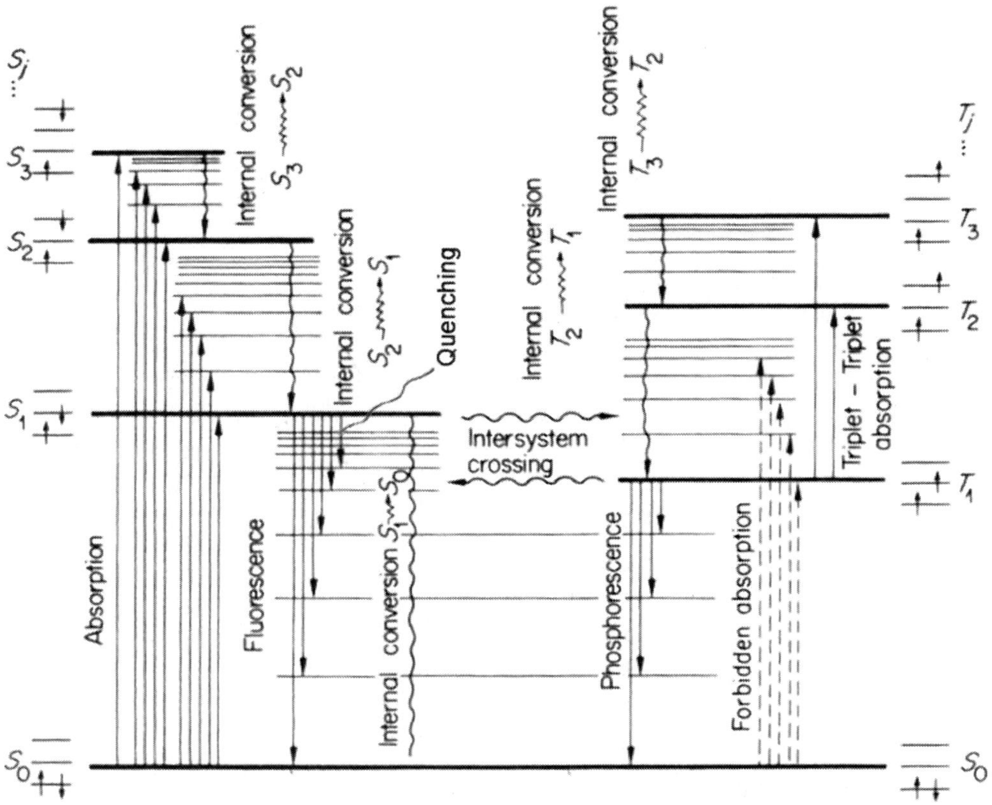

Figure 2. Modified Jablonski diagram [38].

UV absorbers are, as a matter of fact, a special type of fluorescent whitening agents and have the same or similar effect [6, 40]. Molecules of UV absorbers, such as benzotriazole and phenyl benzotriazole, are able to absorb the damaging UV-R range of 290 nm to 360 nm, and convert it into harmless heat energy. Therefore, they are even more effective than fluorescent whitening agents [3]. The impact of fluorescent whitening agents on the whiteness degree of cotton fabrics, as well as PES/cotton blends, in multiple washing cycles, has been comprehensively investigated together with the UV protection abilities. [26, 29-33]. Recently, there has been an systematic investigation of the UV absorber resistance to light since the final effect of fluorescent whitening agents is affected by the exposal to sunlight and by drying after washing. Exposing the materials treated with fluorescent compounds to sunlight can cause various photochemical reactions as they are prone to absorb UV radiation [32, 41].

Since the latest research declare that FWAs and UV absorbers can be applied in washing process as well, the UV protective properties of cotton and cotton/polyester blend fabrics achieved by light conversion in textile finishing and care was researched in this chapter. UV protection was determined *in vitro* through Ultraviolet protection factor, UPF. Additionally the influence to fabric whiteness was researched. Since the fabric properties change in wet state, the discrepancy in whiteness and UV protection was research in distilled water as well as Adriatic Sea water.

EXPERIMENTAL

Materials

Two fabrics, cotton (C) and polyester/cotton (65/35) blend (P/C), such are frequently used during summer time, were used in the investigation. Both fabrics were pre-bleached, in plain weave, with the following properties: Cotton fabric surface mass of 175.6 g/m^2 and yarn density of (warp/weft 25/25 yarns/cm), and P/C blend fabric surface mass 155.1 g/m^2 and yarn density of (warp/weft 26/25 yarns/cm).

Three fluorescent compounds of stilbene type were used (Table 1): one fluorescent whitening agent (FWA) commonly used in textile finishing (F1), one FWA commonly used in textile care in detergent formulation (F2), and UV absorber (F3).

Table 1. Characteristics and structural formula of applied fluorescent compounds

Compound characteristic	Structural formula
F1 Fluorescent whitening agent (FWA) - stilbene type CI Fluorescent Brightener 336 Uvitex BAM (Ciba-Geigy AG) For textile finishing	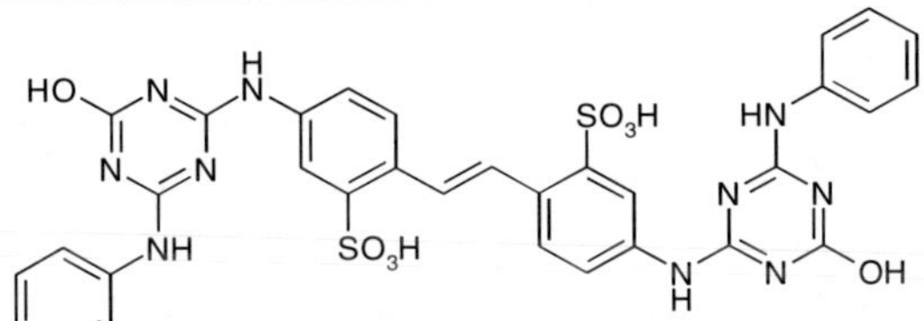 bis(4,4'-triazinylamino)-stilbene-2,2'-disulfonic acid derivative
F2 Fluorescent whitening agent (FWA) - stilbene type Optiblanc 2MG/LT Extra (Sigma 3V) In detergent formulation	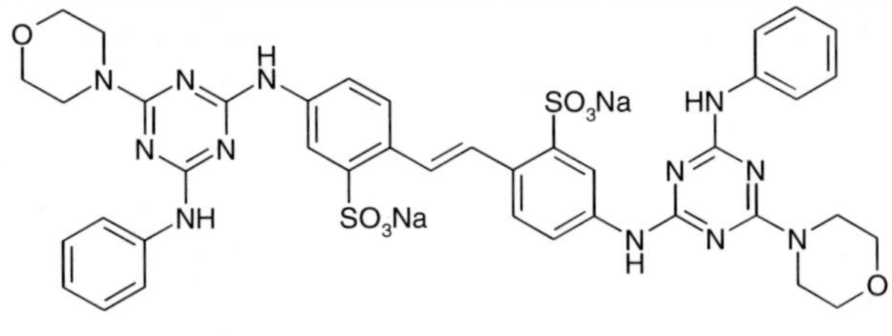 disodium 4.4’-bis[(4-anylino-6-morpholino-1.3.5-triazine-2-yl) amino]-stilbene-2.2’-disulphonate

F3 UV absorber - stilbene type Tinosorb FD (Ciba-Geigy AG)	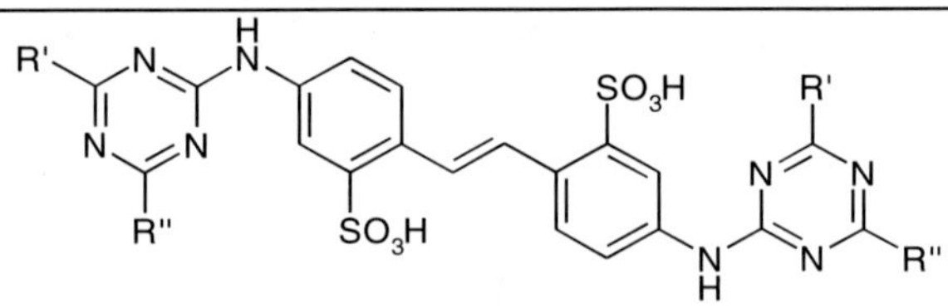 R', R'' - differently substituted amines stilbene disulphonic acid triazine derivative

Procedure

In this chapter, fluorescent compounds – two FWAs and UV absorber, all stilbene derivatives, were applied to cotton and cotton/polyester blend fabrics in textile finishing and care.

Textile Finishing

Fluorescent compounds were applied in wide concentration range (c_1 = 0.004 % owf (over weight of fiber); c_2 = 0.006 % owf; c_3 = 0.0125 % owf; c_4 = 0.1 % owf; c_5 = 0.5% owf; c_6 = 1 % owf, c_7 = 10 % owf, c_8 = 50 % owf) by exhaustion procedure at 60 °C for 30 minutes to achieve the best whiteness and UV protection. Afterwards, the discrepancy in whiteness and UV protection was research in distilled and Adriatic Sea water.

Textile Care - Laundering

In textile care fluorescent compounds were applied through 9 washing cycles with ECE reference detergent 77 for color fastness, without optical brightener, phosphate based, for application in ISO 105-C06:2010, ISO 6330:1984; and commercial detergent. Formulations of detergents are given in Table 2.

Table 2. Formulations of detergents

ECE reference detergent	Commercial detergent
- 8% Linear sodium alkyl benzene sulphonate (mean length of alkane chain $C_{11.5}$) - 2,9% Ethoxylated tallow alcohol (14 EO) - 3,5% Sodium soap, (chain length C_{12-16} 13% - 26% : C_{18-22} 74% - 87%) - 43,8% Sodium tripolyphosphate - 7,5% Sodium silicate (SiO_2:Na_2O = 3.3 : 1) - 1,9% Magnesium silicate - 1,2% Carboxy methyl cellulose (CMC) - 0,2% Etylene diamine tetra acetic acid, tetra sodium salt (TAED) - 21,2% Sodium sulphate - 9,8% Water *Added 1 g/l of sodium perborate	- 5% Anionic sufractant - 1% Nonionic sufractant - 2% Sodium soap - 20% Sodium tripolyphosphate - 5% Sodium silicate - 12% Sodium carbonate - 11% Sodium perborate - 1,2% Carboxy methyl cellulose (CMC) - 2% Etylene diamine tetra acetic acid, tetra sodium salt (TAED) - 0,6% Enzymes - up to 100 %: Sodium sulphate and Water

The samples were laundered in the Linitest apparatus, Original Hanau, in the bath of a 5 g/l of detergent. The laundering bath was prepared in the ratio of 1:15, heated from the initial temperature of 25°C for 15 minutes to 60°C. The fabrics were laundered at 60°C for 15 minutes up to 9 laundering cycles. The samples were rinsed and dried in a Scholl drier for 45 minutes at 40°C. For the purpose of better visibility and review of the results, only the results after the 1st, 3rd, 6th and 9th laundering cycle are presented. Laundering was done with the addition of fluorescent whitening agent and UV absorber in different concentration over weight of detergent. FWA was applied in concentrations of 0.08 %, 0.16 % and 0.25 %; UV absorber in concentration of 0.20 %, and in combination 0.10 % of each.

Methods

The fabric UV protection was determined according to AS/NZS 4399:1996 *Sun Protective Clothing: evaluation and classification.* UV-A and UV-B transmission through fabric were measured on Spectrophotometer Cary 50 (Varian). This instrument measures sunlight transmission in the range from 280 to 400 nm. The irradiation applied is a simulation of a part of sunlight spectrum, as measured at noon on January 17th 1990 in Melbourne, Australia, while the results obtained indicate the degree of protection offered by the fabric when worn directly to the skin.

The *ultraviolet protection factor* (*UPF*) was calculated automatically according to:

$$UPF = \frac{\sum_{\lambda=280}^{400} E(\lambda)\cdot\varepsilon(\lambda)\cdot\Delta\lambda}{\sum_{\lambda=280}^{400} E(\lambda)\cdot T(\lambda)\cdot\varepsilon(\lambda)\cdot\Delta\lambda} \qquad (1)$$

where:

$E(\lambda)$ = Solar radiation [W m^{-2} nm^{-1}]
$\varepsilon(\lambda)$ = relative erythemal spectral effectiveness
$T(\lambda)$ = spectrum permeability at wavelength λ
$\Delta\lambda$ = measured wavelength interval [nm]

UPF indicate the ability of fabrics to protect the skin against sun burning saying how much longer a person can stay in the sun with the fabric covering the skin as compared with the uncovered skin to obtain same erythemal response [3-20] According to the standards excellent protection is if UPF is higher 40 (Table 3). However, for the countries with UV index 7-10 as Mediterranean countries, Australia and USA, the UPF should be 15 times higher than UV index [17]. Therefore, it is recommended for people who spend eight hours in the open to use UV clothing with UPF between 105 and 150 if they want excellent UV protection.

Table 3. UV protection rating according to AS/NZS 4399:1996

UPF range	UPF rating	UV-R protection category	UV-R blocking [%]
< 14	0, 5, 10	non-rateable	<93,3
15-24	15, 20	good	93,3-95,8
25-39	25, 30, 35	very good	95,9-97,4
> 40	40, 45, 50, 50+	excellent	> 97,5

Remission spectrophotometer SF 600 PLUS CT (Datacolor) was used for measuring spectral characteristics of cotton and PES/cotton blend fabrics. CIE whiteness degree (W_{CIE}) was calculated automatically according to ISO 105-J02:1997 *Textiles - Tests for colour fastness - Part J02: Instrumental assessment of relative whiteness.* The discrepancy in wet state was determined through color differences of color coordinates according to:

$$\Delta E^*_{ab} = \left[(\Delta H^*)^2 + (\Delta L^*)^2 + (\Delta C^*)^2\right]^{\frac{1}{2}} \tag{2}$$

where ΔL* is change in lightness, ΔC* change in chroma and ΔH* change in hue.

The relative intensity of fluorescence (Φ_{rel}) was calculated from measured fluorescence on adapted spectrophotometer Specol SV (Carl Zeiss). Illuminant is high voltage Hg bulb (λ_{max} = 366 nm). Fluorescent Reference Standard (Datacolor) was used for $\Phi_{rel.\ standard} = 40$, with amplifying of 200x.

RESULTS AND DISCUSSION

The UV protective properties of cotton and cotton/polyester blend fabrics achieved by light conversion of fluorescent compounds applied in textile finishing and care was researched in this chapter. For that purpose, three stilbene derivatives fluorescent compounds were selected: FWA for cellulosic materials – one commonly used in textile finishing and the other in detergent formulations; and UV absorber. UV protection was determined *in vitro* through Ultraviolet protection factor, UPF. Additionally the influence to fabric whiteness was researched. Main characteristics of fabrics are collected in Table 4.

Table 4. Main characteristics of cotton (C) and polyester/cotton blend (P/C) fabrics: Mean UPF, UV-A and UV-B transmission, UV protection rating according to AS/NZS 4399:1996, CIE whiteness (W_{CIE}), relative intensity of fluorescence (Φ_{rel}), maximum of remission (R_{max}) and wavelength (λ_{max})

Fabric	**Mean UPF**	τ_{UVA}	τ_{UVB}	**UPF rating**
C	7.276	16.714	11.969	5: Non-rateable
P/C	18.426	17.148	3.289	15: Good
Fabric	W_{CIE}	Φ_{rel}	R_{max} [%]	λ_{max} [nm]
C	74.3	0	86.51	700
P/C	70.7	0	85.34	700

In textile finishing process fluorescent compounds were applied by exhaustion procedure in wide concentration range. Since the fabric properties change in wet state, the discrepancy in whiteness and UV protection was research in distilled water as well as Adriatic Sea water. The UV protective properties of cotton and PES/cotton blend fabric achieved by light conversion of fluorescent compounds are presented in Tables 5-7.

The discrepancy of UV protection in wet state by distilled (DW) and sea (SW) water is shown in Figures 3-8. Remission curves of cotton fabric treated with FWA - disodium 4.4'-bis[(4-anylino-6-morpholino-1.3.5-triazine-2-yl)amino]-stilbene-2.2'-disulphonate (F2) in wide concentration range as example of Stokes law are presented in Figure 9.

CIE whiteness (W_{CIE}), relative intensity of fluorescence (Φ_{rel}), maximum of remission (R_{max}) and wavelength (λ_{max}), and the discrepancy of whiteness in wet state of cotton fabrics treated with all fluorescent compounds are collected in Tables 8-13.

Table 5. Mean UPF, UV-A and UV-B transmission, and UV protection rating according to AS/NZS 4399:1996 of cotton and PES/cotton fabrics treated with fluorescent whitening agent - bis(4,4'-triazinylamino)-stilbene-2,2'-disulfonic acid derivative (F1)

Sample	Mean UPF	τ_{UVA}	τ_{UVB}	UPF rating	
C-F1-0,004	9,502	9,472	12,219	5	Non-rateable
C-F1-0,006	9,605	9,407	12,738	5	Non-rateable
C-F1-0,0125	9,379	9,501	11,251	5	Non-rateable
C-F1-0,1	14,005	6,490	5,513	10	Non-rateable
C-F1-0,5	16,219	5,635	4,005	15	Good
C-F1-1	30,061	3,230	2,032	30	Very good
C-F1-10	125,094	0,776	0,439	50+	Excellent
C-F1-50	203,793	0,503	0,333	50+	Excellent
P/C -F1-0,004	35,797	1,366	11,160	30	Very good
P/C -F1-0,006	35,493	1,517	10,231	30	Very good
P/C -F1-0,0125	36,606	1,504	10,185	30	Very good
P/C -F1-0,1	38,589	1,221	9,901	35	Very good
P/C -F1-0,5	45,006	1,383	5,862	45	Excellent
P/C -F1-1	45,122	1,526	4,899	45	Excellent
P/C -F1-10	62,291	1,258	2,883	50+	Excellent
P/C -F1-50	88,355	0,842	1,926	50+	Excellent

Table 6. Mean UPF, UV-A and UV-B transmission, and UV protection rating according to AS/NZS 4399:1996 of cotton and PES/cotton fabrics treated with fluorescent whitening agent - disodium 4.4'-bis[(4-anylino-6-morpholino-1.3.5-triazine-2-yl) amino]-stilbene-2.2'-disulphonate (F2)

Sample	Mean UPF	τ_{UVA}	τ_{UVB}	UPF rating	
C-F2-0,004	9,245	9,776	10,985	5	Non-rateable
C-F2-0,006	9,459	9,600	9,901	5	Non-rateable
C-F2-0,0125	9,690	9,539	8,468	5	Non-rateable
C-F2-0,1	18,578	5,179	2,673	15	Good

Table 6. (Continued)

Sample	Mean UPF	τ_{UVA}	τ_{UVB}	UPF rating	
C-F2-0,5	62,023	1,554	0,656	50+	Excellent
C-F2-1	63,339	1,589	0,585	50+	Excellent
C-F2-10	497,005	0,268	0,214	50+	Excellent
C-F2-50	548,558	0,208	0,158	50+	Excellent
P/C -F2-0,004	28,589	2,221	9,901	25	Very good
P/C -F2-0,006	31,578	1,833	10,012	30	Very good
P/C -F2-0,0125	32,950	1,552	11,193	30	Very good
P/C -F2-0,1	34,161	2,185	6,341	30	Very good
P/C -F2-0,5	66,276	1,607	0,651	40	Excellent
P/C -F2-1	180,311	0,660	0,291	50+	Excellent
P/C -F2-10	606,725	0,225	0,426	50+	Excellent
P/C -F2-50	98,540	0,836	1,408	50+	Excellent

Table 7. Mean UPF, UV-A and UV-B transmission, and UV protection rating according to AS/NZS 4399:1996 of cotton and PES/cotton fabrics treated with fluorescent UV absorber -stilbene disulphonic acid triazine derivative (F3)

Sample	Mean UPF	τ_{UVA}	τ_{UVB}	UPF rating	
C-F3-0,004	12,078	7,389	8,518	10	Non-rateable
C-F3-0,006	11,338	8,118	7,936	10	Non-rateable
C-F3-0,0125	11,022	8,151	9,663	10	Non-rateable
C-F3-0,1	37,246	2,649	2,667	20	Good
C-F3-0,5	90,434	1,057	0,984	50+	Excellent
C-F3-1	122,067	0,867	0,803	50+	Excellent
C-F3-10	424,074	0,260	0,285	50+	Excellent
C-F3-50	1000,000	0,100	0,100	50+	Excellent
P/C –F3-0,004	31,038	1,906	10,376	30	Very good
P/C –F3-0,006	33,758	1,714	9,321	30	Very good
P/C –F3-0,0125	34,136	1,679	9,896	30	Very good
P/C –F3-0,1	41,600	1,470	6,699	40	Excellent
P/C –F3-0,5	81,291	0,773	2,960	50+	Excellent
P/C –F3-1	70,671	1,040	2,671	50+	Excellent
P/C –F3-10	161,614	0,486	1,170	50+	Excellent
P/C –F3-50	160,207	0,536	1,105	50+	Excellent

In textile care fluorescent compounds were added to ECE referent detergent or commercial detergent. It was applied separately or in combination through 9 washing cycles at 60°C. The achieved UV protections of cotton and PES/cotton blend fabric are presented through Mean UPF, UV-A and UV-B transmission in Tables 14-17. CIE whiteness (W_{CIE}), relative intensity of fluorescence (Φ_{rel}), maximum of remission (R_{max}) and wavelength (λ_{max}) achieved by repeated laundering are shown in Tables 18-21.

The impact of fluorescent compounds – FWAs and UV absorber on the UV protection of cotton and polyester/cotton blend fabrics was monitored by the UV-A and UV-B transmission and UPF.

	C	F1-0,004	F1-0,006	F1-0,0125	F1-0,1	F1-0,5	F1-1	F1-10	F1-50
■ Dry	7,28	9,50	9,61	9,38	14,01	16,22	30,06	125,09	203,79
DW	3,79	4,31	4,03	4,37	5,68	7,95	11,02	75,11	713,58
■ SW	4,34	4,40	4,21	4,32	5,92	7,69	10,94	48,25	633,69

Figure 3. The discrepancy of UV protection in wet state by distilled (DW) and sea (SW) water of cotton fabric treated with FWA - bis(4,4'-triazinylamino)-stilbene-2,2'-disulfonic acid derivative (F1).

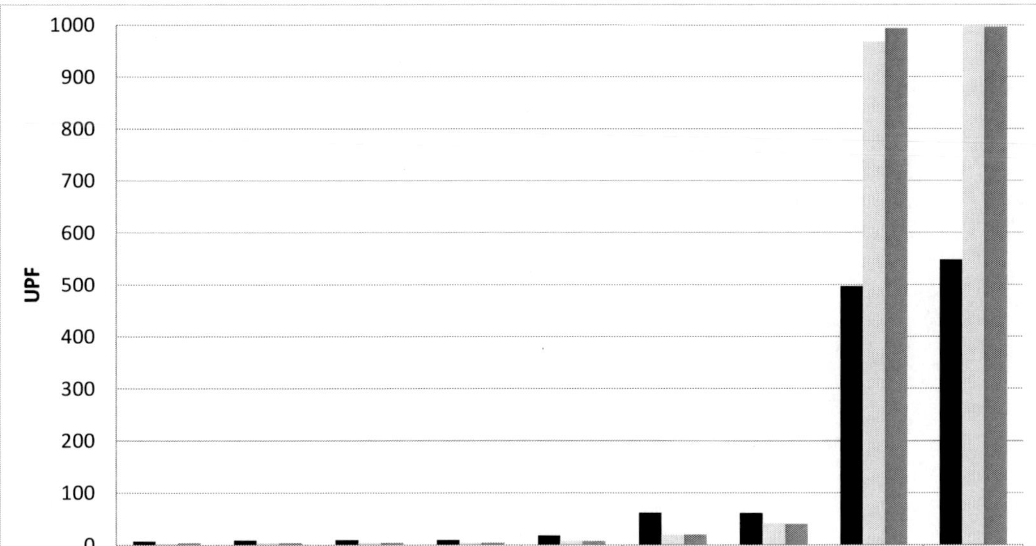

	C	F2-0,004	F2-0,006	F2-0,0125	F2-0,1	F2-0,5	F2-1	F2-10	F2-50
■ Dry	7,28	9,25	9,46	9,69	18,58	62,02	61,34	497,01	548,56
DW	3,79	4,35	4,20	4,32	7,74	18,87	41,65	967,38	1000,00
■ SW	4,34	4,24	4,50	4,48	7,75	20,19	40,20	993,92	996,99

Figure 4. The discrepancy of UV protection in wet state by distilled (DW) and sea (SW) water of cotton fabric treated with FWA - **disodium 4.4'**-bis[(4-anylino-6-morpholino-1.3.5-triazine-2-yl) amino]-stilbene-2.2'-disulphonate (F2).

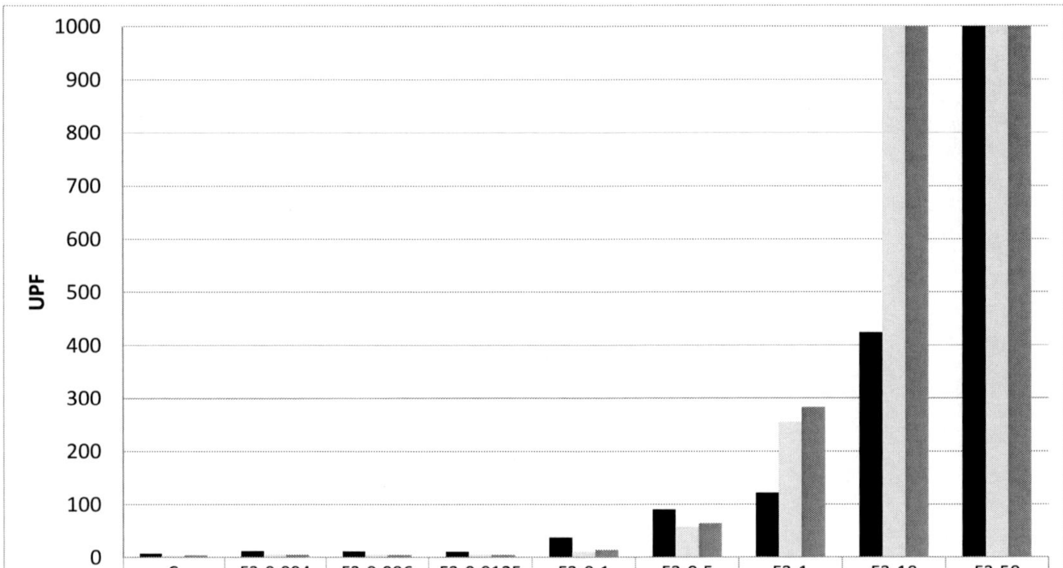

	C	F3-0,004	F3-0,006	F3-0,0125	F3-0,1	F3-0,5	F3-1	F3-10	F3-50
Dry	7,28	12,08	11,34	11,02	37,25	90,43	122,07	424,07	1000,00
DW	3,79	5,35	5,30	4,56	10,34	58,49	255,49	1000,00	1000,00
SW	4,34	5,32	4,78	5,05	14,49	64,24	282,84	999,70	1000,00

Figure 5. The discrepancy of UV protection in wet state by distilled (DW) and sea (SW) water of cotton fabric treated with UV absorber - stilbene disulphonic acid triazine derivative (F3).

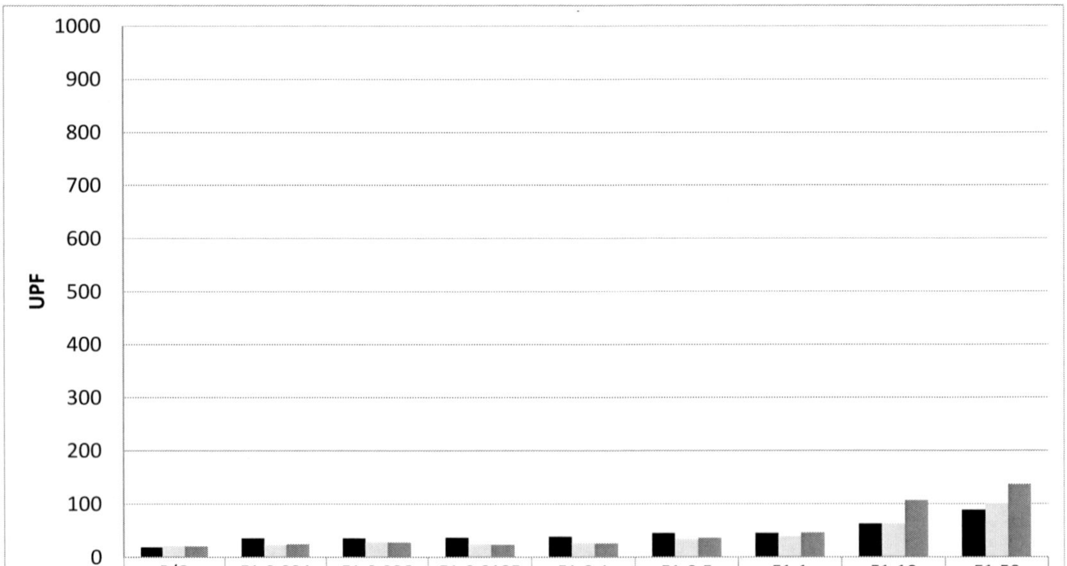

	P/C	F1-0,004	F1-0,006	F1-0,0125	F1-0,1	F1-0,5	F1-1	F1-10	F1-50
Dry	18,43	35,80	35,49	36,61	38,59	45,01	45,12	62,29	88,36
DW	20,58	22,53	27,54	24,44	27,27	32,98	39,93	62,49	100,96
SW	20,48	25,02	27,44	23,43	25,68	36,12	45,82	106,86	136,90

Figure 6. Discrepancy of UV protection in wet state – distilled (DW) and sea (SW) water of polyester/cotton blend fabric treated with fluorescent whitening agent - bis(4,4'-triazinylamino)-stilbene-2,2'-disulfonic acid derivative (F1).

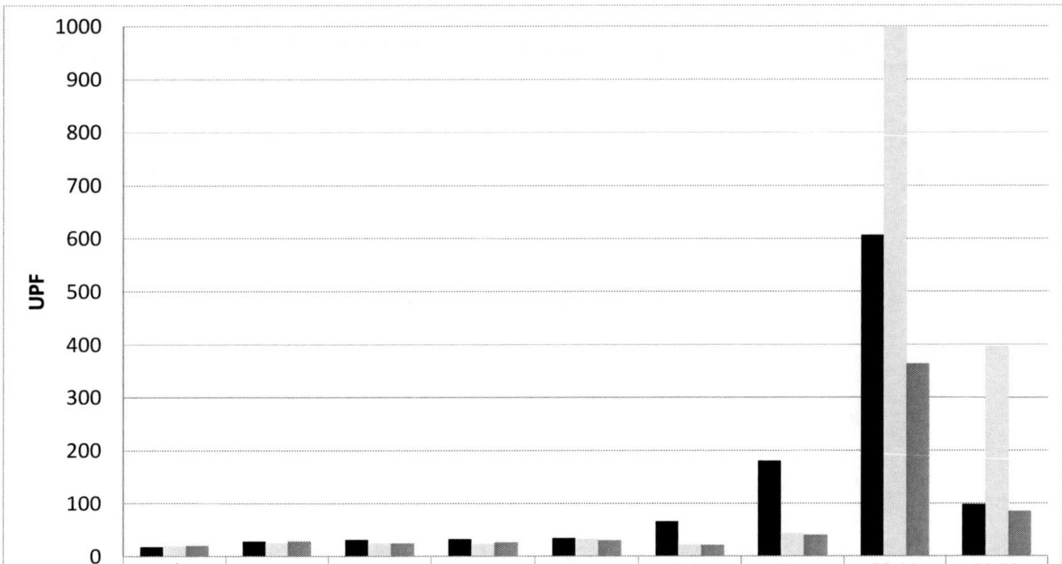

	P/C	F2-0,004	F2-0,006	F2-0,0125	F2-0,1	F2-0,5	F2-1	F2-10	F2-50
■ Dry	18,43	28,589	31,578	32,95	34,161	66,276	180,311	606,725	98,54
DW	20,58	24,66	24,63	24,31	31,98	22,20	43,92	1000,00	395,65
SW	20,48	29,14	24,49	26,46	30,23	21,74	40,21	364,71	85,73

Figure 7. The discrepancy of UV protection in wet state by distilled (DW) and sea (SW) water of polyester/cotton fabric treated with FWA - **disodium** 4.4'-bis[(4-anylino-6-morpholino-1.3.5-triazine-2-yl) amino]-stilbene-2.2'-disulphonate (F2).

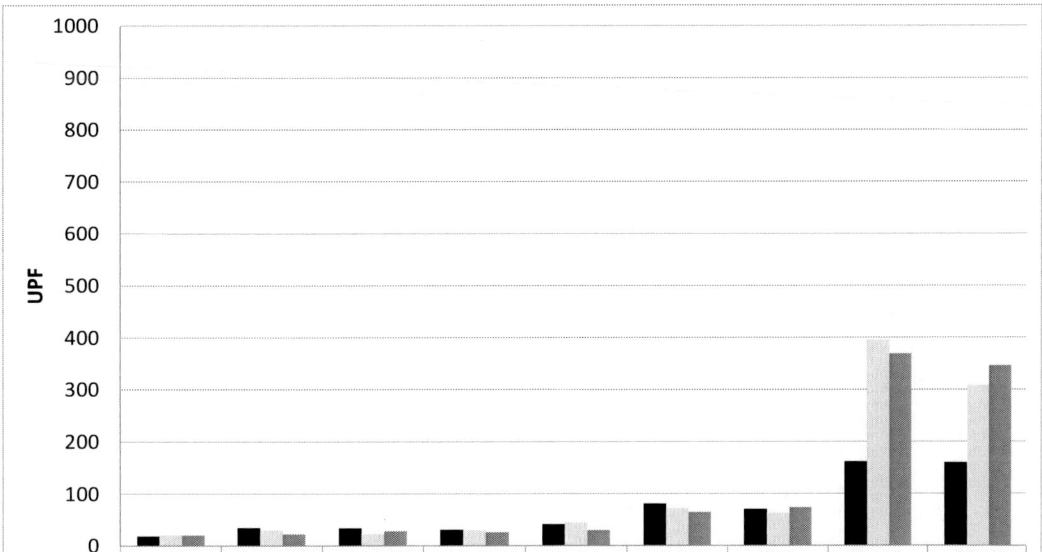

	P/C	F3-0,004	F3-0,006	F3-0,0125	F3-0,1	F3-0,5	F3-1	F3-10	F3-50
■ Dry	18,43	34,14	33,76	31,04	41,60	81,29	70,67	161,61	160,21
DW	20,58	30,70	23,55	29,42	44,02	72,35	63,51	394,42	308,80
SW	20,48	22,88	28,00	25,95	30,29	65,13	74,02	369,08	346,25

Figure 8. The discrepancy of UV protection in wet state by distilled (DW) and sea (SW) water of polyester/cotton fabric treated with UV absorber - stilbene disulphonic acid triazine derivative (F3).

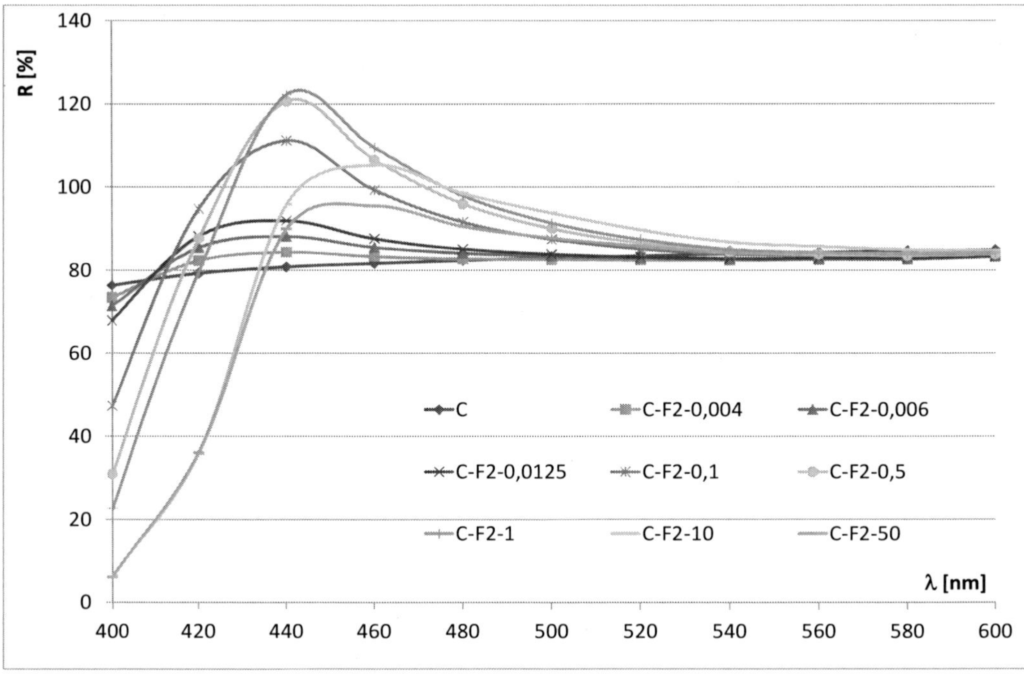

Figure 9. Remission curves of cotton fabric treated with FWA - disodium 4.4'-bis[(4-anylino-6-morpholino-1.3.5-triazine-2-yl) amino]-stilbene-2.2'-disulphonate (F2) in wide concentration range.

From Table 7 it is evident that high effects in textile cleaning of genetic and added impurities such are waxes, protein substances, pectin and other during scouring and bleaching in peroxide baths, where pigments are removed [42-44], leads to white cotton. On the other hand, it leads to low UV protection as well (Table 4). Therefore, chemically bleached cotton fabric (C) is non-rateable for UV protection since UPF is 7.28. Polyester/cotton blend (P/C) fabric gives off good UV protection (UPF=18.43 due to the present benzene ring in PES fibres that absorbs UV radiation.

Table 8. CIE whiteness (W_{CIE}), relative intensity of fluorescence (Φ_{rel}), maximum of remission (R_{max}) and wavelength (λ_{max}), and the discrepancy of whiteness in wet state of cotton fabrics treated with FWA - bis(4,4'-triazinylamino)-stilbene-2,2'-disulfonic acid derivative (F1)

Fabric	W_{CIE}	Φ_{rel}	R_{max}[%]	λ_{max} [nm]	dE*	Discrepancy
C	74.3	0	86.51	700	-	-
C-DW	61.7	0	83.25	700	2.633	Darker yellow
C-SW	62.9	0	83.47	700	2.413	Darker yellow
C-F1-0.004	77.4	0	85.83	700	-	-
C-F1-0.004-DW	67.4	0	83.28	700	2.147	Darker yellow
C-F1-0.004-SW	66.7	0	82.95	700	2.428	Darker yellow
C-F1-0.006	79.0	4.56	85.95	700	-	-
C-F1-0.006-DW	69.8	4.23	83.32	700	2.072	Darker yellow
C-F1-0.006-SW	69.7	4.25	83.31	700	2.107	Darker yellow
C-F1-0.0125	83.4	8.85	85.88	700	-	-

Fabric	W_{CIE}	Φ_{rel}	R_{max} [%]	λ_{max} [nm]	dE*	Discrepancy
C-F1-0.0125-DW	76.3	7.28	83.42	700	1.787	Darker less blue
C-F1-0.0125-SW	73.6	7.02	82.78	700	2.336	Darker redder less blue
C-F1-0.1	109.1	27.72	96.84	440	-	-
C-F1-0.1-DW	109.4	27.99	95.29	440	2.021	Darker redder bluer
C-F1-0.1-SW	109.4	27.90	95.45	440	1.855	Darker redder bluer
C-F1-0.5	127.1	38.18	106.37	440	-	-
C-F1-0.5-DW	127.6	37.80	105.35	440	1.895	Darker redder bluer
C-F1-0.5-SW	130.2	39.32	107.18	440	1.999	Darker redder bluer
C-F1-1	135.9	40.98	112.60	440	-	-
C-F1-1-DW	139.1	45.99	113.26	440	2.306	Darker redder bluer
C-F1-1-SW	138.8	45.31	113.43	440	2.146	Darker redder bluer
C-F1-10	143.4	51.53	118.55	440	-	-
C-F1-10-DW	146.0	55.15	120.55	440	1.598	Darker redder bluer
C-F1-10-SW	143.0	50.53	118.73	440	1.470	Darker bluer
C-F1-50	132.2	48.73	114.07	440	-	-
C-F1-50-DW	134.3	49.29	115.02	440	1.855	Darker redder bluer
C-F1-50-SW	126.7	43.37	110.89	440	1.689	Darker less red less blue

Table 9. CIE whiteness (W_{CIE}), relative intensity of fluorescence (Φ_{rel}), maximum of remission (R_{max}) and wavelength (λ_{max}), and the discrepancy of whiteness in wet state of cotton fabrics treated with FWA - disodium 4.4'-bis[(4-anylino-6-morpholino-1.3.5-triazine-2-yl) amino]-stilbene-2.2'-disulphonate (F2)

Fabric	W_{CIE}	Φ_{rel}	R_{max} [%]	λ_{max} [nm]	dE*	Discrepancy
C-F2-0.004	84.7	4.64	85.95	700		
C-F2-0.004-DW	77.5	4.22	83.47	700	1.798	Darker less blue
C-F2-0.004-SW	76.1	4.20	83.36	700	2.304	Darker redder less blue
C-F2-0.006	93.0	16.67	88.16	440	-	-
C-F2-0.006-DW	86.2	14.44	83.59	440	1.787	Darker redder bluer
C-F2-0.006-SW	84.4	12.98	83.55	700	1.576	Darker redder bluer
C-F2-0.0125	100.5	27.22	91.95	440	-	-
C-F2-0.0125-DW	97.1	22.24	88.97	440	1.833	Darker redder bluer
C-F2-0.0125-SW	94.5	17.76	87.88	440	2.152	Darker redder bluer
C-F2-0.1	134.3	47.07	111.15	440	-	-
C-F2-0.1-DW	136.0	49.93	111.15	440	1.857	Darker less green bluer
C-F2-0.1-SW	134.6	46.74	110.27	440	1.450	Darker bluer
C-F2-0.5	147.4	60.66	120.68	440	-	-
C-F2-0.5-DW	148.7	62.75	121.00	440	1.756	Darker bluer
C-F2-0.5-SW	147.7	61.53	120.75	440	1.526	Darker less red bluer
C-F2-1	148.1	62.09	122.24	440	-	-
C-F2-1-DW	148.2	62.60	122.25	440	1.623	Darker bluer
C-F2-1-SW	147.9	58.87	122.35	440	2.500	Darker less red bluer
C-F2-10	98.4	39.68	105.29	460	-	-
C-F2-10-DW	104.6	42.32	105.75	460	2.924	Darker less green bluer
C-F2-10-SW	101.3	40.30	105.04	460	2.419	Darker less green bluer
C-F2-50	82.3	20.01	95.51	460	-	-
C-F2-50-DW	72.8	19.93	91.63	460	2.148	Darker less green yellow
C-F2-50-SW	60.0	14.78	87.41	460	4.283	Darker yellow

Table 10. CIE whiteness (W_{CIE}), relative intensity of fluorescence (Φ_{rel}), maximum of remission (R_{max}) and wavelength (λ_{max}), and the discrepancy of whiteness in wet state of cotton fabrics treated with UV absorber - stilbene disulphonic acid triazine derivative (F3)

Fabric	W_{CIE}	Φ_{rel}	R_{max} [%]	λ_{max} [nm]	dE*	Discrepancy
C-F3-0.004	93.1	12.20	88.73	440	-	-
C-F3-0.004-DW	91.7	11.61	86.49	440	1.916	Darker redder bluer
C-F3-0.004-SW	85.4	9.65	83.76	440	1.945	Darker less blue
C-F3-0.006	96.4	13.72	92.96	440	-	-
C-F3-0.006-DW	89.0	11.42	89.69	440	1.721	Darker redder
C-F3-0.006-SW	90.5	12.79	88.24	440	1.922	Darker redder less blue
C-F3-0.0125	102.0	17.27	90.17	440	-	-
C-F3-0.0125-DW	98.4	13.75	85.48	440	1.887	Darker redder bluer
C-F3-0.0125-SW	95.6	13.23	85.66	440	1.809	Darker redder bluer
C-F3-0.1	130.0	39.39	107.87	440	-	-
C-F3-0.1-DW	131.6	40.61	107.83	440	1.595	Darker redder bluer
C-F3-0.1-SW	131.5	40.60	107.87	440	1.697	Darker redder bluer
C-F3-0.5	146.9	56.95	120.13	440	-	-
C-F3-0.5-DW	147.0	58.68	120.21	440	1.411	Darker bluer
C-F3-0.5-SW	144.2	55.55	118.37	440	1.559	Darker less red
C-F3-1	149.2	62.49	122.80	440	-	-
C-F3-1-DW	147.1	59.66	121.67	440	1.385	Darker less red
C-F3-1-SW	144.9	56.55	120.59	440	1.579	Darker less red less blue
C-F3-10	99.9	24.20	105.67	460	-	-
C-F3-10-DW	66.3	17.44	96.41	460	6.897	Darker greener less blue
C-F3-10-SW	68.1	19.50	97.00	460	6.509	Darker greener less blue
C-F3-50	71.8	13.66	100.18	460	-	-
C-F3-50-DW	16.3	4.48	85.38	460	11.017	Darker greener yellow
C-F3-50-SW	15.3	3.83	84.91	460	11.173	Darker greener yellow

Table 11. CIE whiteness (W_{CIE}), relative intensity of fluorescence (Φ_{rel}), maximum of remission (R_{max}) and wavelength (λ_{max}), and the discrepancy of whiteness in wet state of polyester/cotton blend fabrics treated with FWA - bis(4,4'-triazinylamino)-stilbene-2,2'-disulfonic acid derivative (F1)

Fabric	W_{CIE}	Φ_{rel}	R_{max} [%]	λ_{max} [nm]	dE*	Discrepancy
P/C	70.7	0	85.34	700	-	-
P/C-DW	62.1	0	83.38	700	1.766	Darker yellow
P/C-SW	61.5	0	83.33	700	1.880	Darker greener yellow
P/C-F1-0.004	75.1	5.23	85.36	700	-	-
P/C-F1-0.004-DW	68.5	5.00	83.52	700	1.627	Darker less red yellow
P/C-F1-0.004-SW	67.9	4.93	83.30	700	1.743	Darker less red yellow
P/C-F1-0.006	76.4	6.86	85.28	700	-	-
P/C-F1-0.006-DW	67.4	5.55	83.29	700	1.928	Darker less red yellow
P/C-F1-0.006-SW	69.1	5.85	83.45	700	1.661	Darker yellow
P/C-F1-0.0125	77.8	7.65	85.47	700	-	-
P/C-F1-0.0125-DW	71.1	7.23	83.45	700	1.617	Darker yellow
P/C-F1-0.0125-SW	70.6	6.92	83.62	700	1.593	Darker yellow

Fabric	W_{CIE}	Φ_{rel}	R_{max} [%]	λ_{max} [nm]	dE*	Discrepancy
P/C-F1-0.1	91.6	17.76	86.76	440	-	-
P/C-F1-0.1-DW	90.3	15.43	85.09	440	1.152	Darker redder bluer
P/C-F1-0.1-SW	89.3	15.09	84.92	440	0.935	Darker redder
P/C-F1-0.5	106.3	18.98	94.12	440	-	-
P/C-F1-0.5-DW	106.2	18.82	93.28	440	1.046	Darker redder bluer
P/C-F1-0.5-SW	107.5	19.54	93.45	440	1.524	Darker redder bluer
P/C-F1-1	112.6	20.48	98.07	440	-	-
P/C-F1-1-DW	115.1	25.74	98.51	440	1.438	Darker redder bluer
P/C-F1-1-SW	114.7	23.91	98.02	440	1.629	Darker redder bluer
P/C-F1-10	126.9	51.51	107.92	440	-	-
P/C-F1-10-DW	132.4	50.14	109.86	440	1.984	Darker redder bluer
P/C-F1-10-SW	132.5	49.53	110.28	440	1.937	Darker redder bluer
P/C-F1-50	124.7	48.73	107.95	440	-	-
P/C-F1-50-DW	130.7	49.29	111.29	440	2.196	Darker redder bluer
P/C-F1-50-SW	128.9	38.67	110.00	440	2.103	Darker redder bluer

Table 12. CIE whiteness (W_{CIE}), relative intensity of fluorescence (Φ_{rel}), maximum of remission (R_{max}) and wavelength (λ_{max}), and the discrepancy of whiteness in wet state of polyester/cotton blend fabrics treated with FWA - disodium 4.4'-bis[(4-anylino-6-morpholino-1.3.5-triazine-2-yl) amino]-stilbene-2.2'-disulphonate (F2)

Fabric	W_{CIE}	Φ_{rel}	R_{max} [%]	λ_{max} [nm]	dE*	Discrepancy
P/C-F2-0.004	78.3	4.44	85.30	700	-	-
P/C-F2-0.004-DW	72.4	4.01	83.57	700	1.401	Darker yellow
P/C-F2-0.004-SW	72.3	3.86	83.70	700	1.421	Darker yellow
P/C-F2-0.006	92.8	14.63	87.55	440	-	-
P/C-F2-0.006-DW	83.6	11.98	83.36	700	2.035	Darker less red less blue
P/C-F2-0.006-SW	86.2	12.78	83.32	440	1.743	Darker less red less blue
P/C-F2-0.0125	98.2	17.65	85.40	440	-	-
P/C-F2-0.0125-DW	93.8	15.24	83.77	440	1.315	Darker less blue
P/C-F2-0.0125-SW	94.0	15.66	83.69	440	1.374	Darker less blue
P/C-F2-0.1	112.2	43.07	97.78	440	-	-
P/C-F2-0.1-DW	114.1	44.43	97.88	440	1.266	Darker redder bluer
P/C-F2-0.1-SW	113.1	45.01	97.31	440	1.290	Darker redder bluer
P/C-F2-0.5	148.7	60.52	121.66	440	-	-
P/C-F2-0.5-DW	148.5	59.74	121.14	440	1.626	Darker less red bluer
P/C-F2-0.5-SW	148.1	58.53	120.84	440	1.882	Darker less red bluer
P/C-F2-1	148.6	57.22	122.66	440	-	-
P/C-F2-1-DW	148.6	57.30	122.67	440	1.710	Darker bluer
P/C-F2-1-SW	147.2	53.77	121.92	440	1.623	Darker less red bluer
P/C-F2-10	97.1	49.68	101.34	460	-	-
P/C-F2-10-DW	100.3	42.02	104.18	460	1.915	Darker less green bluer
P/C-F2-10-SW	100.4	41.33	99.60	460	2.309	Darker less green bluer
P/C-F2-50	80.7	23.01	91.92	460	-	-
P/C-F2-50-DW	85.6	29.18	92.98	460	1.933	Darker less green less yellow
P/C-F2-50-SW	80.2	22.73	91.91	460	1.140	Darker less green less yellow

Table 13. CIE whiteness (W_{CIE}), relative intensity of fluorescence (Φ_{rel}), maximum of remission (R_{max}) and wavelength (λ_{max}), and the discrepancy of whiteness in wet state of polyester/cotton blend fabrics treated with UV absorber - stilbene disulphonic acid triazine derivative (F3)

Fabric	W_{CIE}	Φ_{rel}	R_{max} [%]	λ_{max} [nm]	dE*	Discrepancy
P/C-F3-0.004	82.2	11.00	85.19	700	-	-
P/C-F3-0.004-DW	75.5	9.63	83.29	700	1.552	Darker yellow
P/C-F3-0.004-SW	75.6	9.90	83.18	700	1.547	Darker yellow
P/C-F3-0.006	89.5	13.31	86.02	440	-	-
P/C-F3-0.006-DW	85.5	12.27	83.59	700	1.432	Darker redder less blue
P/C-F3-0.006-SW	86.3	12.75	83.66	700	1.244	Darker redder less blue
P/C-F3-0.0125	96.3	14.28	84.41	440	-	-
P/C-F3-0.0125-DW	90.3	13.35	83.85	700	1.321	Darker less blue
P/C-F3-0.0125-SW	91.7	13.86	83.58	700	1.392	Darker redder less blue
P/C-F3-0.1	107.6	22.38	95.51	440	-	-
P/C-F3-0.1-DW	106.9	20.64	94.39	440	1.170	Darker redder bluer
P/C-F3-0.1-SW	106.5	18.59	94.28	440	1.016	Darker redder bluer
P/C-F3-0.5	123.7	36.93	105.18	440	-	-
P/C-F3-0.5-DW	127.2	45.60	106.43	440	1.565	Darker redder bluer
P/C-F3-0.5-SW	125.7	43.59	106.21	440	1.297	Darker redder bluer
P/C-F3-1	126.5	47.42	107.63	440	-	-
P/C-F3-1-DW	129.4	46.44	109.47	440	1.317	Darker bluer
P/C-F3-1-SW	131.2	46.53	110.52	440	1.430	Darker bluer
P/C-F3-10	95.2	23.42	99.07	460	-	-
P/C-F3-10-DW	76.7	17.44	93.96	460	3.807	Darker greener less blue
P/C-F3-10-SW	67.0	15.43	92.22	460	5.810	Darker greener less blue
P/C-F3-50	74.6	16.66	95.52	460	-	-
P/C-F3-50-DW	39.9	7.83	87.61	460	7.130	Darker greener yellow
P/C-F3-50-SW	32.3	5.82	84.86	460	8.490	Darker greener yellow

Table 14. Mean UPF, UV-A and UV-B transmission of cotton fabrics treated with fluorescent compounds in laundering - 1st, 3rd, 6th and 9th washing cycle with ECE referent detergent

Sample	Mean UPF	τ_{UVA}	τ_{UVB}	Mean UPF	τ_{UVA}	τ_{UVB}
	1st			3rd		
C-ECE	7.134	17.056	12.270	7.441	15.515	11.754
C-F2-0.08	8.326	11.694	10.601	11.038	5.972	8.038
C-F2-0.12	8.929	9.575	10.054	14.078	3.978	6.369
C-F2-0.25	9.943	7.762	9.292	19.314	2.468	4.568
C-F3-0.2	14.674	8.196	5.955	41.424	2.380	2.057
C-F2-0.1+F3-0.1	11.498	8.356	7.539	30.264	2.382	2.845
	6th			9th		
C-ECE	7.135	15.660	12.253	6.970	15.750	12.765
C-F2-0.08	17.575	3.404	5.284	20.845	2.601	4.406
C-F2-0.12	22.768	2.178	3.772	29.965	1.437	2.959
C-F2-0.25	48.240	1.229	1.958	61.834	0.859	1.484
C-F3-0.2	89.895	1.450	0.982	124.911	0.823	0.652
C-F2-0.1+F3-0.1	57.638	1.484	1.474	85.133	0.935	1.093

Table 15. Mean UPF, UV-A and UV-B transmission of PES/cotton fabrics treated with fluorescent compounds in laundering - 1st, 3rd, 6th and 9th washing cycle with ECE reference detergent

Sample	Mean UPF	τ_{UVA}	τ_{UVB}	Mean UPF	τ_{UVA}	τ_{UVB}
	1st			3rd		
P/C-ECE	21.034	15.818	2.641	23.013	23.66	13.709
P/C-F2-0.08	27.411	10.643	2.336	39.416	5.812	1.717
P/C-F2-0.12	23.645	10.781	2.938	29.857	6.367	2.451
P/C-F2-0.25	27.319	8.069	2.515	48.332	3.522	1.558
P/C-F3-0.2	34.295	8.223	1.848	37.759	4.895	1.898
P/C-F2-0.1+F3-0.1	24.039	9.200	2.662	42.915	4.271	1.689
	6th			9th		
P/C-ECE	25.368	13.096	2.207	23.729	13.600	2.423
P/C-F2-0.08	45.893	4.579	1.558	43.958	4.100	1.704
P/C-F2-0.12	30.475	5.503	2.474	30.483	5.108	2.560
P/C-F2-0.25	50.035	3.401	1.542	51.041	2.961	1.601
P/C-F3-0.2	51.245	4.092	1.449	48.923	3.657	1.610
P/C-F2-0.1+F3-0.1	47.058	3.926	1.582	44.036	3.736	1.786

Table 16. Mean UPF, UV-A and UV-B transmission of cotton fabrics treated with fluorescent compounds in laundering - 1st, 3rd, 6th and 9th washing cycle with commercial detergent

Sample	Mean UPF	τ_{UVA}	τ_{UVB}	Mean UPF	τ_{UVA}	τ_{UVB}
	1st			3rd		
C-commerc.	9.742	12.351	8.893	10.914	8.708	8.236
C-F2-0.08	11.315	8.921	7.369	16.066	3.990	5.589
C-F2-0.12	10.342	8.923	8.249	16.677	3.415	5.416
C-F2-0.25	13.350	6.175	6.166	29.390	1.564	2.932
C-F3-0.2	18.551	7.473	4.627	49.628	2.042	1.610
C-F2-0.1+F3-0.1	13.189	7.980	6.527	57.378	1.488	1.576
	6th			9th		
C-commerc.	11.797	7.255	7.584	15.753	6.233	5.739
C-F2-0.08	25.343	2.038	3.704	35.565	2.348	2.562
C-F2-0.12	28.376	1.608	3.197	43.904	2.431	2.038
C-F2-0.25	55.566	0.768	1.601	95.917	1.630	0.926
C-F3-0.2	172.094	0.599	0.509	233.725	1.486	0.329
C-F2-0.1+F3-0.1	101.630	0.711	0.879	175.466	1.579	0.473

From the results in Tables 5 and 6 can be seen that fluorescent whitening agent applied even in small concentration leads to higher whiteness and higher UPF. By absorbing UV-A radiation optical brightened fabrics transform this radiation to blue fluorescence what leads to excellent UV protection in higher concentrations. Optical brightening due to its fluorescence contributes to the fabric high whiteness and beauty in optimal range of concentration. That is the concentration of fluorescent compound at which the maximum of Φ_{rel} or W_{CIE} are observed [16,39]. From the results of the whiteness and fluorescence of FWA treated cotton fabrics it can be seen that FWA concentration of 1 % (up to 10 % owf) in relation to mass of material is the optimum concentration for bis(4,4'-triazinylamino)-stilbene-2,2'-disulfonic acid derivative (F1), whilst for polyester/cotton blend fabric is 10 % owf. In the case of disodium 4.4'-bis[(4-anylino-6-morpholino-1.3.5-triazine-2-yl)amino]-stilbene-2.2'-disulphonate (F2) optimal concentration for cotton and polyester/cotton fabric is 0.5-1 % owf.

Table 17. Mean UPF, UV-A and UV-B transmission of PES/cotton fabrics treated with fluorescent compounds in laundering - 1st, 3rd, 6th and 9th washing cycle with commercial detergent

Sample	Mean UPF	τ_{UVA}	τ_{UVB}	Mean UPF	τ_{UVA}	τ_{UVB}
	1st			3rd		
P/C-commerc.	27.308	13.774	2.036	27.408	11.821	2.288
P/C-F2-0.08	26.200	11.901	2.156	32.072	7.495	1.995
P/C-F2-0.12	31.386	10.127	1.801	34.703	6.213	1.744
P/C-F2-0.25	35.318	7.956	1.844	34.593	5.138	2.033
P/C-F3-0.2	28.711	10.934	2.009	41.130.	5.320	1.629
P/C-F2-0.1+F3-0.1	22.038	11.623	2.802	30.837	6.508	2.492
	6th			9th		
P/C-commerc.	32.068	9.239	1.832	31.309	9.872	2.010
P/C-F2-0.08	40.072	4.893	1.743	40.819	6.003	1.827
P/C-F2-0.12	50.499	3.736	1.343	47.836	5.054	1.528
P/C-F2-0.25	42.789	3.462	1.746	46.379	4.433	1.660
P/C-F3-0.2	60.181	2.974	1.209	51.863	4.583	1.483
P/C-F2-0.1+F3-0.1	38.520	4.092	1.964	43.131	4.655	1.896

Table 18. CIE whiteness (W_{CIE}), relative intensity of fluorescence (Φ_{rel}), maximum of remission (R_{max}) and wavelength (λ_{max}) of cotton fabrics treated with fluorescent compounds in laundering - 1st, 3rd, 6th and 9th washing cycle with ECE detergent

Sample	W_{CIE}	Φ_{rel}	R_{max} [%]	λ_{max} [nm]	W_{CIE}	Φ_{rel}	R_{max} [%]	λ_{max} [nm]
	1st				3rd			
C-ECE	80,00	-	82,71	700	81,39	-	82,49	700
C-F2-0,08	103,23	-	92,39	440	127,49	-	101,85	440
C-F2-0,12	115,32	-	95,03	440	135,94	-	105,17	440
C-F2-0,25	128,11	-	102,88	440	147,45	-	112,33	440
C-F3-0,2	116,75	-	98,65	440	142,34	-	110,13	440
C-F2-0,1+F3-0.1	124,05	-	99,55	440	145,22	-	111,54	440
	6th				9th			
C-ECE.	80,04	-	85,58	700	79,79	-	85,58	700
C-F2-0,08	138,28	-	115,59	440	146,86	-	122,07	440
C-F2-0,12	147,59	-	121,95	440	154,64	-	127,95	440
C-F2-0,25	156,35	-	129,59	440	160,66	-	134,63	440
C-F3-0,2	149,03	-	123,42	440	155,42	-	129,31	440
C-F2-0,1+F3-0.1	153,87	-	127,45	440	157,67	-	131,52	440

Table 19. CIE whiteness (W_{CIE}), relative intensity of fluorescence (Φ_{rel}), maximum of remission (R_{max}) and wavelength (λ_{max}) of polyester/cotton fabrics treated with fluorescent compounds in laundering - 1st, 3rd, 6th and 9th washing cycle with ECE detergent

Sample	W_{CIE}	Φ_{rel}	R_{max} [%]	λ_{max} [nm]	W_{CIE}	Φ_{rel}	R_{max} [%]	λ_{max} [nm]
	1st				3rd			
P/C-ECE	76,20	-	82,71	700	76,83	-	82,49	700
P/C-F2-0,08	101,41	-	92,39	440	117,12	-	101,85	440
P/C-F2-0,12	106,36	-	95,03	440	122,28	-	105,17	440
P/C-F2-0,25	119,11	-	102,88	440	131,97	-	112,33	440
P/C-F3-0,2	112,22	-	98,65	440	129,40	-	110,13	440
P/C-F2-0,1+F3-0.1	114,09	-	99,55	440	131,61	-	111,54	440
	6th				9th			
P/C-ECE	80,50	-	83,44	700	83,73	-	83,19	700
P/C-F2-0,08	125,37	-	106,77	440	129,06	-	109,45	440
P/C-F2-0,12	130,51	-	110,62	440	134,05	-	113,44	440
P/C-F2-0,25	136,24	-	115,58	440	136,88	-	116,52	440
P/C-F3-0,2	133,57	-	112,64	440	135,36	-	112,75	440
P/C-F2-0,1+F3-0.1	134,90	-	113,70	440	135,80	-	115,18	440

Table 20. CIE whiteness (W_{CIE}), relative intensity of fluorescence (Φ_{rel}), maximum of remission (R_{max}) and wavelength (λ_{max}) of cotton fabrics treated with fluorescent compounds in laundering - 1st, 3rd, 6th and 9th washing cycle with commercial detergent

Sample	W_{CIE}	Φ_{rel}	R_{max} [%]	λ_{max} [nm]	W_{CIE}	Φ_{rel}	R_{max} [%]	λ_{max} [nm]
	1st				3rd			
C-commerc.	95.36	0	86,32	700	103.80	0	86,04	700
C-F2-0,08	105.33	3,58	96,92	440	124.14	18,83	108,06	440
C-F2-0,12	110.91	8,60	99,93	440	129.88	24,60	111,66	440
C-F2-0,25	123.44	17,25	107,43	440	139.14	39,30	118,46	440
C-F3-0,2	112.33	13,99	100,36	440	136.64	28,16	115,86	440
C-F2-0,1+F3-0.1	110.83	17,99	99,84	440	138.50	32,59	117,95	440
	6th				9th			
C-commerc.	112.45	32,91	86,56	700	115.24	27,38	86,72	700
C-F2-0,08	140.66	65,63	116,47	440	143.88	45,22	120,53	440
C-F2-0,12	147.56	78,30	121,27	440	150.06	46,50	125,55	440
C-F2-0,25	153.36	89,43	126,91	440	154.34	51,64	130,55	440
C-F3-0,2	150.25	76,55	125,49	440	153.24	44,81	129,06	440
C-F2-0,1+F3-0.1	151.67	82,79	126,78	440	154.83	54,03	130,34	440

Since this UV absorber is fluorescent compound as well, having similar chemical composition (stilbene disulphonic acid derivative) as FWA, optimum concentration for UV absorber was determined as well, and it is 0.5-1 % owf (Table 7). At the low concentrations of all fluorescent compounds – FWAs and UV absorber, blue fluorescence neutralizes the yellowness of bleached fabric giving the high luminosity and "most beautiful" white.

Table 21. CIE whiteness (W_{CIE}), relative intensity of fluorescence (Φ_{rel}), maximum of remission (R_{max}) and wavelength (λ_{max}) of polyester/cotton fabrics treated with fluorescent compounds in laundering - 1st, 3rd, 6th and 9th washing cycle with commercial detergent

Sample	W_{CIE}	Φ_{rel}	R_{max} [%]	λ_{max} [nm]	W_{CIE}	Φ_{rel}	R_{max} [%]	λ_{max} [nm]
	1st				3rd			
P/C-commerc.	85.85	0	85,51	700	96.83	0	85,19	700
P/C-F2-0,08	100.20	2.06	93,26	440	115.28	9,61	102,34	440
P/C-F2-0,12	103.79	2,14	95,21	440	118.81	12,56	104,37	440
P/C-F2-0,25	112.37	12,76	100,39	440	125.70	22,03	109,75	440
P/C-F3-0,2	102.39	4,15	97,39	440	121.77	16,82	105,85	440
P/C-F2-0,1+F3-0.1	105.22	4,62	94,57	440	122.91	18,83	106,53	440
	6th				9th			
P/C-commerc.	109.52	18,43	85,84	700	104.23	21,17	86,13	700
P/C-F2-0,08	136.60	49,08	108,71	440	129.32	34,23	111,80	440
P/C-F2-0,12	143.16	51,90	111,89	440	133.67	38,54	115,46	440
P/C-F2-0,25	149.62	63,29	116,25	440	135.73	40,06	118,91	440
P/C-F3-0,2	146.44	64,06	116,16	440	135.71	44,91	118,35	440
P/C-F2-0,1+F3-0.1	147.27	53,86	115,28	440	136.31	45,12	118,57	440

Applied in the higher concentration than optimal one, from results of remission and wavelength maximums can be seen that the change in emission spectrum occurred. It is a consequence of well-known bathochromic shift of the remission spectrum (see Figure 9). It comes to a reduction of remission intensity with FWA and/or UV absorber's concentrations causing the extinction of fluorescence by quenching phenomenon, with a consequence of yellowness.

Cotton fabrics of the highest FWAs concentration have the highest UPF in dry state. Similar to the results of the cotton fabrics whiteness and fluorescence, at the optimal concentration of FWA excellent UV protection has been achieved. For bis(4,4'-triazinylamino)-stilbene-2,2'-disulfonic acid derivative (F1), UPF > 50 was achieved at concentration 10 % owf ($UPF_{F1-0.5}$=125.094); whilst in the case of disodium 4.4'-bis[(4-anylino-6-morpholino-1.3.5-triazine-2-yl)amino]-stilbene-2.2'-disulphonate (F2) at 0.5% owf ($UPF_{F2-0.5}$=62.023). More benzene rings in the structure of the stilbene-type contribute to better UV protection. That confirms that FWA insures high protection of UV radiation.

By treating cotton fabric with an UV absorber in the wide concentration range protective effect is more enhanced. UV absorber offers excellent UV protection if applied in optimal concentration of 0.1 % owf or higher. That is because UV absorbers absorb damaging UV-R range of 290 nm to 360 nm, and convert it into harmless heat energy. For difference of FWA's UV absorbers offer UV-B protection as well. However, the fabrics with the highest intensity of fluorescence do not show the highest UPF values. In dry state, UV protection increase with fluorescent compound concentration, regardless of quenching phenomenon.

Treatment of the polyester/cotton blend fabric with fluorescent compounds shows similar behavior as cotton ones. The presence of benzene ring in PES fibres results in good UV protection of polyester/cotton blend (P/C) fabric. For that reason, treatment of the polyester/cotton blend fabric results in very good UV protection for even smallest concentrations of fluorescent compounds applied. Since these applied fluorescent compounds are primary for the cellulosic fibers, only the cotton in the blend absorbed it. Therefore, in the higher concentrations of applied compounds, excellent UV protection has been achieved, but UPF value is lower than for cotton fabrics.

Washing fabrics with only the detergent, UPF stays mainly the same, and fabrics are non-rateable UV protection (Tables 14-17). Since commercial detergent contained the soap that fluorescence as well (can be seen after 6th cycle – Tables 20-21), UPF is little bit higher, but fabrics are still without UV protection.

UPF significantly grows when washed in a detergent containing fluorescent compounds. The influence of fluorescent whitening agent in initial launderings on the UPF shows that cotton fabrics are non-rateable for UV protection after the first laundering cycle regardless of applied detergent with fluorescent whitening agents added, and even when an UV absorber is added to the detergent as well. However, even small addition of disodium 4.4'-bis[(4-anylino-6-morpholino-1.3.5-triazine-2-yl)amino]-stilbene-2.2'-disulphonate (F2) increase UPF from 7.28 to UPF = 8.32 for ECE detergent and to UPF = 11.31 for commercial detergent. Application of UV absorber (F3) results in UPF of 14.67 for ECE detergent and to UPF = 18.55 for commercial one.

To obtain better UV protection the treatment should be performed in the course of finishing. UV absorber offers excellent UV protection (UPF>40) after three laundering cycles regardless of applied detergent, whilst for achieving excellent UV protection with the fluorescent whitening agent six cycles are necessary.

Polyester/cotton blend fabric shows similar behaviour as cotton ones. The growth of UPF is not so much prominent as with cotton fabrics, as the fluorescent compounds used act on the cotton part of the PES/cotton blend only. However, very good UV protection can be achieved after 1 laundering cycle regardless of applied detergent. The excellent UV protection can be achieved applying stilbene type FWA (F2) after 6 laundering cycles and/or UV absorber (F3).

The obtained results confirm the well-known fact that fluorescent whitening agents applied in textile finishing or added into detergents in laundering manage to keep and even improve basic whiteness degree. This phenomenon is present even when lower concentration of fluorescent whitening agent is used than recommended. Obviously, whiteness degree grows with higher concentration. In the case of laundered samples with no fluorescent whitening agents, it can be seen that basic whiteness degree is somewhat higher, which is due to the perborate degradation of residual pigments on the cotton fabric. This occurs after the first laundering cycle already and is more prominent with every succeeding laundering cycle. It can be seen that higher remission is obtained after the 9th laundering cycle when higher concentration of fluorescent whitening agent is employed (0.25%), as compared to lower concentration (0.08%). High whiteness degrees are achieved in the combination of UV absorbers and fluorescent whitening agents. From the Tables 18-21 it can be seen that the wavelength of R_{max} did not changed after multiple laundering. Stilbene fluorescent whitening agent, as well as stilbene UV absorber, showed remission maximum at 440 nm. After repeated laundering and accumulation did not occur bathochromic shift, which confirmed that the whiteness and UV protective effects stay retain.

Somewhat lower degrees of whiteness are achieved on PES/cotton fabrics than on cotton fabric. The reason for that is in the fact that PES fibres cannot be optically brightened with applied FWAs. Since in this research stilbene derivatives were applied in laundering and finishing, PES fibres were not brightened, and the positive effects are achieved on the cotton component only. Therefore, the achieved effects on PES/cotton blend cannot compare to the ones achieved on 100% cotton fabric.

Considering the results of discrepancy of whiteness shown in Tables 9-11 it can be observed that all fabrics get darker when wet and in general bluer and redder. The reason for that is lower reflection of light from the fabric. In dry fabric, some of the photons of light are absorbed, but some are reflected and land on the eye's retina what gives the sensation of seeing a certain level of brightness. But when the fabric gets wet, the water fills in the interyarn spacing. When the light falls on the wet fabric, some of it enters the water at one angle and refracts at other because the light waves travel at a slower speed in water than it does in air. Fewer photons of light get back to the eyeball, and therefore the wet fabric "appears" darker than the dry one. When the water gradually evaporates, more and more light is reflected back to the eyeball, and can be seen brighter again. The amount of refraction, referred to as the refractive index, is affected by both the salinity and temperature of the water, and therefore there is a difference between fabrics treated with sea and distilled water. It is to point out that the salts in Sea water act as quenchers of fluorescence as well. Therefore, for the highest concentration of applied FWAs - disodium 4.4'-bis[(4-anylino-6-morpholino-1.3.5-triazine-2-yl)amino]-stilbene-2.2'-disulphonate (F2) 50 % owf, degree of whiteness falls from 82.3 to 60.0. This phenomenon is even more evident for UV absorber applied in concentrations higher than optimal one. The whiteness for applied 10 % owf decreases from 99.9 to 77.9, and for 50 % owf from 71.8 to low 15.3.

Considering the different refractive index in water and in the air it is differently reflected from the surface as explained before. Because of higher and scattered reflection, transmission is lower for both water applied, distilled and sea water, resulting in higher UPF values (Figures 3-8). It can be said that in wet state cotton knit fabrics treated with fluorescent compounds give off better UV protection than in dry state regardless of the concentration and type of fluorescent compound applied.

This phenomenon is more enhanced for Sea water, since the refractive index increases with salinity increment and decrease of temperature. That can be explained by that some of the Sun's radiant energy is reflected from the water surface; it is not absorbed, but additionally scattered by molecules suspended in the water, whilst the other part penetrates the water's surface, absorb and converse to other forms of energy, such as heat that warms or evaporates water, or is used by plants to fuel photosynthesis. Considering the applied concentrations, in general it can be said that higher concentration of fluorescent compound applied to cotton and polyester/cotton blend fabrics, better UV protection was achieved in wet state. It was observed that for the concentrations lower than optimal one, UV protection in wet state is lower or similar, whilst for the higher concentrations it gets significantly higher. The achieved UV protection is excellent regardless of the drop and can even obey that request regarding UV index during the summer time in Mediterranean countries, as well as Australia and USA, which acquire UPF>UV index*15.

The concentration of 0.08 % addition to detergent is the same amount as 0.004 % owf applied in textile finishing, etc. The concentration of fluorescent compound accumulated in 9 laundering cycles is similar to the concentration of 0.1% owf in textile finishing. Therefore, the comparison of two procedures was done and it is shown in Figures 10 and 11.

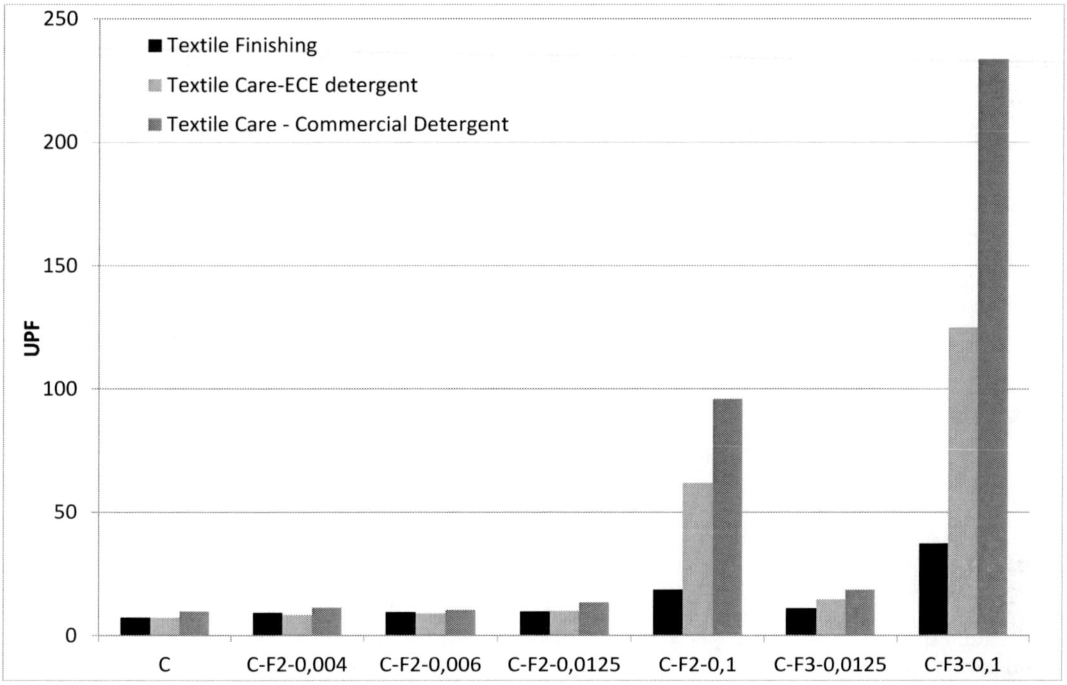

Figure 10. The differences in UV protection of cotton fabrics (C) as a result of different application of fluorescent compounds – FWA (F2) and UV absorber (F3) in textile finishing or textile care.

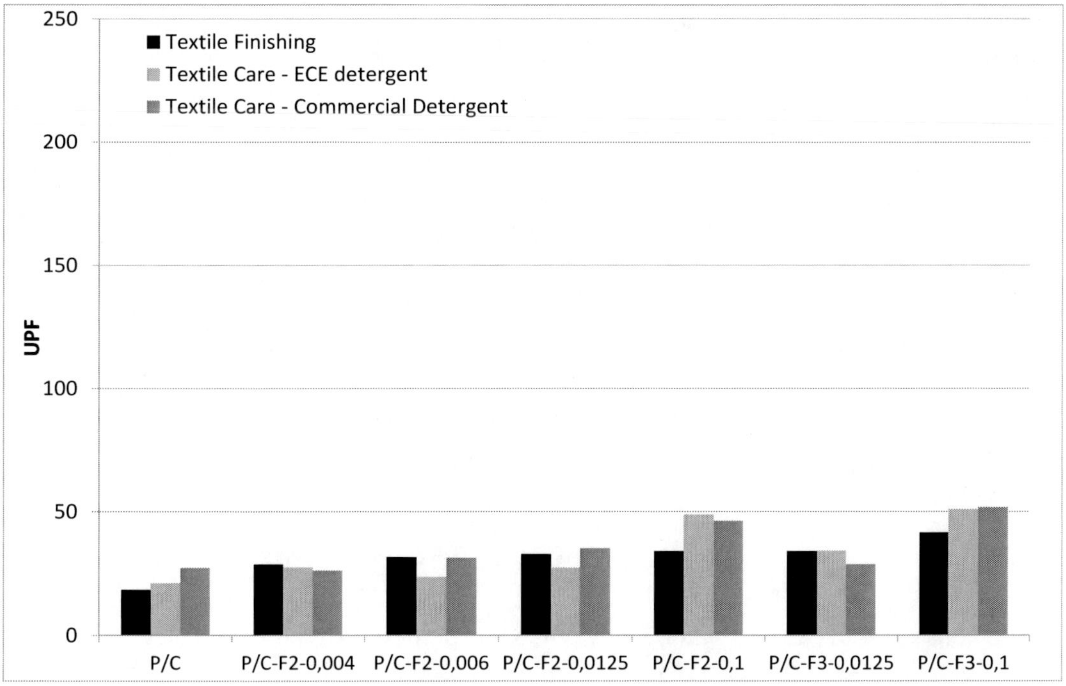

Figure 11. The differences in UV protection of polyester/cotton blend fabrics (P/C) as a result of different application of fluorescent compounds – FWA (F2) and UV absorber (F3) in textile finishing or textile care.

As it can be seen in Figure 10, UV protection of cotton fabrics treated with fluorescent whitening agent - disodium 4.4'-bis[(4-anylino-6-morpholino-1.3.5-triazine-2-yl)amino]-stilbene-2.2'-disulphonate (F2) is similar regardless of procedure. However, if UV absorber was applied as addition to laundry detergent it is more efficient, than if applied in the same concentration in textile finishing.

Considering 9x higher concentration and/or accumulation through 9 washing cycles it is evident that in accumulation UV protection gets significantly higher. It is to point out that application to commercial detergent resulted in higher UPF than if applied ECE reference detergent, as a result of fluorescence of the soap in commercial detergent composition. On the other hand, the differences in UV protection of polyester/cotton blend fabrics (P/C), shown in Figure 11, are not so enhanced. The reason for that is in chemical composition of applied fluorescent compounds. All of them are stilbene derivatives, which are for application to cellulosic fibers, and therefore, only cotton absorbed it.

CONCLUSION

Primary prevention and early detection are essential regarding deduction of melanoma incidence. Considering prevention, especially in childhood and adolescence, it is necessary to apply sunscreening lotions and wear adequate clothing. Chemically bleached cotton and polyester/cotton blend fabrics are non-rateable for UV protection. Treatment with fluorescent compounds, FWA and UV absorber leads to its multifunctionality - high whiteness, neutralization of yellowness, giving to the fabric the high luminosity and protection against UV radiation. The fluorescence contributes to the high whiteness and beauty in optimal concentration.

In the range of higher concentration quenching of fluorescence occurs, resulting in fabric yellowness. In wet state, regardless of applied water – sea or distilled, fabrics get darker, lowering its whiteness, but because of reflection from water, better UV protection is achieved. This phenomenon is more evident for Sea water, because of additional light scattering since it contains about 40 % of inorganic salts.

UV protection and optical effects of fabrics laundered in ECE and commercial detergent containing fluorescent compounds of stilbene type has been achieved by light conversion and cumulative addition through 9 washing cycles. For that reason, it is to suggest application of these compounds for prevention of skin cancer incidence, especially in commercial detergent formulation for protection of wider population.

ACKNOWLEDGMENTS

The authors would like to acknowledge the University of Zagreb for financial support to research "Optical and Protective Potential of Fluorescent Compounds in Cotton Material Finishing and Care" (KFPI 1, TP1.89).

REFERENCES

[1] Robins P, and Perez M. (1966). *Understanding melanoma*; *The Skin Cancer Foundation,* New York.

[2] Šitum M. (2012) Melanoma. Chapter 57 in Guidliness in common dermatoses and skin cancers diagnostics and treatments (in Croatian: Smjernice u dijagnostici i liječenju najčešćih dermatoza i tumora kože). Naklada Slap, Jastrebarsko.

[3] Tarbuk, A., Grancarić A. M., Šitum, M. and Martinis M: UV Clothing and Skin Cancer, *Collegium Antropologicum*. 34 (2010) 179-183.

[4] Armstrong, B. K., Kricker, A. (1993). How much melanoma is caused by sun exposure? *Melanoma Res* 3 (6), 395-401.

[5] Berwick, M., Armstrong, B. K., Ben-Porat, L., Fine, J., Kricker, A., Eberle, C., Barnhill, R. (2005) Sun exposure and mortality from melanoma. *J Natl Cancer Inst* 97(3), 195-199.

[6] Tarbuk, A., Grancarić A. M., and Šitum, M. (2014). Discrepancy of Whiteness and UV Protection in Wet State. *Collegium antropologicum*. 38, 4; 1110-1117.

[7] Lugović Mihić, L.; Bulat, V.; Šitum, M.; Čavka, V.; Krolo, I. (2008). Allergic hypersensitivity skin reactions following sun exposure. *Collegium antropologicum* 32 (suppl 2); 153-157.

[8] Šitum, M.; Buljan, M.; Čavka, V.; Bulat, V.; Krolo, I.; Lugović Mihić, L. (2008). Skin changes in the elderly people--how strong is the influence of the UV radiation on skin aging? *Collegium antropologicum* 32 (suppl 2); 9-13.

[9] Diffey, B. L. (1991). Solar ultraviolet radiation effects on biological systems. *Physics in Medicine and Biology* 36(3), 299-328.

[10] Eckhardt, C., H. Rohwer (2000). UV protector for cotton fabrics. *Textile Chemist and Colorist,* 32(4), 21-23.

[11] Hoffmann, K., Laperre, J., Avermaete, A., Altmeyer, P., Gambichler, T. (2001). Defined UV protection by apparel textiles, *Arch Dermatol.* 137(8),1089-1094.

[12] Gambichler, T., Rotterdam, S., Altmeyer, P., Hoffmann, K. (2001). Protection against ultraviolet radiation by commercial summer clothing: need for standardised testing and labelling, *BMC Dermatology* 1 (6).

[13] Reinert, G., Fuso, F., Hilfiker, R., Schmidt, E. (1997). UV-protecting properties of textile fabrics and their improvement. *Textile Chemist and Colorist* 29(12), 36-43.

[14] Gies, P. H., Roy, C. R., Toomey, S., Mclennan, A. (1998). Protection against solar ultraviolet radiation, *Mutation Research* 422, 15-22.

[15] Grancarić, A.M., Tarbuk, A., and Botteri, L. (2014). Light Conversion and Scattering in UV Protective Textiles. *AUTEX research journal.* 14 (4), 1-12.

[16] Grancarić, A. M., Tarbuk, A., Dumitrescu, I., Bišćan J. (2006). UV Protection of Pretreated Cotton – Influence of FWA's Fluorescence, *AATCC Review* 6(4), 44-48.

[17] Tarbuk, A., Grancarić, A.M., Jančijev, I., Sharma, S. (2006). Protection against UV radiation using a modified polyester fabric, *Tekstil* 55 (8), 383-394.

[18] Hilfiker, R., Kaufmann, W., Reinert, G., Schmidt, E. (1996). Improving sun protection factors of fabrics by applying UV- absorbers. *Text. Res. J.* 66(2), 61-70.

[19] Algaba, I., Riva, A., Crews, P. C. (2004). Influence of Fiber Type and Fabric Porosity on the UPF of Summer Fabrics, *AATCC Review*, 4(2), 26-31.

[20] Dobnik Dubrovski P., Dumitrescu J., Zabetakis A. (2004). Special Finishing Treatments and UPF improvement; in Book of Proceedings, 2nd International Textile, Clothing & Design conference – Magic World of Textiles, (Ed. Z. Dragčević), Dubrovnik, 3-6 October 2004, 340-346.

[21] Grancarić, A.M., Penava, Ž., Tarbuk, A. (2005) UV Protection of Cotton – the Influence of Weaving Structure, Hemijska industrija (*Serbian Society of Chemical Industry Journal*) 59(9-10), 230-234.

[22] Grancarić, A. M.; Tarbuk, A.; Marković, L. (2007). UV Protection with Zeolite Treated Cotton Knitted Fabric - The Influence of Yarn Linear Density; Buletinul Institutului Politehnic din Iasi. LIII (LVII) (5); 441-446.

[23] Grancarić, A. M., Tarbuk, A. (2009). EDA Modified PET Fabric Treated with Activated Natural Zeolite Nanoparticles, Materials Technology: *Advan. Performance Materials,* 24 (1); 58-63.

[24] Grancarić, A. M., Tarbuk, A., Kovaček, I. (2009). Nanoparticles of Activated Natural Zeolite on Textiles for Protection and Therapy, *Chem. Ind. & Chem. Engineering Quarterly.* 15(4), 203-210.

[25] Cox Crews P., Zhou Y. (2004). The effect of wetness on the UVR transmission of woven fabrics. *AATCC. Review*, 4(8), 41-43.

[26] Riva, A., Algaba, I., Prieto, R. (2007). Optical Brightening Agents Based on Stilbene and Distyryl Biphenyl for the Improvement of Ultraviolet Protection of Cotton Fabrics, *Tekstil* 56 (1), 1-6

[27] Saravanan, D.: UV protection textile materials, *AUTEX Research Journal* 7 (2007) 53-62.

[28] Grancarić, A. M., Tarbuk, A. and McCall D. (2007). Surface Modification of Polyester Fabric with Tribomechanical-activated Natural Zeolite (TMAZ) Nanoparticles, *Polimeri* 28 (4); 219-224.

[29] Zhou Y., Cox Crews P., (1998). Effect of OBAs and repeated launderings on UVR transmission through fabrics. *Textile Chemist and Colorist* 30 (11), 19-24.

[30] Das, B. R. (2010) UV Radiation Protective Clothing. *The Open Textile Journal* 3, 14-21.

[31] Kim, J., Stone, J., Crews, P., Shelley, M. and Hatch, K. L. (2004). Improving Knit Fabric UPF Using Consumer Laundry Products: A Comparison of Results Using Two Instruments, *Family and Consumer Sciences Research Journal* 3, 141-158.

[32] Dekanić, T., Pušić, T., Soljačić I. Impact of artificial light on optical and protective effects of cotton after washing with detergent containing fluorescent compounds, *Tenside Surf. Det.* 51 (2014) 5, 451-459, doi: TS110329 – 16.7.14 dk/stm köthen

[33] Stanford, D. G., Georgouras, K. E. and Pailthorpe, M. T. (1995). The effect of laundering on the sun protection afforded by a summer weight garment, *Journal of the European Academy of Dermatology and Venereology* 5, 28-30.

[34] Tang, E., Cheng, G., Pang, X., Ma, X., Xing, F. (2006). Synthesis of nano-ZnO/poly(methyl methacrylate) composite microsphere through emulsion polymerization and its UV-shielding property, *Colloid and Polymer Science* 284 (4), 422-428.

[35] Farouk, A., Textor, T. Schollmeyer, E. Tarbuk, A. Grancarić, A. M. (2010). Sol-gel Derived Inorganic-organic Hybrid Polymers Filled with ZnO Nanoparticles as Ultraviolet Protection Finish for Textiles, *AUTEX research journal* 10 (8); 58-63.

[36] Sundaresan, K., Sivakumar A., Vigneswaran, C., Ramachandran, T. (2012). Influence of nano titanium dioxide finish, prepared by sol-gel technique, on the ultraviolet protection, antimicrobial, and self-cleaning characteristics of cotton fabrics, *Journal of Industrial Textiles* 41 (3), 259-277.

[37] Xin, J. H., Daoud, W. A., Kong, Y. Y. (2004). A new approach to UV-blocking treatment for cotton fabrics. *Text Res* J 74:97–10.

[38] Ranby, B., Rabek, J. F. (1975). *Photodegradation, Photo-oxidation and Photostabilization of Polymers,* John Wiley, (London, New York, Sydney and Toronto), 6-27.

[39] Grancarić A. M., Soljačić, I. (1980). Einflus der Konzentration optischer Aufheller auf Fluorescenz und Weissgrad von Baumwollgeweben, *Melliand Textilberichte* 61, 242-245.

[40] Lautenschlager, S., Wulf, H.. and Pittelkow, M. R.: Photoprotection, *The Lancet* 370 (2007) 528-537.

[41] Dekanić, T.; Pušić, T.; Soljačić, I. (2014). Light fastness of cotton optical and UV protection effects, *Book of Proceedings of the 7th International Textile*, Clothing & Design Conference, Zagreb, University of Zagreb, *Faculty of Textile Technology*, 183-188.

[42] Pušić, T.; Tarbuk, A.; Dekanić, T. (2015). Bio-innovation in cotton scouring - acid and neutral pectinases. *Fibres & Textiles in Eastern Europe*. 23 (109), 1; 98-103.

[43] Tarbuk, A., Grancarić, A.M. Leskovac M. (2014). Novel cotton cellulose by cationisation during the mercerisation process - *Part 1: Chemical and morphological changes, Cellulose* 21 (3); 2167-2179.

[44] Tarbuk, A.; Pušić, T.; Jukić, M. Optimizing in cotton bioscouring with acid and neutral pectinases. *Tekstil* 62 (2013) 9-10; 353-360.

In: Sunscreens
Editors: Sean Henry Sharp

ISBN: 978-1-63482-160-5

Chapter 9

THE POTENTIAL OF MYCOSPORINE-LIKE AMINO ACIDS AS UV-SUNSCREENS

***Rajesh P. Rastogi*[1], *Ravi R Sonani*[1], *Datta Madamwar*[1] *and Aran Incharoensakdi*[2,*]**

[1]BRD School of Biosciences, Vadtal Road, Satellite Campus, Sardar Patel University, Anand, Gujarat, India

[2]Laboratory of Cyanobacterial Biotechnology, Department of Biochemistry, Faculty of Science, Chulalongkorn University, Bangkok, Thailand

ABSTRACT

Strong ultraviolet (UV) radiation is one of the most lethal and carcinogenic exogenous agents that can interact with and alter the normal life processes by means of its direct or indirect damaging effects. Mycosporine-like amino acids (MAAs) are important 'multipurpose' small biomolecules that provide protection from intense UV radiation without producing the reactive oxygen species (ROS). A number of MAAs have been reported from different taxonomic groups. MAAs have great potential in photoprotection and genome maintenance by minimizing the cellular damage from UV-induced ROS and thymine dimer formation. Moreover, due to strong UV-absorbing/screening function, photo-induction, strong antioxidant properties and resistance to abiotic stressors, MAAs are considered as natural photoprotectants that may be biotechnologically exploited in cosmetics and other pharmaceutical industries. In the present article, an attempt has been made to critically review and highlight the recent updates on various MAAs with respect to their function as potential UV-sunscreens.

Keywords: Mycosporine-like amino acids, UV radiation, oxidative stress, photoprotectants, sunscreens

[*] Corresponding author: Tel.: +66 2 218 5422; fax: +66 2 218 5418 (A. Incharoensakdi), E-mail: aran.i@chula.ac.th (A. Incharoensakdi).

1. INTRODUCTION

The increase in short wavelength solar ultraviolet (UV) radiation on the Earth's atmosphere due to anthropogenically increased ozone depleting substances has aroused tremendous concern about its negative impacts on living organisms in both aquatic as well as terrestrial ecosystems. UV radiation (280-400 nm) may affect several biochemical and physiological processes leading to loss of normal life functionality of photosynthetic and non-photosynthetic organisms including human beings (Rastogi and Sinha, 2011a). It has been established that solar UV-A radiation (315-400 nm) has less direct effects on living systems since native DNA of living organisms cannot absorb UV-A. However, UV-A can indirectly affect the cellular function by the generation of reactive oxygen species (ROS) via photosensitizing reactions. In contrast, UV-B (280-315 nm) radiation has direct effects on key cellular machinery such as proteins and nucleic acids (Rastogi et al., 2010a). The short wavelength solar UV radiation may cause protein modification, membrane disruption, enzyme inactivation, generation of DNA lesions, alteration of transcription and translation process, mutagenesis and several other external effects such as sunburn and skin cancer (Bruce and Brodland, 2000; Rastogi et al., 2010a).

Moreover, several defense mechanisms have been reported in diverse organisms to counteract the harmful effects of UV radiation (Rastogi and Sinha, 2011b). Biosynthesis of certain UV-absorbing/screening compounds in different organisms is considered as an effective mode of defense mechanisms to reduce the damaging effects of solar UV radiation (Karentz et al., 1991; Rastogi et al., 2010b; Carreto and Carignan, 2011). Mycosporine-like amino acids (MAAs) are considered as prominent photoprotectants that provide photoprotection against harmful UV radiation (Cockell and Knowland, 1999; Oren and Gunde-Cimerman, 2007). In the present chapter, we summarize the eco-biological importance of the biologically relevant molecules MAAs, with special emphasis on their UV-screening or photoprotective functions.

2. SOLAR ULTRAVIOLET RADIATION AND BIOLOGICAL EFFECTS

In the past few decades, loss in stratospheric ozone layer due to anthropogenically released ozone depleting substances such as chlorofluorocarbons (CFCs) and reactive nitrogen species such as nitrous oxide (N_2O) has generated tremendous concern about the increasing level of short wavelength UV radiations reaching the Earth's atmosphere (Ravishankara et al., 2009; Manney el., 2011; Cabrol et al., 2014; Williamson et al., 2014). In all the groups of UV radiation (280–400 nm), UV-B radiation produces more adverse effects on diverse habitats, despite the fact that most of the extraterrestrial UV-B is absorbed by the stratospheric ozone layer (McKenzie et al., 2003). It has been established that UV-C (100-280 nm) radiation is quantitatively absorbed by oxygen and ozone in the Earth's atmosphere, and does not show any harmful effects on our ecosystems. Furthermore, UV-A (315-400 nm) radiation has low efficacy in inducing the DNA damage, as it is not absorbed by native DNA molecules; however, it can damage DNA via indirect photosensitizing reactions by the formation of reactive oxygen species (Rastogi et al., 2010a). The data obtained from European Light Dosimeter Network (Eldonet) dosimeters (Häder et al., 1999) have revealed the extreme UV-B irradiance in different parts of the Earth (Jacovides et al., 2009; Cabrol et al., 2014). Several other environmental factors such as aerosols and various tropospheric pollutants, cloud cover, sun-angle and surface reflectants also affect the intensity of UV-B radiation reaching the Earth's surface to a certain extent (Madronich et al., 1998). UV radiation also induces single- and/or double-strand DNA breaks in various organisms (Rastogi et al., 2010a; Rastogi and Sinha, 2011a). Moreover, the global climate change and increase in harmful short wavelength UV radiation can affect the normal life processes of all organisms inhabiting the aquatic or terrestrial habitats (Häder et al., 2014, 2015). In addition to UV effects on photosynthetic life (Rastogi et al., 2013; Rastogi et al., 2014a), a number of UV-induced effects such as occurrence of melanoma and non-melanoma skin cancer, sunburn, photo-allergy, eye disorders and immune suppression have also been reported in humans (McAteer et al., 1998; Lima-Bessa et al., 2008) (Figure 1). Solar UV-B radiation damages cellular DNA inducing mainly cyaclobutane purine/pyrimidine dimers (CPDs) and pyrimidine (6–4) pyrimidone photoproducts (6–4 PPs) and their Dewar isomers (Rastogi et al., 2010a). DNA double strand breaks (DSBs) may lead to loss of genetic information. Increased production of UV-induced ROS may alter the configuration of cell structure, lipids, proteins and DNA molecules, all of which are the cause of a number of human diseases (Valko et al., 2007). It has been shown that CPDs inhibit the progress of microbial and mammalian DNA polymerases (Britt, 1999). Moreover, UV-A-induced production of CPDs has also been observed in bacteria as well as in eukaryotic cells (Douki et al., 2003; Courdavault et al., 2004; Rastogi et al., 2014b). In response to detrimental effects of UV radiation, some organisms have developed certain defense mechanisms such as DNA repair and synthesis of UV-protective compounds to mitigate the harmful effects of short wavelength solar radiation (Rastogi et al., 2014c).

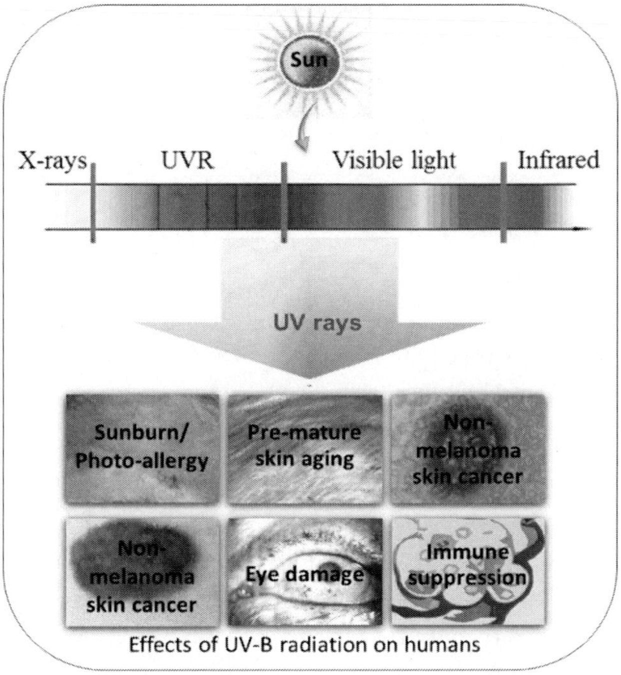

Figure 1. Effects of solar UV radiation on human health (details in text).

3. UV-Absorbing Compounds

A number of UV-absorbing/screening biomolecules such as mycosporines/mycosporine-like amino acids (MAAs), scytonemin, melanins, carotenoids, flavonoids, parietin and usnic acid, have been reported to be synthesized by diverse organisms (Figure 2) to counteract the detrimental effects of solar UV-B radiation (Rastogi et al., 2010b). There have been a number of reviews about diverse classes of photoprotective compounds from natural sources (Karsten et al., 2000; Bjerke et al., 2002; Gauslaa and McEvoy, 2005; Rastogi et al., 2010b; Rastogi and Incharoensakdi, 2013; 2014a, 2014b, 2014c); however, their application as photoprotectants and development of cosmeceutical products has only partially been elucidated. In the present review, we focus on the occurrence, biosynthesis and commercial application as potential sunscreens of the important UV-absorbing/screening compounds, MAAs from various sources.

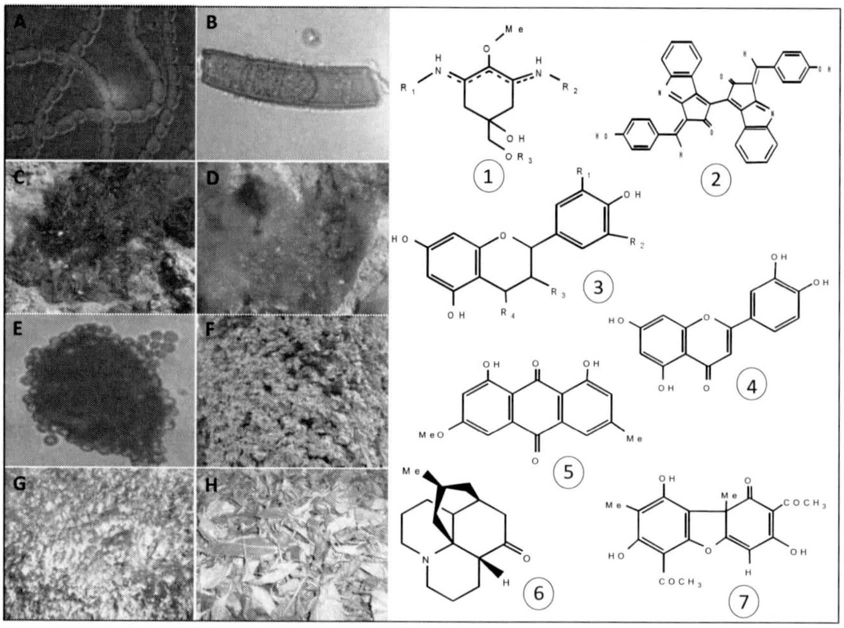

Figure 2. UV-absorbing/screening compounds (1 to 7) from different plant sources (A, B-The cyanobacterium *Anabaena* sp. and *Lynnbya* sp., respectively; C-Brown algae; D-Green algae; E-Fungi; F-Lichens; G-Bryophytes; H-tea leaves) [1 to 7: general structure of MAA, scytonemin, higher plant flavonoid, luteolin, parietin, lycopodine, and usnic acid, respectively].

3.1. Mycosporine-like Amino Acids

Mycosporine-like amino acids are small, colorless and highly hydrophilic compounds. They consist of cyclohexenone or cyclohexenimine chromophores, conjugated with the nitrogen substituent of an amino acid or its imino alcohol. The ring system of MAA includes a glycine subunit at the 3C atom, though some MAAs also contain sulfate esters or glycosidic linkages through the imine substituents (Wu Won et al., 1997). The UV absorption spectra of different MAAs differ due to variations in the attached side groups and nitrogen substituents (Böhm et al., 1995; Wu Won et al., 1997). Moreover, the precise stereostructure of MAAs (except palythine and palythene), including amino acids substituents is not completely elucidated. MAAs are extremely hydrophilic due to their zwitter ionic form derived from the amino acid substitution. Further hydrophilicity can also be increased by modification with sulfonic acids or sugar molecules (Böhm et al., 1995; Wu Won et al., 1997). Presently, more than 25 MAAs (Figure 3) have been reported from diverse organisms; however, a number of other UV-absorbing/screening compounds with potential application as UV photoprotectants remain to be explored from nature.

3.2. Occurrence and Distribution of MAAs

Among various UV-photoprotectant biomolecules, the biosynthesis of different MAAs has been reported from diverse taxonomic groups (Sinha et al., 2007; Rastogi et al., 2010b) (Table 1). Cyanobacteria are the most dominant photoautotrophs that can synthesize a range of different MAAs (Shibata, 1969). The MAAs shinorine and porphyra-334 have been found to be the most dominant MAAs in several species of terrestrial or fresh/marine water cyanobacteria (Karsten and Garcia-Pichel, 1996; Sinha et al., 2003; Volkmann et al., 2006; Rastogi et al., 2010b; Chuang et al., 2014; Rastogi et al., 2012). Rastogi and Incharoensakdi (2014a, b, c) have isolated and characterized some primary MAAs from different cyanobacteria inhabiting diverse habitats (Figure 4). Several MAAs were isolated from different species/strains of cyanobacteria inhabiting the hot springs (Rastogi et al., 2012). Two novel glycosylated MAAs such as a pentose-bound porphyra-334 derivative (MW 478 Da; UVλ_{max}: 335 nm) and other MAAs (MW1050 Da; UVλ_{max}: 312 and 340 nm) consisting of two distinct chromophores of 3-aminocyclohexen-1-one and 1,3-diaminocyclohexen and two pentose and hexose sugars were identified in *Nostoc commune* (Matsui et al., 2011). Recently, the glycosylated MAAs such as glycosylated porphyra-334 (MW 508 Da; UVλ_{max}: 334 nm) and palythine-threoninehave (MW 612 Da; UVλ_{max}: 322 nm) have also been reported in the cyanobacterium *Nostoc commune* (Nazifi et al., 2013).

Besides cyanobacteria, a range of MAAs have also been reported in cyanobacterial lichens (Coba et al., 2009), micro/macro algae and animals (Sinha et al., 2007) Table 1). A number of microalgae/phytoplankton such as diatoms (Riegger and Robinson, 1997; Hernando et al., 2002; Ingalls et al., 2010), dinoflagellates (Klisch and Häder, 2000; Banaszack and Trench, 2001; Laurion et al., 2004; Banaszak et al., 2006; Laurion and Roy, 2009), chlorophytes (Gröniger and Häder, 2002; Llewellyn and Airs, 2010; Rastogi and Incharoensakdi, 2013), and prymnesiophytes (Marchant et al., 1991; Riegger and Robinson, 1997; Hannach and Sigleo, 1998) have been found to produce different MAAs. Several species of macroalgae (Karsten et al., 1998a; Hoyer et al., 2002) belonging to chlorophyceae (Han and Han, 2005), rhodophyceae (Kräbs et al., 2004; Coba et al., 2009; Yuan et al., 2009; Cardozo et al., 2011) and phaeophyceae have been reported to synthesize an array of MAAs and other UV-absorbing compounds.

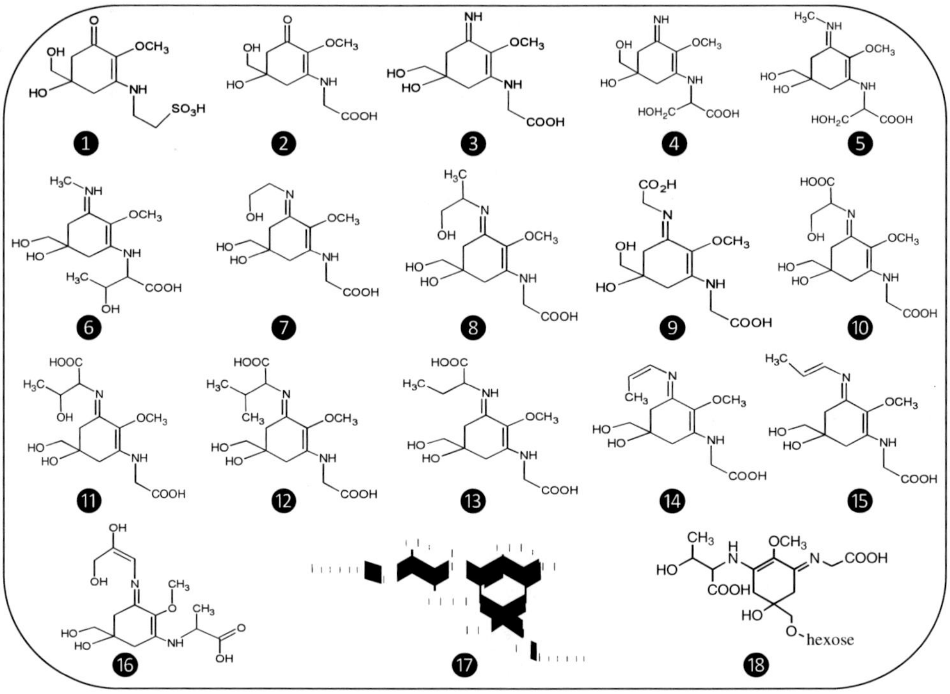

Figure 3. Chemical structure of some important MAAs found in different taxonomic groups. [1 to 18: Mycosporine-taurine, Mycosporine-glycine, Palythine, Palythine-serine, Mycosporine-methylamine-serine, Mycosporine-methylamine-threonine, Asterina-330, Palythinol, Mycosporine-2-glycine, Shinorine, Porphyra-334, Mycosporine-glycine-valine, Palythenic acid, Usujirene, Palythene, Euhalothece-362, Glycosylated palythine-threonine and Glycosylated porphyra-334, respectively].

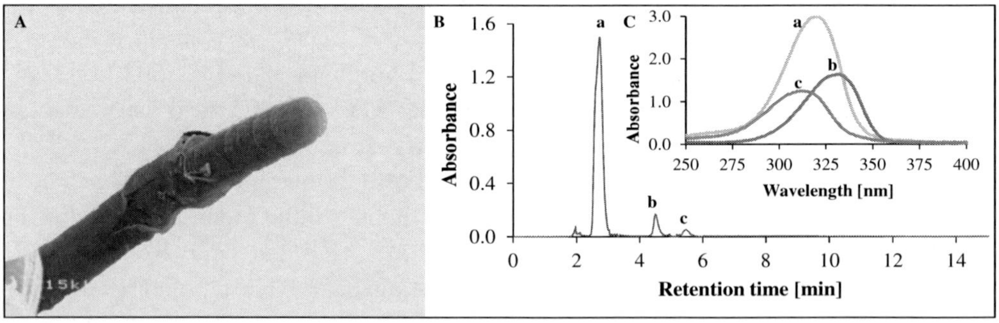

Figure 4. The cyanobacterium *Lyngbya* sp. (A) and high performance liquid chromatograph (B) showing the UV-absorption maxima (B-inset) of some MAAs such as palythine (a, UV λ_{max}: 320 nm), asterina-330 (b, UV λ_{max}: 330 nm) and an unknown MAA, M-312 (c, UV λ_{max}: 312) (Adapted from Rastogi and Incharoensakdi, 2014c).

The accumulation of several MAAs have also been reported in different animals such as arthropods, rotifers, molluscs, fishes, cnidarians, tunicates, eubacteriobionts, poriferans, nemertineans, echinodermates, platythelminthes, polychaetes, bryozoans and protozoans (Sinha et al., 2007). However, it has been thought that MAAs are not directly synthesized by animals, but rather accumulated in these animals as a result of dietary food acquisition (Carroll and Shick, 1996; Newman et al., 2000).

Table 1. Occurrence and distribution of some common MAAs in different taxonomic groups

Taxonomic groups	Mycosporine-like amino acids												
	AS	MG	M2G	MT	MGV	PE	PR	PL	PT	SH	US	DL	PS
Cyanobacteria	+	+	+	+		+	+	+	+	+		+	
Green algae	+	+					+	+	+	+			
Brown algae	+	+					+	+	+	+			
Red algae	+	+				+	+	+	+	+			
Microalgae/phytoplankton	+	+	+	+	+	+	+	+	+	+	+		+
Copepods	+	+				+	+	+	+	+	+		
Corals	+	+	+			+	+	+	+	+			
Krill	+	+			+	+	+	+	+	+			
Amphipod	+	+			+	+	+	+	+	+			
Molluscs	+	+	+			+	+	+	+	+			
Fish	+	+			+	+	+	+	+	+			
Sea Anemones	+	+	+	+	+	+	+		+	+			
Sponge	+	+	+				+	+	+	+			

(For details please see the references, Sinha et al., 2007; Rastogi et al., 2014c; Rastogi et al., 2014 a, Rastogi et al., 2010b for details and references therein) [AS, asterina-330; MG,mycosporine-glycine; M2G, mycosporine-2-glycine; MT, mycosporine-taurine; MGV, mycosporineglycine-valine; PE, palythene; PR, porphyra-334; PL, palythinol; PT, palythine; SH, shinorine; US, usurijene; DL, dehydroxylusujirene; PS, palythine-serine].

3.3. Regulation of MAAs Biosynthesis

The biosynthesis of MAAs in fungi and cyanobacteria are supposed to occur via the first part of the shikimate pathway, 3-dehydroquinate (DHQ) formed during the early part of the shikimate pathway. The DHQ molecule is assumed to act as a precursor for the synthesis of primary MAA, via gadusol or deoxygadusol (Portwich and Garcia-Pichel, 2003). Moreover, the main steps of the MAAs biosynthetic pathway and their genetic basis have recently been elucidated in *Anabaena variabilis* ATCC 29413 (Balskus and Walsh, 2010). A cluster of four genes (Ava_3858-3855) was found in the cyanobacterium *Anabaena variabilis*, responsible for the biosynthesis of a MAA shinorine using the common pentose-phosphate-pathway intermediate sedoheptulose-7-phosphate via 4-deoxygadusol (Balskus and Walsh, 2010; Spence et al., 2012). The dehydroquinate synthase homologue Ava_3858 and the O-methyltransferase Ava_3857 was found to convert the precursor into 4-deoxygadusol (4-DG), and the ATP-grasp homologue Ava_3856 converts the 4-DG as well as glycine into mycosporine-glycine (M-Gly) (Figure 5). The MAA M-Gly is converted into shinorine with addition of serine molecule catalyzed by a nonribosomal peptide synthetase (NRPS) encoded by Ava_3855 (Figure 5). Recently, the MAA biosynthetic gene cluster has also been reported in some other cyanobacteria such as *Nostoc punctiforme* (Gao and Garcia-Pichel, 2011) and *Aphanothece halophytica* (Waditee-Sirisattha et al., 2014). In *Nostoc punctiforme* ATCC

29133, the four gene cluster such as NpR5600, NpR5599, NpR5598, and NpF5597 was shown to catalyze the biosynthesis of M-Gly in a similar manner as was found in *A. variabilis*. However, the NpF5597 was found to encode D-Ala-D-Ala ligase and the direction of transcription of NpF5597 was opposite to those of NpR5600 and NpR5598 (Gao and Garcia-Pichel, 2011). In the halotolerant cyanobacterium *Aphanothece halophytica*, the MAA gene cluster was capable of synthesizing mycosporine-2-glycine. A unique MAA core 4-DG-synthesizing gene was separated from three other genes. The identified genes, Ap3857, Ap3856, and Ap3855, were homologous to Ava_ 3857/NpR5599, Ava_3856/NpR5598, and NpF5597, respectively. It was found that *A. halophytica* does not contain a gene homologous to Ava_3855 encoding NRPS, but contains a gene homologous to NpF5597 encoding D-Ala-D-Ala ligase (Waditee-Sirisattha et al., 2013).

3.4. MAA Biosynthesis under Different Abiotic Factors

A number of abiotic factors, such as short wavelength UV radiations, temperature, desiccation, light/dark periods, salt concentrations and various nutrients affect the biosynthesis of MAAs in cyanobacteria and other organisms (Rastogi et al., 2010b). Several studies have established the increased production of MAAs under different wavebands of UV radiation in cyanobacteria (Sinha et al., 2003; Singh et al., 2008a; Rastogi et al., 2010c; Rastogi and Incharoensakdi, 2014a, b, c; Rastogi and Incharoensakdi, 2013, 2015) and micro/macroalgae or phytoplanktons (Riegger and Robinson, 1997; Klisch and Häder, 2002). The production of MAAs in various organisms are highly responsive to UV-B radiation (Sinha et al., 2001; Singh et al., 2008a; Rastogi and Incharoensakdi, 2015; 2014a, c) (Figure 6); howevr, UV-A induced production of MAAs has also been reported in different organisms (Kräbs et al., 2004; Rastogi et al., 2010c). Korbee et al. (2005a) studied the accumulation of MAAs in *Porphyra leucosticte* and found the favorable role of blue light in the accumulation of porphyra-334, palythine and asterina-330 in contrast to the accumulation of shinorine which was observed under white, green, yellow or red light. Contrary to light period, the biosynthesis of MAAs was found to decrease under dark period (Rastogi et al., 2010c; Rastogi and Incharoensakdi, 2015), suggesting an energy-dependent process of MAA synthesis.

The biosynthesis of MAAs is also affected under different nutrient conditions (Rastogi et al., 2010b). A remarkable decrease in MAA content was found under nitrogen limitations in the marine dinoflagellates (Litchman et al., 2002). Induction of some MAAs in *Anabaena variabilis* PCC 7937 was caused by salt and ammonium in a concentration-dependent manner (Singh et al., 2008b). Increased biosynthesis of certain photoprotective compounds under enriched ammonium concentrations was also found in the red alga *Porphyra* sp. (Korbee et al., 2005b, Peinado et al., 2004). Bio-conversion of a primary MAA into a secondary MAA was found under sulfur deficiency in *A. variabilis* PCC 7937 (Singh et al., 2010). High concentration of certain UV-absorbing compounds has also been reported under desiccation (Jiang et al., 2008) and warm temperature (Karsten et al., 1998) in the Rhodophytes *Chondrus crispus* and *Porphyra haitanensis*, respectively. Moreover, MAAs biosynthetic pathway may be regulated by multiple environmental signals.

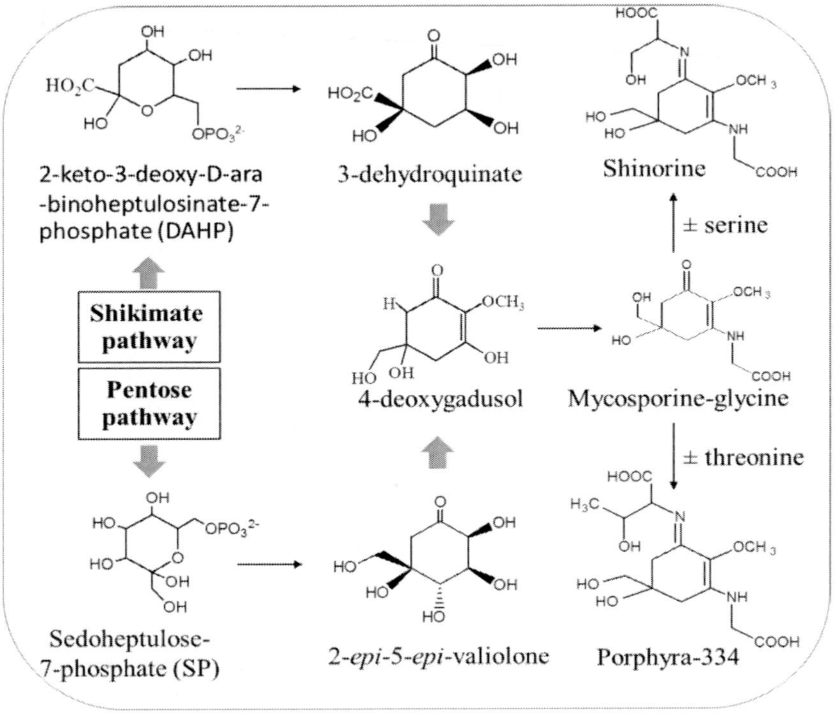

Figure 5. A proposed pathway of the biosynthesis of some primary MAAs (Adapted from Balskus and Walsh, Rastogi et al., 2010b, 2010; Spence et al., 2012) (details in text).

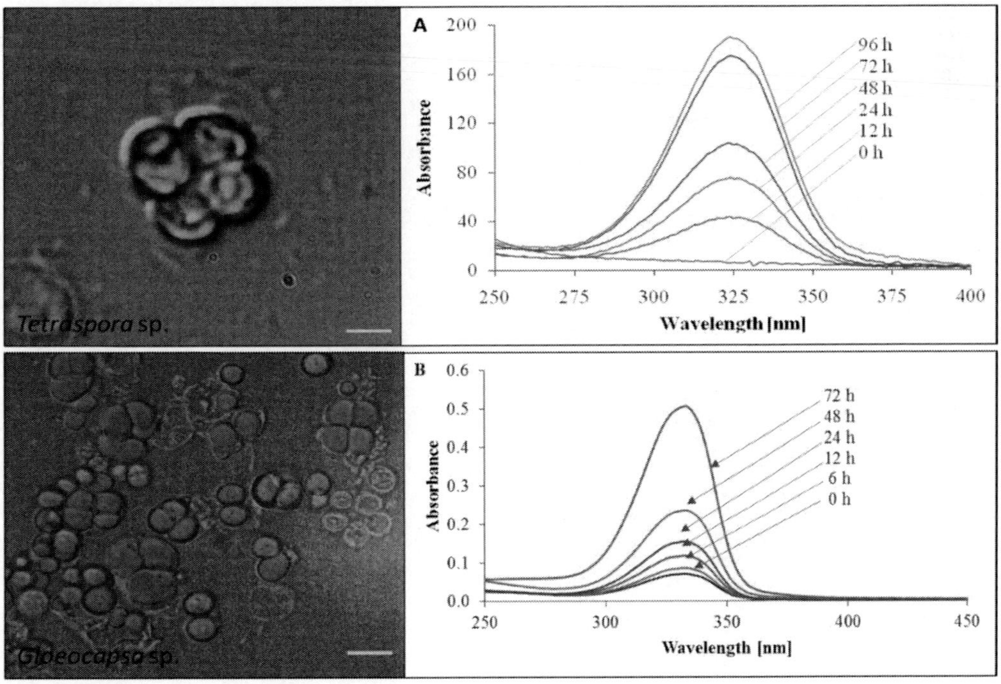

Figure 6. Induction of a 324 nm-MAA (A) and shinorine (B) after different durations of UV-B irradiation in the green alga *Tetraspora* sp. and Gloeocapsa sp. (Adapted from Rastogi and Incharoensakdi, 2013, 2014a).

4. MAAs as Sunscreens: Dominant Role in Photoprotection

Mycosporine-like amino acids (MAAs) are well-known UV-absorbing/screening compounds for their crucial role in photoprotection. Several properties such as strong UV-absorption maxima, high molar extinction coefficients, competence to dissipate absorbed radiation as heat without producing reactive oxygen species (ROS), UV-induction and stability under different physicochemical factors such as UV radiation, heat, pH, strong oxidizing agent and different organic solvents strongly support the MAAs as photoprotective compounds (Gröniger and Häder, 2000; Whitehead and Hedges, 2005; Conde et al., 2007; Rastogi and Incharoensakdi, 2014a, 2014c). It has been shown that MAAs provide protection from UV radiation not only to their producers, but also to primary and secondary consumers through the food chain (Helbling et al., 2002), and may be considered as a broad-spectrum UV absorbers/protectors. As discussed above, UV radiation can promote the occurrence of sunburn on skin cells; the application of UV-absorbing compound may provide protection against intense solar radiation or sunburns (Drolet and Connor, 1992). MAAs may protect the skin cells from UV-induced cell death. Recently, Rastogi and Incharoensakdi (2013) investigated for the first time the photoprotective activities of 324 nm-MAA and 322 nm-MAA isolated from a green microalga, *Tetraspora* sp., against UV radiation. It was found that the MAA porphyra-334 along with shinorine can suppress UV-induced aging in human skin (Daniel et al., 2004). The MAAs were found to protect eggs of the sea hare *Aplysia dactylomela* from UV radiation (Carefoot et al., 1998). The MAAs such as shinorine (SH), porphyra-334 (P-334) and mycosporine-glycine were found to protect the human fibroblast cells from UVR-induced cell death (Oyamada et al., 2008).

Some MAAs have been reported to have strong antioxidant or free radical scavenging capacity (Coba et al., 2007a, 2007b; Oren and Gunde-Cimerman, 2007) (Figure 7A). The MAA mycosporine-glycine (MG) was found to protect biological systems against photodynamic damage by quenching singlet oxygen with a high efficiency (Suh et al., 2003). Some MAAs such as porphyra-334 and shinorine showed high antioxidant activity against free radicals (Coba et al., 2007a, 2007b) generated from UV radiation (Oren and Gunde-Cimerman, 2007).

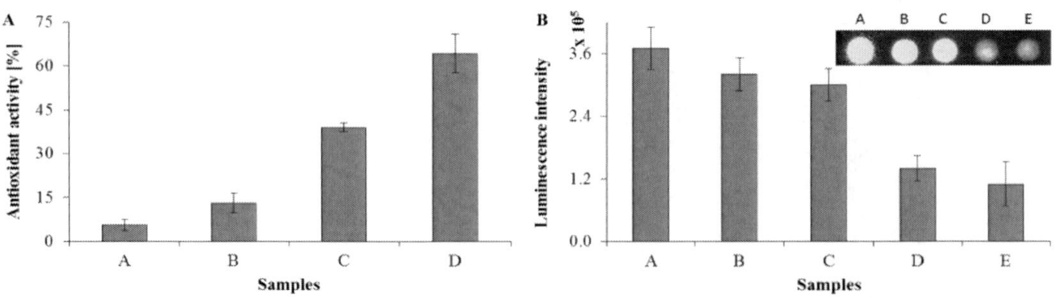

Figure 7. Free radical scavenging capacity of MAAs shinorine + M-307 (panel A) (adapted from Rastogi and Incharoensakdi, 2014a) and inhibition of thymine dimer formation (panel B: data not published). [in panel A; the samples contain 0.2(A), 0.4(B), 0.83(C) and 1.6 (D) mg/ml MAAs; in panel B; Control cells exposed to UV without (A) and with 0.05 (B), 0.1 (C), 0.25 (D) and 0.5 (E) mg/ml M-gly].

The antioxidant activities of the MAAs M-gly and usujilene have also been reported to inhibit lipid peroxidation (Nakayama et al., 1999; Suh et al., 2003). The presence of the glycosylated MAAs with radical scavenging activity has been reported in the cyanobacterium *Nostoc commune* (Matsui et al., 2011). Recently, Rastogi and Incharoensakdi (2014a) have found the efficacy of MAAs (shinorine + M-307) from *Gloeocapsa* sp. as a potential sunscreen. The MAAs (palythine + asterina + M-312) isolated from *Lyngbya* sp. were found to act as strong radical scavenger (Rastogi and Incharoensakdi, 2014c).

Recently, some MAAs have been investigated for their potential role in genome maintainance (Rastogi, 2010). The UV-absorbing compound isolated from a red alga *Porphyra yezoensis* was found to block the production of thymine dimer (T<>T) (Misonou et al., 2003). Recently, Rastogi (2010) has also found the great efficacy of MAAs in reducing the most genotoxic and cytotoxic DNA lesions, CPD T<>T (Figure 7B). Moreover, some synthetic analogues of MAAs, such as tetrahydropyridine derivatives, have been developed for commercial application as suncare products (Bird et al., 1987; Chalmers et al., 1990; Coba et al., 2007b). Moreover, due to potent UV protecting capacity, MAAs can be a potential candidate for the commercial development of suncare products.

Conclusion

MAAs are multipurpose secondary compounds reported in a number of taxonomic groups. These compounds are highly stable against a number of physicochemical factors, act as strong antioxidants, and are able to prevent cellular as well as genomic damage resulting from UV-induced ROS. Several studies have established the anti-aging role of MAAs, minimizing the risk of skin cancer. Overall, MAAs can be considered as high value compounds that have great potential applications as natural photoprotectants and antioxidants that can be exploited in cosmetics and pharmaceutical industries for the development of novel cosmeceuticals.

Acknowledgments

Rajesh P. Rastogi is thankful to the University Grant Commission (UGC), New Delhi, India, for financial support in the form of Dr. D. S. Kothari Postdoctoral grant. Aran Incharoensakdi thanks Chulalongkorn University Ratchadaphiseksomphot Endowment Fund for financial support on the project "Value-added products and bioenergy from microalgae".

References

Balskus, EP; Walsh, CT. The genetic and molecular basis for sunscreen biosynthesis in cyanobacteria. *Science*, 2010, 329, 1653-1656.

Banaszack, AT; Trench, RK. Ultraviolet sunscreens in dinoflagellates. *Protist*, 2001, 152, 93-101.

Banaszak, AT; Santos, MG; LaJeunesse, TC; Lesser, MP. The distribution of mycosporine-like amino acids (MAAs) and the phylogenetic identity of symbiotic dinoflagellates in cnidarian hosts from the Mexican Caribbean. *J. Exp. Mar. Biol. Ecol.*, 2006, 337, 131-146.

Bird, G; Fitzmaurice, N; Dunlap, WC; Chalker, BE; Bandaranayake, WM. Sunscreen compositions and compounds for use therein. International patent application PCT/AU87/00330, publication no. WO 88/02251, 1987. Australian patent 595075. ICI Australia Operations Pty Ltd and Australian Institute of Marine Science, Townsville.

Bjerke, JW; Lerfall, K; Elvebakk, A. Effects of ultraviolet radiation and PAR on the content of usnic and divaricatic acids in two arctic-alpine lichens. *Photochem. Photobiol. Sci.*, 2002, 1, 678–685.

Böhm, GA; Pfleiderer, W; Böger, P; Scherer, S. Structure of a novel oligosaccharide-mycosporine-amino acid ultraviolet A/B sunscreen pigment from the terrestrial cyanobacterium *Nostoc* commune. *J. Biol. Chem.*, 1995, 270, 8536-8539.

Britt, AB. Molecular genetics of DNA repair in higher plants. *Trends Plant Sci.*, 1999, 4, 20-25.

Bruce, AJ; Brodland, DG. Overview of skin cancer detection and prevention for the primary care physician. *Mayo Clin. Ptoc.*, 2000, 75, 491-500.

Cabrol, NA; Feister, U; Häder, DP; Piazena, H; Grin, EA; Klein, A. Record solar UV irradiance in the Tropical Andes. *Environ. Toxicol.*, 2014, 2, 19.

Cardozo, KHM; Marques, LG; Carvalho VM; Carignan MO; Pinto E; Marinho-Soriano, E; Colepicolo, P. Analyses of photoprotective compounds in red algae from the Brazilian coast. *Braz. J. Pharmacogn.*, 2011, 21, 202-208.

Carefoot, TH; Harris, M; Taylor, BE; Donovan, D; Karentz, D. Mycosporine-like amino acids: possible UV protection in eggs of the sea hare *Aplysia dactylomela*. *Mar. Biol.*, 1998, 130, 389-396.

Carreto, JI; Carignan, MO. Mycosporine-Like amino acids: Relevant secondary metabolites. Chemical and ecological aspects. *Mar. Drugs*, 2011, 9, 387-446.

Carroll, AK; Shick, JM. Dietary accumulation of mycosporine-like amino acids (MAAs) by the green sea urchin (*Strongylocentrus droebachiensis*). *Mar. Biol.*, 1996, 124, 561–569.

Chalmers, PJ; Fitzmaurice, N; Rigg, DJ; Thang, SH; Bird, G. UV absorbing compounds and compositions. International Patent Application PCT/AU90/00078, publication no. WO 90/09995, 1990. Australian patent 653495. ICI Australia Operations Pty Ltd and Australian Institute of Marine Science, Townsville.

Chuang, LF; Chou, HN; Sung, PJ. Porphyra-334 isolated from the marine algae *Bangia atropurpurea*: Conformational performance for energy conversion. *Mar. drugs*, 2014 12, 4732-4740.

Coba, FDL; Aguilera, J; Figueroa, FL. Use of mycosporine-type amino acid porphyra-334 as an antioxidant. *Intl Patent WO2007/026035 A2* 2007a.

Coba, FDL; Aguilera, J; Figueroa, FL. Use of mycosporine-type aminoacid shinorine as an antioxidant. *Intl Patent WO2007/026038 A2* 2007b.

Coba, FDL; Aguilera, J; Figueroa, FL; de Gàlvez, MV; Herrera, E. Antioxidant activity of mycosporine-like amino acids isolated from three red macroalgae and one marine lichen. *J. Appl. Phycol.*, 2009, 21, 161-169.

Cockell, CS; Knowland, J. Ultraviolet radiation screening compounds. *Biol. Rev.*, 1999, 74, 311-345.

Conde, FR; Churio, MS; Previtali, CM. Experimental study of the excited-state properties and photostability of the mycosporine-like amino acid palythine in aqueous solution. *Photochem. Photobiol. Sci.*, 2007, 6, 669-674.

Courdavault, S; Baudouin, C; Charveron, M; Favier, A; Cadet, J; Douki, T. Larger yield of cyclobutane dimers than 8-oxo-7, 8-dihydroguanine in the DNA of UVA-irradiated human skin cells. *Mutation Res.*, 2004, 556, 135-142.

Daniel, S; Cornelia, S; Fred, Z. UV-A sunscreen from red algae for protection against premature skin aging. *Cosmet. Toilet. Manuf. Worldw.*, 2004, 139-143.

Douki, T; Reynaud-Angelin, A; Cadet, J; Sage, E. Bipyrimidine photoproducts rather than oxidative lesions are the main type of DNA damage involved in the genotoxic effects of solar UVA radiation. *Biochemistry*, 2003, 42, 9221-9226.

Drolet, BA; Connor, MJ. Sunscreens and the prevention of ultraviolet radiation-induced skin cancer. *J. Dermatol. Surg. Oncol.*, 1992, 18, 571-576.

Gao, Q; Garcia-Pichel, F. An ATP-grasp ligase involved in the last biosynthetic step of the iminomycosporine shinorine in *Nostoc punctiforme* ATCC 29133. *J. Bacteriol.*, 2011 193, 5923-5928.

Gauslaa, Y; McEvoy, M. Seasonal changes in solar radiation drive acclimation of the sun-screening compound parietin in the lichen *Xanthoria parietina. Basic. Appl. Ecol.*, 2005, 6, 75-82.

Gröniger, A; Häder, DP. Stability of mycosporine-like amino acids. *Recent Res. Devel. Photochem. Photobiol.*, 2000, 4, 247-252.

Gröniger, A; Häder, DP. Induction of the synthesis of an UVabsorbing substance in the green alga *Prasiola stipitata. J. Photochem. Photobiol. B.*, 2000, 66, 54-59.

Häder, DP; Williamson, CE; Wängberg, SÅ; Rautio, M; Rose, KC; Gao, K; Helbling, EW; Sinha RP; Worrest, R. Effects of UV radiation on aquatic ecosystems and interactions with other environmental factors. *Photochem. Photobiol. Sci.*, 2015, DOI: 10.1039/c4pp90035a.

Häder, DP; Villafañe, VE; Helbling, EW. Productivity of aquatic primary producers under global climate change. *Photochem. Photobiol. Sci.*, 2014, DOI: 10.1039/c3pp50418b.

Häder, DP; Lebert M; Marangoni R; Colombetti, G. ELDONET-European Light Dosimeter Network hardware and software. *J. Photochem. Photobiol. B.*, 1999, 52, 51-58.

Han, YS; Han, T. UV-B induction of UV-B protection in *Ulva pertusa* (chlorophyta). *J. Phycol.*, 2005, 41, 523-530.

Hannach, G; Sigleo, AC. Photoinduction of UV-absorbing compounds in six species of marine phytoplankton. *Mar. Ecol. Prog. Ser.*, 1998, 174, 207-222.

Helbling, EW; Menchi, CF; Villafañe, VE. Bioaccumulation and role of UV-absorbing compounds in two marine crustacean species from Patagonia, Argentina. *Photochem. Photobiol. Sci.*, 2002, 1, 820–825.

Hernando, M; Carreto, JI; Carignan, MO; Ferreyra, GA; Gross, C. Effects of solar radiation on growth and mycosporine-like amino acids content in *Thalassiosira* sp., an Antarctic diatom. *Polar Biol.*, 2002, 25, 12-20.

Hoyer, K; Karsten, U; Wiencke, C. Induction of sunscreen compounds in Antarctic macroalgae by different radiation conditions. *Mar. Biol.*, 2002, 141, 619-627.

Ingalls, AE; Whitehead, K; Bridoux, MC. Tinted windows: the presence of the UVabsorbing compounds called mycosporine-like amino acids embedded in the frustules of marine diatoms. *Geochim. Cosmochim. Acta*, 2010, 74, 104-115.

Jacovides, DO; Tymvios, FS; Asimakopoulos, DN; Kaltsounides, NA; Theoharatos, GA; Tsitouri, M. Solar global UVB (280-315 nm) and UVA (315-380nm) radiant fluxes and their relationships with broad- band global radiant flux at an eastern Mediterranean site. *Agr. Forest. Met.*, 2009, 149, 1188-1200.

Jiang, H; Gao, K; Helbling, EW. UV-absorbing compounds in *Porphyra haitanensis* (*Rhodophyta*) with special reference to effects of desiccation. *J. Appl. Phycol.*, 2008, 20, 387-395.

Karentz, D; McEuen, ES; Land, MC; Dunlap, WC. Survey of mycosporine-like amino acid compounds in Antarctic marine organisms: potential protection from ultraviolet exposure. *Mar. Biol.*, 1991, 108, 157-166.

Karsten, U; Garcia-Pichel, F. Carotenoids and mycosporine-like amino acid compounds in members of the genus *Microcoleus* (cyanobacteria): a chemosystematic study. *Syst. Appl. Microbiol.*, 1996, 19, 285-294.

Karsten, U; Sawall, T; West, J; Wiencke, C. Ultraviolet sunscreen compounds in epiphytic red algae from mangroves. *Hydrobiology*, 2000, 432, 159-171.

Karsten, U; Sawall, T; Wiencke, C. A survey of the distribution of UV absorbing substances in tropical macroalgae. *Phycol. Res.*, 1998a, 46, 271-279.

Klisch, M; Häder DP. Wavelength dependence of mycosporine-like amino acid synthesis in Gyrodinium dorsum. *J. Photochem. Photobiol. B.*, 2002, 66, 60-66.

Klisch, M; Häder, DP. Mycosporine-like amino acids in the marine dinoflagellate *Gyrodinium dorsum*: induction by ultraviolet irradiation. *J. Photochem. Photobiol. B.*, 2000, 55, 178-182.

Korbee, N; Figueroa, FL; Aguilera, FJ. Effect of light quality on the accumulation of photosynthetic pigments, proteins and mycosporine-like amino acids in the red alga *Porphyra leucosticta* (*Bangiales, Rhodophyta*). *J. Photochem. Photobiol. B.*, 2005a, 80, 71-78.

Korbee, N; Huovinen, P; Figueroa, FL; Aguilera, J; Karsten, U. Availability of ammonium influences photosynthesis and the accumulation of mycosporine-like amino acids in two *Porphyra* species (*Bangiales, Rhodophyta*). *Mar. Biol.*, 2005b, 146, 645-654.

Kräbs, G; Watanabe, M; Wiencke, C. A monochromatic action spectrum for the photoinduction of the UV-absorbing mycosporine-like amino acid shinorine in the red alga *Chondrus crispus*. *Photochem. Photobiol.*, 2004, 79, 515-519.

Laurion, I; Roy, S. Growth and photoprotection in three dinoflagellates (including two strains of *Alexandrium tamarense*) and one diatom exposed to four weeks of natural and enhanced UVB radiation. *J. Phycol.*, 2009, 45, 16-33.

Laurion, I; Blouin, F; Roy, S. Packaging of mycosporine-like amino acids in dinoflagellates. *Mar. Ecol. Prog. Ser.*, 2004, 279, 297-303.

Lima-Bessa, KMD; Armelini, MG; Chiganças, V; Jacysyn, JF; Amarante-Mendes, GP; Sarasin, A; Menck, CFM. CPDs and 6–4PPs play different roles in UV-induced cell death in normal and NER-deficient human cells. *DNA Repair*, 2008, 7, 303-312.

Litchman, E; Neale, PJ; Banaszak, AT. Increased sensitivity to ultraviolet radiation in nitrogen-limited dinoflagellates: photoprotection and repair. *Limnol. Oceanogr.*, 2002, 47, 86-94.

Llewellyn, CA; Airs, RL. Distribution and abundance of MAAs in 33 species of microalgae across 13 classes. *Mar. Drugs*, 2010, 8, 1273-1291.

Madronich, S; McKenzie, RL; Björn, LO; Caldwell, MM. Changes in biologically active ultraviolet radiation reaching the Earth's surface. *J. Photochem. Photobiol. B.*, 1998, 46, 5-19.

Manney, GL; Santee, ML; Rex, M; Livesey, NJ; Pitts, MC; Veefkind, P; et al. Unprecedented Arctic ozone loss in 2011, *Nature*, 2011, 478, 469-475.

Marchant, HJ; Davidson, AT; Kelly, GJ. UV-B protecting compounds in the marine alga *Phaeocystis pouchetii* from Antarctica. *Mar. Biol.*, 1991, 109, 391-395.

Matsui, K; Nazifi, E; Kunita, S; Wada, N; Matsugo, S; Sakamoto, T. Novel glycosylated mycosporine-like amino acids with radical scavenging activity from the cyanobacterium *Nostoc commune*. *J. Photochem. Photobiol. B.*, 2011, 105, 81-89.

McAteer, K; Jing, Y; Kao, J; Taylor, JS; Kennedy, MA. Solution-state structure of a DNA dodecamer duplex containing a cis-syn thymine cyclobutane dimer, the major UV photoproduct of DNA. *J. Mol. Biol.*, 1998, 282, 1013-1032.

McKenzie, RL; Aucamp, PJ; Bais, AF; Björn, LO; Ilyas, M. Changes in biologically active ultraviolet radiation reaching the Earth's surface. *Photochem. Photobiol. Sci.*, 2003, 2, 5-15.

Misonou, T; Saitoh, J; Oshiba, S; Tokitomo, Y; Maegawa, M; Inoue, Y; Hori, H; Sakurai, T; UV-absorbing substance in the red alga *Porphyra yezoensis* (Bangiales, Rhodophyta) block thymine dimer production. *Mar. Biotechnol.*, 2003, 5, 194-200.

Nakayama, R; Tamura, Y; Kikuzaki, H; Nakatani, N. Antioxidant effect of the constituents of susabinori (*Porphyra yezoensis*). *JAOCS*, 1999, 76, 649-653.

Nazifi, E; Wada, N; Yamaba, M; Asano, T; Nishiuchi, T; Matsugo, S; Sakamoto, T. Glycosylated porphyra-334 and palythine-threonine from the terrestrial cyanobacterium *Nostoc commune*. *Mar. Drugs*, 2013, 11, 3124-3154.

Newman, SJ; Dunlap, WC; Nicol, S; Ritz, D. Antarctic krill (*Euphausia superba*) acquire a UV-absorbing mycosporine-like amino acid from dietary algae. *J. Exper. Mar. Biol. Ecol.*, 2000, 255, 93-110.

Oren, A; Gunde-Cimerman, N. Mycosporines and mycosporine-like amino acids: UV protectants or multipurpose secondary metabolites? *FEMS Microbiol. Lett.*, 2007, 269, 1-10.

Oyamada, C; Kaneniwa, M; Ebitani, K; Murata, M; Ishihara, K. Mycosporine-like amino acids extracted from Scallop (*Patinopecten yessoensis*) ovaries: UV protection and growth stimulation activities on human cells. *Mar. Biotechnol.*, 2008, 10, 141-150.

Peinado, NK; Abdala Díaz, RT; Figueroa, FL; Helbling, EW. Ammonium and UV radiation stimulate the accumulation of mycosporine-like amino acids in *Porphyra columbina* (Rhodophyta) from Patagonia, Argentina. *J. Phycol.*, 2004, 40, 248-259.

Portwich, A; Garcia-Pichel, F. Biosynthetic pathway of mycosporines (mycosporine-like amino acids) in the cyanobacterium *Chlorogloeopsis* sp. strain PCC 6912. *Phycologia*, 2003, 42, 384-392.

Rastogi, RP. UV-B-induced DNA damage and repair in cyanobacteria, *PhD Thesis* 2010, Banaras Hindu University, Varanasi, India.

Rastogi, RP; Richa; Kumar, A; Tyagi, MB; Sinha, RP. Molecular mechanisms of ultraviolet radiation-induced DNA damage and repair. *J. Nucleic Acids*, 2010a. http://dx.doi.org/10.4061/2010/592980 (Article ID 592980).

Rastogi, RP; Richa; Sinha, RP; Singh, SP; Häder, DP. Photoprotective compounds from marine organisms. *J. Ind. Microbiol. Biotechnol.*, 2010b, 37, 537-558.

Rastogi, RP; Richa; Singh, SP; Häder, DP; Sinha, RP. Mycosporine-like amino acids profile and their activity under PAR and UVR in a hot-spring cyanobacterium *Scytonema* sp. HKAR-3. *Aust. J. Bot.*, 2010c, 58, 286-293.

Rastogi, RP; Sinha, RP. Genotoxin-Induced DNA Damage: Detection, Recovery and Influence on Human Health. In: Sinha RP, Sharma NK, Rai AK (eds). *Recent Advances in Life Sciences. India*: IK International Publishing House Pvt. Ltd., New Delhi, India, 2011a, pp. 275-309.

Rastogi, RP; Sinha, RP. Solar ultraviolet radiation-induced DNA damage and protection/repair strategies in cyanobacteria. *Inter. J. Phar. Bio Sci.*, 2011b, 2, B271–B288.

Rastogi, RP; Kumari, S; Richa; Han, T; Sinha, RP. Molecular characterization of hot spring cyanobacteria and evaluation of their photoprotective compounds. *Can. J. Microbiol.*, 2012, 58, 719-727.

Rastogi RP; Incharoensakdi A. UV radiation-induced accumulation of photoprotec-tive compounds in the green alga *Tetraspora* sp. CU2551. *Plant Physiol. Biochem.*, 2013, 70, 7-13.

Rastogi, RP; Incharoensakdi, A; Madamwar, D. Responses of a rice-field cyanobacterium *Anabaena siamensis* TISTR-8012 upon exposure to PAR and UV radiation. *J. Plant Physiol.*, 2014a, 171, 1545-1553.

Rastogi, RP; Singh, SP; Incharoensakdi, A; Häder, DP; Sinha, RP. Ultraviolet radiation-induced generation of reactive oxygen species, DNA damage and induction of UV-absorbing compounds in the cyanobacterium *Rivularia* sp. HKAR-4. *South Afr. J. Bot.*, 2014b, 90, 163-169.

Rastogi, RP; Madamwar, D; Incharoensakdi, A. Multiple defense systems in cyanobacteria in response to solar UV radiation. In: Davison D (ed). Cyanobacteria: Ecological Importance, Biotechnological Uses and Risk Management. USA: Nova Science Publishers 2014c, In Press.

Rastogi, RP; Incharoensakdi, A. UV radiation-induced biosynthesis, stability and antioxidant activity of mycosporine-like amino acids (MAAs) in a unicellular cyanobacterium *Gloeocapsa* sp. CU2556. *J. Photochem. Photobiol. B.*, 2014a, 130, 287-292.

Rastogi, RP; Incharoensakdi, A. Analysis of UV-absorbing photoprotectant mycosporine-like amino acid (MAA) in the cyanobacterium *Arthrospira* sp. CU2556. *Photochem. Photobiol. Sci.*, 2014b, 13, 1016-1024.

Rastogi, RP; Incharoensakdi, A. Characterization of UV-screening compounds, mycosporine-like amino acids, and scytonemin in the cyanobacterium *Lyngbya* sp. CU2555. *FEMS Microbiol. Ecol.*, 2014c, 87, 244-256.

Rastogi, RP; Incharoensakdi, A. Occurrence and induction of a ultraviolet-absorbing substance in the cyanobacterium *Fischerella muscicola* TISTR8215. *Phycol. Res.*, 2015. doi: 10.1111/pre.12069.

Ravishankara, AR; Daniel, JS; Portmann, RW. Nitrous oxide (N_2O): The dominant ozone-depleting substance emitted in the 21st century. *Science*, 2009, 326, 123-125.

Riegger, L; Robinson, D. Photoinduction of UV-absorbing compounds in Antarctic diatoms and *Phaeocystis Antarctica. Mar. Ecol. Prog. Ser.*, 1997, 160, 13-5.

Shibata, K. Pigments and a UVabsorbing substance in coral and a bluegreen alga living in the Great Barrier Reef. *Plant Cell Physiol.*, 1969, 10, 325-335.

Singh, SP; Sinha, RP; Klisch, M; Häder, DP. Mycosporinelike amino acids (MAAs) profile of a rice-field cyanobacterium *Anabaena doliolum* as influenced by PAR and UVR. *Planta*, 2008a, 229, 225-233.

Singh, SP; Klisch, M; Sinha, RP; Häder, D-P. Effects of abiotic stressors on synthesis of the mycosporine-like amino acid shinorine in the cyanobacterium *Anabaena variabilis* PCC 7937. *Photochem. Photobiol.*, 2008b, 84, 1500-1505.

Singh, SP; Klisch, M; Sinha, RP; Häder, DP. Sulfur deficiency changes mycosporine-like amino acid (MAA) composition of *Anabaena variabilis* PCC 7937: a possible role of sulfur in MAA bioconversion. *Photochem. Photobiol.*, 2010, 86, 862-870.

Sinha, RP; Klisch, M; Helbling, EW; Häder, D-P. Induction of mycosporine-like amino acids (MAAs) in cyanobacteria by solar ultraviolet-B radiation. *J. Photochem. Photobiol. B.*, 2001, 60, 129-135.

Sinha, RP; Ambasht, NK; Sinha, JP; Klisch, M; Häder, D-P. UVB-induced synthesis of mycosporine-like amino acids in three strains of *Nodularia* (cyanobacteria). *J. Photochem. Photobiol. B.*, 2003, 71, 51-58.

Sinha, RP; Singh, SP; Häder, D-P. Database on mycosporines and mycosporine-likeamino acids (MAAs) in fungi, cyanobacteria, macroalgae, phytoplankton and animals. *J. Photochem. Photobiol. B.*, 2007, 89, 29-35.

Spence, E; Dunlap, WC; Shick, JM; Long, PF. Redundant pathways of sunscreen biosynthesis in a cyanobacterium. *ChemBioChem.*, 2012, 13, 531-533.

Suh, HJ; Lee HW; Jung, J. Mycosporine glycine protects biological systems against photodynamic damage by quenching single oxygen with a high efficiency. *Photochem. Photobiol.*, 2003, 78, 109-113.

Valko, M; Leibfritz, D; Moncol, J; Cronin, MTD; Mazur, M; Telser, J. Free radicals and antioxidants in normal physiological functions and human disease. *Int. J. Biochem. Cell Biol.*, 2007, 39, 44-84.

Volkmann, M; Gorbushina, AA; Kedar, L; Oren, A. Structure of euhalothece-362, a novel red-shifted mycosporine-like amino acid, from a halophilic cyanobacterium (*Euhalothece* sp). *Microbiol. Lett.*, 2006, 258, 50-54.

Waditee-Sirisattha, R; Kageyama, H; Sopun, W; Tanaka, Y; Takabe, T. Identification and upregulation of biosynthetic genes required for accumulation of mycosporine-2-glycine under salt stress conditions in the halotolerant cyanobacterium *Aphanothece halophytica*. *App. Env. Microbiol.*, 2014, 80, 1763-1769.

Whitehead, K; Hedges, JI. Photodegradation and photosensitization of mycosporine-like amino acids. *J. Photochem. Photobiol.*, 2005, 80, 115-121.

Williamson, CE; Zepp, RG; Lucas, RM; Madronich, S; Austin, AT; Ballaré, CL; Norval, M; Sulzberger, B; Bais, AF; McKenzie, RL; Robinson, SA; Häder, D-P; Paul, ND; Bornman, JF. Solar ultraviolet radiation in a changing climate. *Nat. Clim. Change*, 2014, 4, 434-441.

Wu Won, JJ; Chalker, BE; Rideout, JA. Two new UVabsorbing compounds from Stylophora pistillata: sulfate esters of mycosporine-like amino acids. *Tetrahedron Lett.*, 1997, 38, 2525-2526.

Yuan, YV; Westcott, ND; Hu, C; Kitts, DD. Mycosporine-like amino acid composition of the edible red alga, *Palmaria palmata* (dulse) harvested from the west and east coasts of Grand Manan Island, New Brunswick. *Food Chem.*, 2009, 112, 321-328.

INDEX

#

A

D

E

F

G

H

N

O

P

Q

R

S